ENZYMES IN METABOLIC PATHWAYS

A Comparative Study of Mechanism, Structure, Evolution, and Control

Milton H. Saier, Jr.
University of California, San Diego

1817

HARPER & ROW, PUBLISHERS, New York
Cambridge, Philadelphia, San Francisco, Washington,
London, Mexico City, São Paulo, Singapore, Sydney

This book is dedicated to:
Hans, Ani and Mandy,
Ada, Mickey, Cathy and Mike,
Tay, Mel, Paula, Greg and Rob,
Michael and Hoyt,
Kari,
and
my biochemistry students
who provided the inspiration for the preparation of this book.

Sponsoring Editor: Lisa S. Berger
Project Editor: Steven Pisano
Cover Design: John Hite
Cover Art: Milton H. Saier, Jr.
Text Art: Kearstie Grenier/Fineline Illustrations, Inc.
Production: Debra Forrest
Compositor: TAPSCO, Inc.
Printer and Binder: R. R. Donnelley & Sons Company

ENZYMES IN METABOLIC PATHWAYS: A Comparative Study of Mechanism, Structure, Evolution, and Control

Library of Congress Cataloging-in-Publication Data

Saier, Milton H.
Enzymes in metabolic pathways.

Includes index.
1. Enzymes. 2. Metabolism. 3. Metabolism—Regulation. I. Title.
QP601.S23 1987 574.19'25 85-31739
ISBN 0-06-045689-2

86 87 88 89 9 8 7 6 5 4 3 2 1

CONTENTS

Wise men have often striven to confer wisdom to those who are to follow. Possibly the student of biochemistry should be aware of the following points of view before embarking on a detailed molecular analysis of biological systems.

It doesn't matter if you fall down as long as you pick up something from the floor while you get up.

—EFRAIM RACKER

If one studies too zealously, one easily loses his pants.

—ALBERT EINSTEIN

Nothing that is worth knowing can be taught.

—OSCAR WILDE

Get your facts first, then you can distort them as much as you please.

—MARK TWAIN

Hofstadter's Law:

It always takes longer than you expect, even when you take into account Hofstadter's Law.

—DOUGLAS HOFSTADTER

It is always the best policy to speak the truth, unless of course you are an exceptionally good liar.

—JEROME K. JEROME

Science is always wrong. It never solves a problem without creating ten more.

—BERNARD SHAW

It is a capital mistake to theorize before one has data. Insensibly one begins to twist facts to suit theories, instead of theories to suit facts.

—SHERLOCK HOLMES

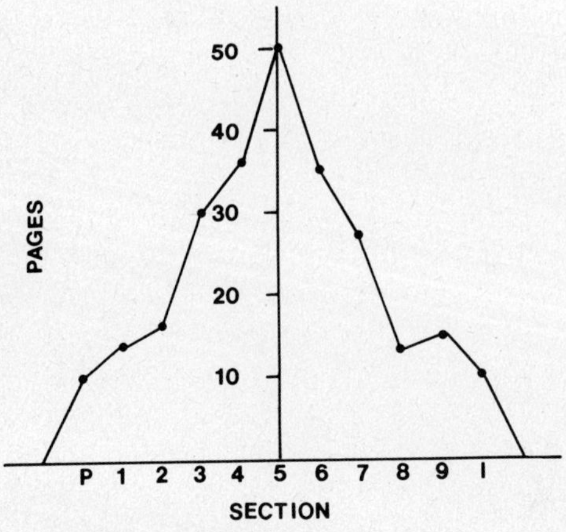

Enzymes in Metabolic Pathways is ordered with approximate bilateral symmetry, as are most living things. Volume is proportional to significance, requisite effort, and expected gain.

PREFACE

> *Apart from the known and the unknown, what else is there?*
> —HAROLD PINTER

In recent years, teachers and students of biochemistry have been faced with the proliferation of massive textbooks, many exceeding a thousand pages in length. These books have attempted to provide a comprehensive review of the field of biochemistry. Among the topics presented in these volumes have been the structures and the biosynthetic and degradative pathways of all the macromolecular precursors (amino acids, sugars, purines, pyrimidines, fatty acids, etc.), all the principal amphibolic pathways responsible for the conversion of simple nutrients into utilizable biosynthetic precursors and energy sources, and the structures of, and biosynthetic pathways for, the major organismal macromolecules (nucleic acids, proteins, polysaccharides, lipids, and conjugated forms of these polymers). Structural and biogenic features of complex cellular constituents (membranes, organelles, contractile systems, viruses, etc.) and specialized processes including neurotransmission, mechanisms of hormone action, and vision, have also been included.

As modern research allows our understanding of each such subject to expand downward to the molecular level, the inclusion of these subjects in a course in biochemistry becomes increasingly appropriate. Distinctions between the disciplines of biochemistry, molecular biology, cell biology, and physiology begin to fade. Consequently, the student of biochemistry is faced with a major dilemma: more subjects must be analyzed biochemically, and more information is available concerning each subject. The tendency is toward exposure to more subjects, away from conceptual understanding, and, consequently, toward superficiality. Most texts present very few of the subjects covered in mechanistic detail. The student is frequently overwhelmed by a large amount of factual information which is not presented in an integrated framework. Consequently, present-day students may be learning and forgetting more than ever before!

In writing this short book, my intent is to initiate reversal of this trend. I believe that students will gain maximal benefit from a more in-depth treatment of fewer subjects. Principles and conceptualization are required if factual materials are to be integrated into a coherent picture. An understanding of the few basic principles and mechanisms utilized by thousands of enzymes makes sense out of and provides unity to otherwise seemingly unrelated details. More complete conceptualization minimizes the need for memorization. What is understood can be remembered.

As a result of these convictions, I attempt in this book to present in concise fashion the most important information currently available about those enzymes that comprise a few of the best-understood metabolic pathways. Mechanistic, structural, regulatory, and evolutionary information are presented in a coherent manner, which should facilitate conceptualization, integration, and utilization of the principles that underlie all of enzyme catalysis. The selected topics serve to exemplify the maze of metabolic pathways which comprise the biochemical machinery of the cell. Emphasis is on quality, not quantity. The whole is greater than the sum of the parts.

This volume was written with several practical purposes in mind. I have attempted to maximize brevity and minimize expense. In so doing, I have assumed that the student already has a fair understanding of the principles of organic chemistry and a rudimentary knowledge of biochemistry and cell and organismal structure. For example, it is assumed that the reader is familiar with molecular orbital structure and chemical bonding theory; with the principles governing ionization and electrostatic interactions; with the nature of hydrogen (enthalpy) bonds and hydrophobic (entropy) interactions; with the significance of dipole moments and bond polarity to both covalent and noncovalent molecular interactions; and with the conventions and principles of stereochemistry. It is further presumed that biologically important molecules such as alcohols, amines, thiols, carboxylic acids, esters, amides, ethers, glycosides, acetals, and hemiacetals are not foreign to the reader.

Because of the restrictive nature of the material presented, many students will find it advantageous to rely on one of the major biochemistry texts for reference and comparative purposes. Those by A. L. Lehninger (Worth Publishing Company), D. E. Meltzer (Academic Press), J. D. Rawn (Harper & Row), E. L. Smith et al. (McGraw-Hill), L. Stryer (Freeman), C. Walsh (Freeman), and G. Zubay (Addison-Wesley) are all appropriate for this purpose.

A quick glance at the table of contents of this book will reveal the scope of the material presented. Properties of the twenty amino acyl residues that comprise proteins will be evaluated in Chapter 1, with emphasis given to those properties that are most relevant to enzyme structure and function. The hydropathy indices, dissociation properties, and reactivities of the side chains will be discussed. In Chapter 2, we shall start with the nature of the peptide bond that links amino acyl residues to one another to give the primary structures of the polypeptide chain. The primary structure of the protein determines the secondary structure, and the nature of the four principal secondary structural elements (α-helix, β-pleated sheet, β-turn, and random coil) will be examined. Specific examples of well-characterized proteins will lead to an appreciation of the tertiary and quaternary structures of proteins.

In Chapter 3, the molecular basis of enzyme catalysis, which can enhance reaction rates as much as 10^{20}-fold, will be discussed. A brief discussion of enzyme kinetics will allow the student to appreciate one of the principal experimental approaches used to study catalytic function. Finally, some discussion will be devoted to the principal mechanisms of enzyme regulation. In Chapter 4, the structures and modes of action of the principal water-soluble coenzymes will be presented in detail. Their biosyntheses from vitamin precursors and the physiological consequences of their deficiencies will also be considered briefly.

In the subsequent three chapters (5–7), the proteins and enzymes that comprise the glycolytic pathway, the pyruvate dehydrogenase complex, the Krebs cycle and the constituents of the electron transport chain and the oxidative phosphorylation system will be studied. Each enzyme will be analyzed in detail with respect to its structure, its coenzyme composition, and its mode of action. For a discussion of the regulatory interactions that allow integration of these amphibolic pathways into the entirety of the cellular metabolic system, two types of organisms, the most primitive and the most complex, will be emphasized. Our two representative taxonomic groups will be enteric bacteria and mammals. It will be seen that similarities in the metabolic processes in these two evolutionarily divergent groups of organisms far outweigh the differences. These subjects will be evaluated in greater detail than in any of the currently available biochemistry textbooks, and the reader will be brought up-to-date with respect to many of the more significant advances of modern-day enzyme research.

Finally, in the last two chapters, the subject matter will be expanded to include illustrative amino acid biosynthetic pathways and the pathways for the oxidation and biosynthesis of saturated fatty acids. In the examples chosen, virtually every major class of enzymes and every common coenzyme will be represented. All the principal regulatory mechanisms will be exemplified, and the probable evolutionary pathways that have given rise to present-day enzyme systems will be presented.

In deriving maximal benefit from exposure to the subject of biochemistry, the student should always attempt to compare, integrate, and distill. First, whenever two enzymes are observed to catalyze similar reactions or utilize the same cofactor, mechanistic parallels should be anticipated. A relatively few well-learned reaction mechanisms allow one to understand the mechanisms of action of literally thousands of enzymes. Second, each fact learned about an enzyme provides insight not only into the functions of that particular protein, but also into the metabolic pathway of which that enzyme is a constituent. This also leads to a more complete understanding of the physiology of the cell and organism in which that enzyme is found. Finally, the careful student will not only compare and integrate, but will also evaluate the material presented. That which is of greater significance must be retained, while less important details should serve to shape the conceptual framework. Nothing should be taken on faith. Only if a new fact makes sense and fits into the overall conceptual picture should it be accepted and allowed to enter into the long-term memory. The processes of comparison, integration, and distillation render biochemistry an active, viable, challenging, and exciting field which should prove meaningful to each student who possesses a desire to understand life at the molecular level.

> *Science is the human activity of finding an order in nature by organizing the scattered, meaningless facts under universal concepts.*
>
> —*J. Bronowski*

I would like to thank my colleagues and friends who contributed to the formulation of this volume: Paula Boerner, Clive Bradbeer, Russ Doolittle, Joe Hatefi, Ron Kaback, Jack Kyte, Kazunobu Matsushita, Donald McCormick, Stanley Mills, Michael Newman, Bill Nunn, Paul Price, F. A. Quiocho, Ef Racker, Lester Reed, Jonathan Reizer, Bob Simoni, and Juan Yguerabide.

Particular thanks are extended to Kari Carlin, who provided excellent technical support and participated in the writing of Chapter 5, to Kearstie Grenier who drew the illustrations, and to Janet Loomis and Jean Mueller who provided secretarial assistance in the preparation of the manuscipt. The contribution of my 200 biochemistry students who proofed the manuscipt during the fall quarter of 1984 is also acknowledged with appreciation. Work in the author's laboratory described in this volume was supported by grants from the National Institutes of Health. David Rawn generously permitted reproduction of figures from his book *Biochemistry* (Harper & Row) without acknowledgement.

MILTON H. SAIER, JR.

Chapter 1

Amino Acyl Residues in Proteins and Their Significance with Respect to Enzyme Structure and Function

> *Everything should be made as simple as possible but not simpler.*
>
> —*A. Einstein*

In order to understand the mechanisms by which enzymes enhance reaction rates, it is necessary to understand the structural features of proteins. These molecules consist of nonbranching chains of the twenty natural amino acids linked to one another via secondary amide bonds called *peptide bonds*. When only a few amino acyl residues are linked to one another, the resultant molecule is called a *peptide*. However, when the number of residues approaches 100, so that the molecular weight is about 10,000 (the average residue molecular weight is about 100), the molecule is referred to as a *protein*. Each protein has a unique amino acid sequence (the primary structure of the protein), and this sequence dictates the secondary structure of the protein: the coiling of the chain. The secondary structure of the molecule in turn determines the tertiary structure of the polypeptide chain: the folding of the coiled chain upon itself. Finally, the tertiary structure determines the quaternary structure: the way in which the folded, coiled chain interacts with other polypeptide chains (Table 1.1). The overall three-dimensional structure of a protein is therefore determined by the thermodynamic stability of amino acyl side-chain interactions.

It can be seen that the primary sequence of the polypeptide chain dictates the three-dimensional structure of a protein complex. The structure of the molecule and its interactions with other cellular constituents are usually determined by the thermodynamic stabilities of the different possible conformational states. For example, some proteins are water soluble and are found in the cellular cytoplasm. Hydrophilic (water loving) residues coat the external surfaces of these molecules, while hydrophobic (water hating) residues project inward. In contrast, proteins that are embedded within membranes frequently (but not always) possess exposed hydrophobic stretches of about 20 residues in length. These stretches have been found to pass through the phospholipid bilayer of biological membranes as a coiled structure called an *α-helix*.

TABLE 1.1 LEVELS OF STRUCTURAL COMPLEXITY IN PROTEINS

1. Primary structure: the amino acyl residue sequence
2. Secondary structure: the coiled chain
3. Tertiary structure: folding of the coiled chain on itself
4. Quaternary structure: interaction of the folded, coiled chain with other polypeptide chains

In order to understand the basic structural features of proteins, characteristics of the constituent amino acyl residue side chains must be evaluated with respect to their polarities, acidities, hydrogen bond-forming capacities, and reactivities. This chapter will deal with these subjects.

1.1 PROPERTIES OF AMINO ACYL RESIDUES IN PROTEINS

The twenty natural amino acids found in proteins (Table 1.2) can be thought of as derivatives of the simplest amino acid, glycine. Glycine possesses an α-amino group joined via a methylene carbon to an α-carboxyl group. Because glycine possesses two identical hydrogen atoms attached to the α-carbon, a plane of symmetry can be drawn through the molecule. Consequently, it is optically inactive. Each of the remaining nineteen natural amino acids possesses a side chain that replaces one of the α-hydrogen atoms in glycine (Table 1.2). The simplest of these side chains is the methyl group of alanine. Because four different groups are bonded to the α-carbon in each of these nineteen amino acids, they are optically active and can rotate plane-polarized light. All optically active amino acyl residues found in proteins are of the L-configuration about the α-carbon. Two and only two of these amino acids, threonine and isoleucine, contain a second chiral center. In proline, the aliphatic side chain cycles back on itself to form a secondary amine involving the α-amino group. The configuration of this amino acyl residue in proteins is constrained so that it cannot easily fit into an α-helical structure. Scanning Table 1.2, it can be seen that there are three branched-chain aliphatic amino acids, four aromatic amino acids, two sulfur-containing amino acids, two aliphatic hydroxy amino acids, two strongly basic and two strongly acidic amino acids, and two amido amino acids derived from the acidic ones by amidation of the side-chain carboxyl groups. It is primarily the properties of the side chains of these amino acids which confer upon a protein its binding and catalytic activities.

Figure 1.1 serves to classify and assign approximate hydropathic character to the twenty amino acyl residue side chains which extend from the backbone of the protein chain. Glycine (*gly*) possesses no side chain and therefore exhibits neutral hydropathic character (it is neither hydrophobic nor hydrophilic). A hydropathy index of zero is assigned to this amino acyl residue. The remaining residues, however, can be classified either as hydrophobic or hydrophilic. The seven hydrophobic residues grouped together in the figure include (in decreasing order of hydrophobicity): isoleucine (*ile*), valine (*val*), leucine (*leu*), phenylalanine (*phe*), methionine (*met*), alanine (*ala*), and proline (*pro*). The side chains of all of these amino acids are inert and cannot form hydrogen-bonded structures, function as nucleophiles, or donate or accept protons during enzyme catalysis. Based on certain criteria, cysteine (*cys*) and the oxidized form of cysteine (*cys–cys*) as well as tryptophan (*trp*), are sometimes grouped with hydrophobic residues. However, the side chains of these amino acids are capable of forming weak hydrogen bonds, and cysteine can dissociate to an anionic species. Consequently, we have grouped these residues with the polar amino acyl residues in Figure 1.1.

The seven polar but neutral (uncharged) amino acids include (in increasing order of hydrophilicity): cysteine (*cys*), tryptophan (*trp*), threonine (*thr*), serine (*ser*), tyrosine (*tyr*), glutamine (*gln*), and asparagine (*asn*). Of these seven amino acids, all possess side chains which can form stable hydrogen bonds, and two of them, cysteine and tyrosine, can dissociate to anionic species within the physiological pH range. Most of these residues can and do function as nucleophiles during catalysis of various enzyme-mediated metabolic reactions.

Two amino acyl residue side chains, those of glutamate (*glu*) and aspartate (*asp*), are strongly acidic. They dissociate to their negatively charged anionic forms at physiological pH in aqueous solution. However, in a hydrophobic environment (i.e., in the interior of a protein) they may remain protonated. These residues can form strong hydrogen bonds, can function as nucleophiles, or can serve as hydrogen donors or acceptors during enzyme catalysis. They also function to neutralize positive charges in substrates, reaction intermediates, and transition states during catalysis.

Finally, the three basic amino acyl residues that can bear a net positive charge at neutral pH are histidine (*his*), lysine (*lys*), and arginine (*arg*). All of these residues form stable hydrogen bonds and can function as hydrogen donors and acceptors. The imidazole ring of histidine is a particularly good nucleophile, and this residue, together with cysteine and serine, most often participates in nucleophilic catalysis. These basic residues can accelerate reaction rates or facilitate substrate binding to the active site of an enzyme by charge neutralization.

In addition to the twenty common amino acids found in proteins, a few rare derivatives of these residues sometimes occur. For example, hydroxyproline and hydroxylysine are found in the structural protein, collagen, while methyl lysine and methyl histidine are found in contractile proteins present in muscle cells. Phosphorylated derivatives of serine, threonine, and tyrosine are common in many proteins, while formylation and acetylation of these and other residues are not uncommon. In some cases, these amino acyl residue modifications alter the activities of enzymes, and in almost all cases the derivatization reactions are catalyzed by enzymes that act on the target proteins as substrates. Only in the case of *N*-formylmethionine, sometimes present at the N-termini of proteins, is the modified amino acyl residue incorporated into the protein during its synthesis.

Finally, many nonprotein amino acids are known to fulfill specialized body or cellular functions. For example, γ-amino butyric acid (GABA) is a neurotransmitter in the central nervous system of higher animals while D-alanine is a common constituent of the cell walls of bacteria. These compounds are never found as constituents of proteins.

TABLE 1.2 NAME, ABBREVIATIONS, STRUCTURE, AND RELATIVE ABUNDANCE OF EACH OF THE NATURAL AMINO ACIDS FOUND IN PROTEINS

Amino acid	3-letter abbreviation	1-letter abbreviation	Abbreviated neutral structure	Relative abundance in proteins (molar %)[a]
Parental				
Glycine	*gly*	G	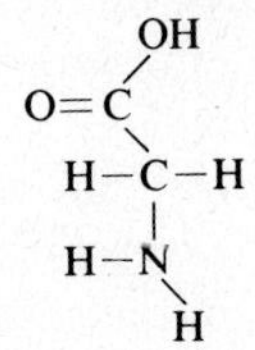	8.3
Aliphatic				
Proline	*pro*	P	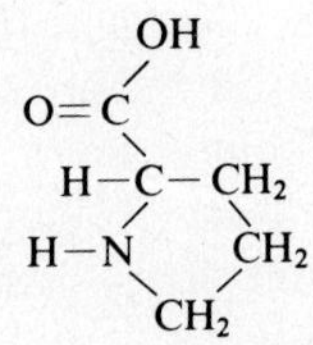	3.4
Alanine	*ala*	A	$\succ\!-CH_3$	9.4
Valine	*val*	V	$\succ\!-CH-(CH_3)_2$	5.8
Leucine	*leu*	L	$\succ\!-CH_2CH-(CH_3)_2$	10.7
Isoleucine	*ile*	I	$\succ\!-\underset{\displaystyle CH_3}{\underset{\vert}{CH}}-CH_2-CH_3$	5.7
Aromatic				
Phenylalanine	*phe*	F	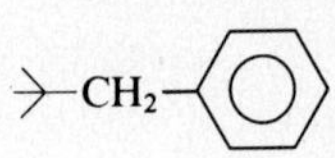	4.8
Tryptophan	*trp*	W	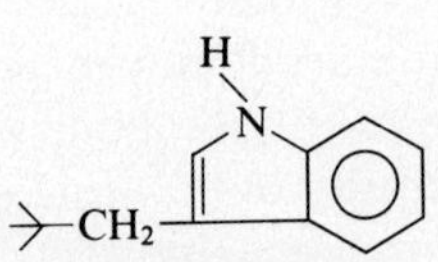	1.1
Tyrosine	*tyr*	Y	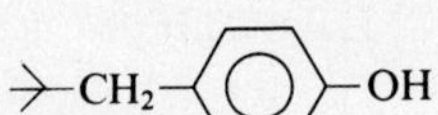	2.9
Histidine	*his*	H	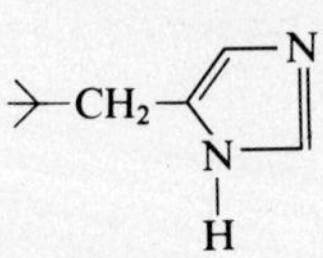	2.1

TABLE 1.2 *(Continued)*

Amino acid	3-letter abbreviation	1-letter abbreviation	Abbreviated neutral structure	Relative abundance in proteins (molar %)[a]
Sulfur				
Cysteine	*cys*	C	$\succ CH_2-SH$	2.5
Methionine	*met*	M	$\succ CH_2-CH_2-S-CH_3$	2.3
Aliphatic hydroxyl				
Serine	*ser*	S	$\succ CH_2-OH$	7.4
Threonine	*thr*	T	$\succ CH(OH)-CH_3$	5.5
Strongly basic				
Lysine	*lys*	K	$\succ (CH_2)_4-NH_2$	5.6
Arginine	*arg*	R	$\succ (CH_2)_3-NH-C(=NH)-NH_2$	4.6
Strongly acidic				
Aspartate	*asp*	D	$\succ CH_2-C(=O)OH$	4.6
Glutamate	*glu*	E	$\succ (CH_2)_2-C(=O)OH$	5.3
Amido				
Asparagine	*asn*	N	$\succ CH_2-C(=O)NH_2$	4.3
Glutamine	*gln*	Q	$\succ (CH_2)_2-C(=O)NH_2$	3.7

[a] The ten proteins analyzed for amino acid composition were: the mannitol permease (*E. coli*); the lactose permease (*E. coli*); the Bence–Jones K protein (human); cytochrome *c* (human); ferridoxin (spinach); glucagon (pig); insulin (bovine); hemoglobin (human); lysozyme (chicken), and wool (sheep).

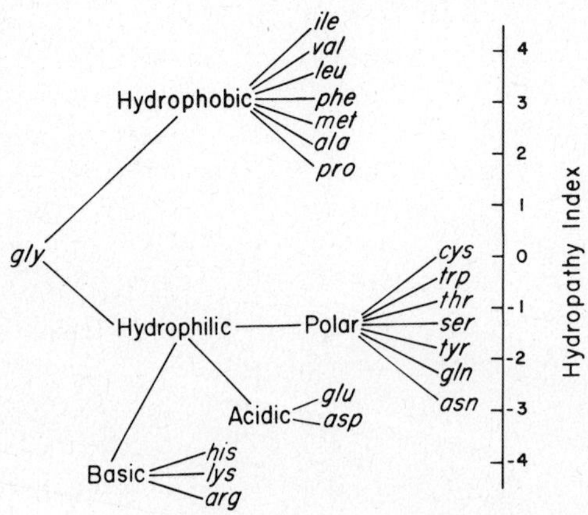

Figure 1.1 Classification and relative hydropathic character of the twenty natural amino acyl residue side chains found in proteins. The amino acyl residue side chains are positioned vertically in the figure in accordance with the degree of their approximate hydrophobic versus hydrophilic character. The hydropathy index is given on the right. Glycine (*gly*), for example, possesses no side chain and has a hydropathy index of zero; isoleucine (*ile*), the most hydrophobic residue found in proteins, has a hydropathy index of +4.5, while arginine (*arg*), the most hydrophilic residue, has a hydropathy index of −4.5. The nineteen optically active amino acyl residues are grouped as either hydrophobic (top) or hydrophilic (bottom), and the latter group is subdivided into polar but neutral residues; acidic, or negatively charged, residues; and basic, or positively charged; residues.

1.2 ACID-BASE PROPERTIES OF AMINO ACYL RESIDUES IN PROTEINS

Most proteins contain a single free α-carboxyl group at the carboxy terminus (or C-terminus) of the protein and a single free α-amino group at the amino terminus (or N-terminus) of the polypeptide chain. Because proteins are large, usually containing between 100 and 1000 amino acyl residues, the two ionizable groups at the chain termini are of minor significance with respect to the charge on the molecule as a whole. Excluding these two dissociable groups, there are only seven amino acyl residues in proteins which normally ionize within the physiological pH range. These residues, in order of decreasing acidity (increasing basicity), are *asp, glu, his, cys, tyr, lys,* and *arg.* These amino acyl residues, the names and structures of their dissociable side chains, and their pKa values in proteins in aqueous solution, are listed in Table 1.3.

All of the dissociable substituents in proteins fall within three classes: (a) carboxyl groups (the C-terminal α-carboxyl group and the side-chain carboxyls of aspartate and glutamate); (b) amino groups or derivatives of them (the N-terminal α-amino group, the ϵ-amino group of lysine, the imidazole ring of histidine, and the guanidyl group of arginine); and (c) hydroxyl and sulfhydryl (thiol) groups (found in tyrosine and cysteine, respectively). The parental compounds with which these three classes of ionizable substituents can be compared are acetate, methylamine, and ethanol, respectively (Table 1.3).

Comparison of the pKa values for the amino acyl derivatives found in proteins with the three parental compounds reveals some similarities as well as differences. For example, the dissociation constants for the side-chain carboxyl groups of *asp* and *glu* in peptides are the same as that of acetic acid; the dissociation constant of the ϵ-amino group of *lys* is essentially the same as that of methylamine; and those of the hydroxyl groups of *ser* and *thr* are essentially the same as that of ethanol. These observations correspond to expectation because in each of these cases (i) there is no electronegative or charged group near the dissociable substituent; (ii) the side-chain substituents do not differ from the parental compounds with respect to their resonance stabilization; and (iii) in all cases, these amino acyl side chains and their parental compounds bind the dissociable proton with the same hybrid sp^3 orbitals (see Table 1.4 for an evaluation of the four principal factors that influence the acid-base properties of molecular substituents). On the other hand, the C-terminal carboxyl group in the peptide chain is more acidic than acetic acid or the side-chain carboxyl group in *glu* or *asp* by an order of magnitude, owing to the electron-withdrawing effect of the acylated α-amino group. Because nitrogen is substantially more electronegative than hydrogen or carbon (Table 1.5), and because the nitrogen atom is separated from the carboxyl group by only one methylene group, displacement of electron density away from the region between the oxygen and hydrogen nuclei in the carboxyl group occurs, and the resultant decrease in electron density between these two atoms facilitates proton dissociation and stabilizes the carboxylate anion.

A similar argument explains the fact that the acidity of the N-terminal amino group in a protein is about three orders of magnitude greater than that of either methylamine or the ϵ-amino group of lysine (Table 1.3). In the former case, the α-carbonyl and the secondary amide bond that links the N-terminal amino acyl residue to the next amino acyl residue in the chain are strongly electron-withdrawing so that electron density is displaced away from the N-terminal amino group, thereby weakening the nitrogen–hydrogen bonds. It is because of these considerations that a proton dissociates from the α-amino group with greater ease than in methylamine or the side chain of lysine.

In the case of the imidazole ring of *his,* three factors influence its acidity relative to methylamine. First, the protonated species is stabilized by resonance:

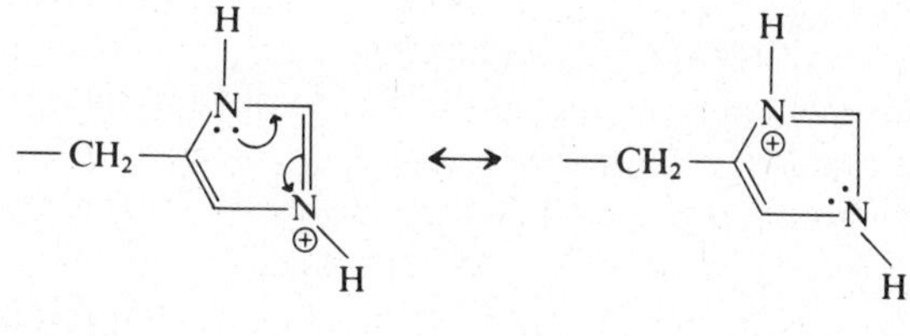

while the neutral species:

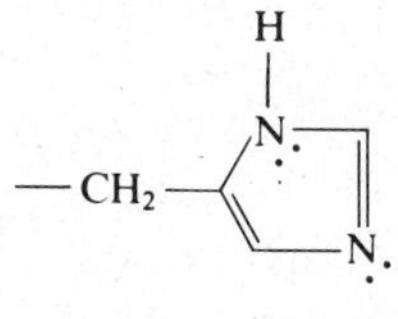

is not. This tends to stabilize the protonated form of the substituent, rendering it more basic. Second, the electron-withdrawing effect of the second ring nitrogen facilitates dissociation of the proton. This tends to render the protonated substituent more acidic.

TABLE 1.3 PROPERTIES OF DISSOCIABLE GROUPS IN PROTEINS

Parental compound	Group	Amino acyl residue	Structure of acid	pKa	Effect on acidity of[a]			
					Polarity	Charge neutralization	Resonance stabilization	Orbital strength
Acetic acid	Carboxyl		$CH_3-C(=O)-OH$	4.7				
	(a) β (or γ)-carboxyl	*asp* (or *glu*)	$-CH_2-C(=O)-OH$	4.7	–	–	–	–
	(b) α-carboxyl	C-terminus	$-C(=O)-NH-CH(R)-C(=O)-OH$	3.7	↑	–	–	–
Methylamine	Amino		$CH_3-NH_3^{\oplus}$	10.5				
	(a) ϵ-amino	*lys*	$-(CH_2)_4-NH_3^{\oplus}$	10.2	–	–	–	–
	(b) α-amino	N-terminus	$-NH-C(=O)-CH(R)-NH_3^{\oplus}$	7.8	↑	–	–	–

	(c) Imidazole	*his*	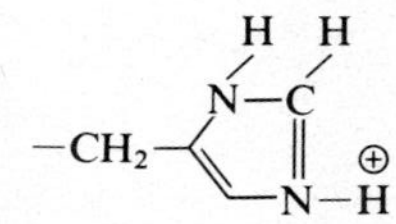	7.0	↑	–	↓	↑
	(d) Guanidinium	*arg*	$-(CH_2)_3-NH-C(=\overset{\oplus}{N}H_2)-NH_2$	12	↑	–	↓	↑
Ethanol	Hydroxyl		CH_3-CH_2-OH	16				
	(a) β-hydroxyl	*ser* (or *thr*)	$-CH_2-OH$	16	–	–	–	–
	(b) Phenolic hydroxyl	*tyr*	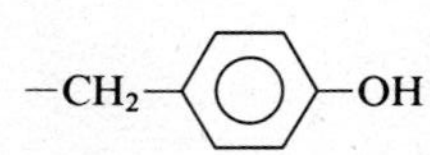	9.6	–	–	↑	–
	(c) Sulfhydryl	*cys*	$-CH_2-SH$	8.5	–	–	–	↑

[a] –, no effect; ↑, increased acidity; ↓, decreased acidity.

TABLE 1.4 THE FOUR MAJOR FACTORS THAT CAN INFLUENCE THE ACID-BASE PROPERTIES OF MOLECULAR SUBSTITUENTS[a]

1. Polarity	The electron-withdrawing effect of an adjacent, more electronegative substituent facilitates proton dissociation.
2. Charge neutralization	A formal charge in the vicinity of the dissociable group stabilizes the form of that substituent which bears a charge of opposite sign, but destabilizes one that bears a charge of the same sign.
3. Resonance stabilization	Resonance stabilizes that form of the substituent for which more equivalent (or nearly equivalent) resonance structures can be drawn.
4. Orbital strength	The nature of the hybrid orbital bonding the dissociable proton to the substituent in question influences acidity in the order: sp^3 (least acidic) < sp^2 < sp (most acidic); or sp^3 < d^2sp^3 (more acidic).

[a] It should be noted that these same factors influence reactivity (i.e. nucleophilicity) and bond strength (heterolytic dissociation) as well as the acidity or basicity (homolytic dissociation) of a protonated substituent.

TABLE 1.5 ELECTRONEGATIVITY VALUES OF ELEMENTS OF BIOLOGICAL SIGNIFICANCE

H 2.1			
C 2.5	N 3.0	O 3.5	F 4.0
Si 1.8	P 2.1	S 2.5	Cl 3.0

Finally, the hybrid orbital bonding hydrogen to nitrogen in methylamine is sp^3, while that associated with the positively charged aromatic ring nitrogen in the imidazole ring is sp^2. Since only one factor (resonance) makes the imidazole ring more basic, while two factors, polarity and the change in hybrid orbital strength, enhance the acidity of the ring, it is not clear what the net effect will be. The fact that the pKa of *his* is 7.0 (more acidic than methylamine) shows that the latter two factors are quantitatively more important than the former.

The considerations discussed above show that polarity effects can increase the acidity of a substituent from one to three orders of magnitude when the electron-withdrawing substituent is separated from the dissociable substituent by only one methylene group. In evaluating the effects of orbital strength, we can compare the acidities of three molecules: ethane, ethylene, and acetylene (Table 1.6). Ethane has a pKa of 43. The pKa of ethylene is 36, and that of acetylene is 26. As the hybrid orbital increases in *s* character, the electron cloud more closely surrounds the positively charged carbon nucleus, and the acidity of the molecule increases by several orders of magnitude. This occurs because effective charge neutralization of the electron cloud by the positively charged nucleus increases the electronegativity of carbon (increases the electron-withdrawing capacity of carbon), thereby facilitating proton dissociation and anion stability.

Concerning the acidity of arginine, notice that the same factors influencing the acidity of the imidazole ring in *his* influence the acidity of the guanidyl group in *arg*,

TABLE 1.6 EFFECT OF ORBITAL STRENGTH ON THE ACIDITIES OF HYDROCARBONS

Compound	Structure	Hybrid orbital	pKa
Ethane	$CH_3{-}CH_3$	*sp*^{3}	43
Ethylene	$CH_2{=}CH_2$	*sp*^{2}	36
Acetylene	$CH{\equiv}CH$	*sp*	26

and in the same directions. However, the net effect is opposite to that observed with *his; arg* is more basic than methylamine. Evidently, resonance stabilization exerts the predominant effect in this case, and the resonance stabilization energy must be larger than the sum of the energies resulting from inductive effects and the change in hybrid orbital strength.

In considering the hydroxy amino acids (within the third group of amino acids in Table 1.3), the phenolic hydroxyl group of *tyr* is more acidic than that of ethanol or *ser* by six orders of magnitude. The sole explanation for this shift in pKa is that the anionic form of this side chain is resonance stabilized

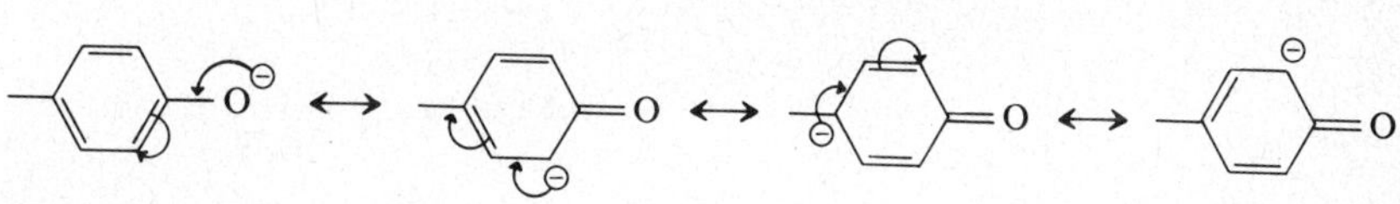

while the neutral form 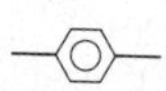 is not.

In evaluating the acidity of the sulfhydryl (thiol) group of *cys,* it will be noted that the principal differences between —OH and —SH are the size of the nucleus and the difference in the electronic configurations. While the oxygen atom possesses sp^3 hybrid orbitals, those of sulfur are d^2sp^3. These octahedral orbitals comprise much more diffuse electron clouds. The diffuse nature of the electron clouds more readily allows dissociation of the proton because the negative charge of the anionic species is spread over a greater volume and is therefore more stable. Additionally, there is less overlap of the bonding orbitals, and oxygen is more electronegative than sulfur. These same considerations render —SH a poor hydrogen-bonder, thus accounting for the greater hydrophobic character of *cys* relative to *ser.* They also explain the fact that the sulfhydryl group is an exceptionally good nucleophile. The malleable nature of the diffuse electron cloud of the thiol group lowers the activation energy for bond formation and bond dissociation during reactions in which the sulfhydryl group functions as a nucleophile or an acid.

The pKa values given in Table 1.3 correspond to experimentally determined values for these peptide substituents. Frequently, the pKa values for specific amino acyl side chains in proteins are the same, or very nearly the same, as those reported in Table 1.3. In other cases the dissociation constants differ markedly, sometimes by as much as two or three orders of magnitude. These differences are usually accounted for by any one of several environmental effects. For example, in a hydrophobic environment a substituent will preferentially exist in its neutral, noncharged form. In hydrophilic environments, the dipole moments of water molecules greatly stabilize charged substituents by allowing the formation of a hydration shell around the ionic residues. No such stabilizing dipole moments are present in a hydrophobic medium. Another factor that may alter pKa values is the proximity of another charged residue or of a metal ion. The presence of an adjacent positive charge will tend to promote the dissociation of an acid while maintaining a base in its neutral state. Other factors such as the availability of hydrogen-bonding residues or aromatic residues capable of π-stacking may also influence acidity. Thus, the pKa value for an amino acyl residue in a protein, particularly one at the active site of an enzyme, may not correspond at all to the expected value based on the data recorded in Table 1.3.

The discussions in this and the previous section have shown that a few fundamental principles of chemistry can help us to understand the acid-base properties and the polar or hydrophilic characteristics of amino acyl residues in proteins. These same principles help to explain the reactivities of amino acyl residues in proteins and their roles in enzyme catalysis. This subject will be considered in the next section.

1.3 REACTIVITIES OF AMINO ACYL RESIDUES IN PROTEINS

Certain amino acyl residues in enzymes participate with high frequency in specific catalytic reactions. For example, *ser* and *cys* residues frequently function as nucleophilic catalysts for the hydrolysis of esters (fats), acetals (carbohydrates), secondary amides (proteins), and phosphodiesters (nucleic acids). The mechanistic principle is usually the same. Consider a protease that utilizes a *cys* residue to hydrolyze the secondary amide bond in a peptide. The *cys* residue functions as a nucleophilic catalyst while a *his* residue may remove the proton from the sulfhydryl group in order to increase its nucleophilicity:

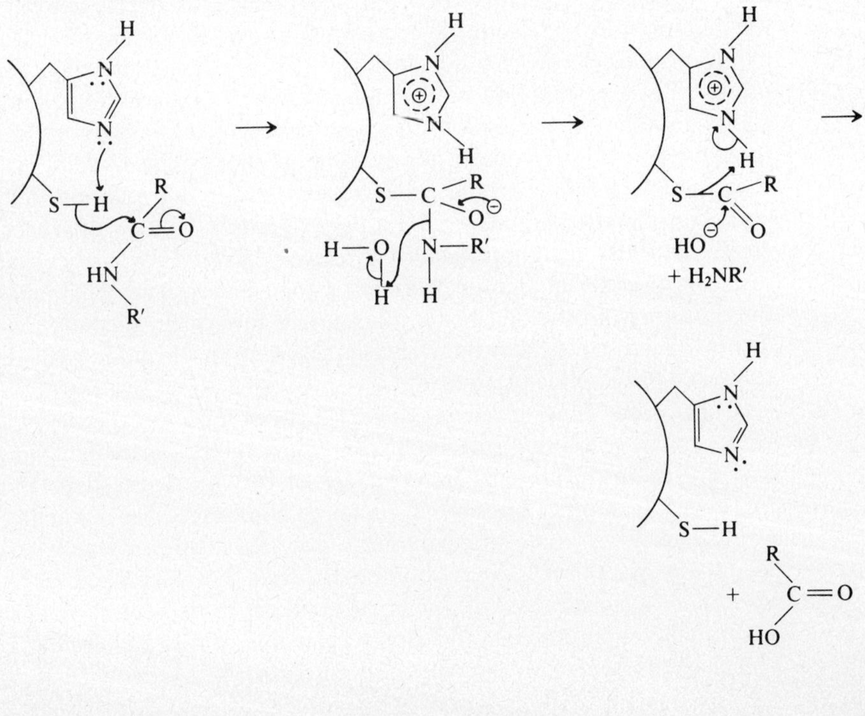

(1.1)

The involvement of a *cys* residue in enzyme catalysis can be ascertained by treating the enzyme with a reagent that specifically reacts with thiol groups and then determining whether the enzyme has retained activity. One such amino acyl-specific reagent that reacts only with *cys* side chains is *N*-ethylmaleimide (NEM). This reagent reacts irreversibly with thiol groups as shown below

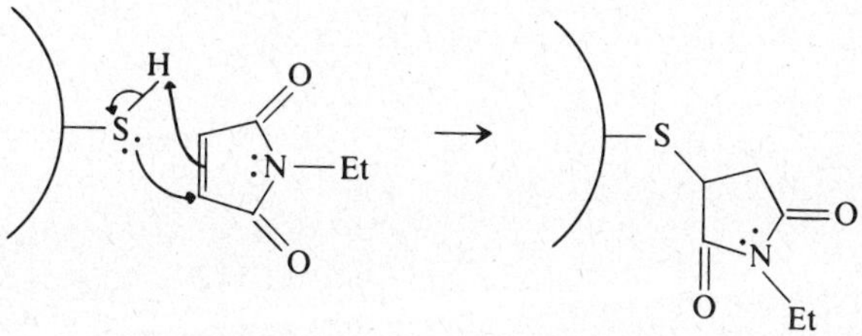

(1.2)

It is the delocalized d^2sp^3 orbitals of sulfur that render it an exceptionally good nucleophile, both for enzyme catalysis and for reaction with *N*-ethylmaleimide.

Active-site *cys* residues are usually very reactive because of the presence of nearby amino acyl substituents which activate them as shown in equation 1.1. However, not all *cys* residues in a protein necessarily react when exposed to NEM. Two observations appear to account for this fact. First, some *cys* residues are buried within the hydrophobic interior of the protein molecule, and they are therefore not accessible to the fairly hydrophilic NEM molecule. Second, although only the reduced form of *cys* is incorporated into newly synthesized proteins, some of the *cys* residues in the protein may be oxidized by molecular oxygen after the protein is biosynthesized. The oxidation reaction proceeds as follows

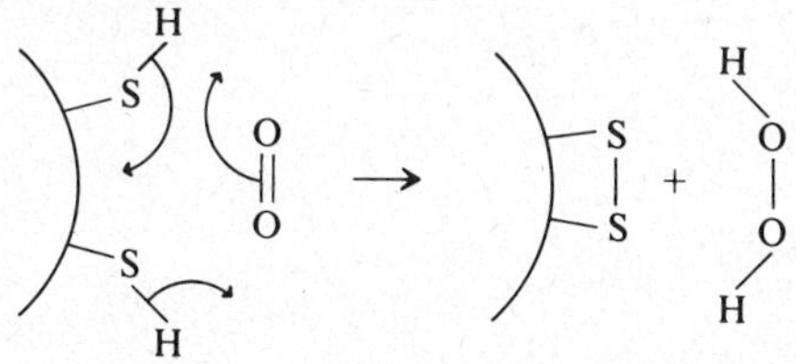

(1.3)

The protein becomes internally cross linked by joining two cysteyl residues in a disulfide bridge. Molecular oxygen is reduced to hydrogen peroxide in this process. The oxidized form of *cys* is resistant to attack by NEM. However, if an essential, active-site *cys* is oxidized, the enzyme invariably loses its activity. Consequently, sulfhydryl-dependent enzymes must be stored in the absence of molecular oxygen or in the presence of an agent that can reduce disulfide bonds to the free sulfhydryl groups. Because of the delocalized d^2sp^3 orbitals of sulfur, the disulfide bond is weak, and the activation energy for its reduction is low. Sulfhydryl oxidation is therefore a readily reversible process, and of all the residue side chains in proteins, only *cys* is readily oxidized by air.

In subsequent chapters, numerous examples will illustrate the involvement of specific amino acyl residues in enzyme catalysis. For almost every polar amino acid, a specific reagent is available that allows the biochemist to determine whether or not the side chain of that particular residue participates in catalysis. However, studies with residue-specific reagents can sometimes be misleading: alteration of a protein at a site distant from the substrate-binding site can change the conformation of the protein to one which is inactive or less active. Such studies have led to the realization that the three-dimensional structure of an enzyme is important to catalysis because each functional residue in the active site must be properly oriented relative to the substrate molecule, and many residues may participate either in substrate binding or in catalysis.

> *The ancient covenant is in pieces; man knows at last he is alone in the universe's unfeeling immensity, out of which he emerged only by chance. His destiny is nowhere spelled out, nor is his duty. The kingdom above or the darkness below: It is for him to choose.*
>
> —JACQUES MONOD

BIBLIOGRAPHY

Asimov, I., *Asimov's New Guide to Science,* Basic Books, New York (1984).

Barker, R., *Organic Chemistry of Biological Compounds,* Prentice-Hall, Englewood Cliffs, NJ (1971).

Blackburn, S., ed., *Amino Acid Determination: Methods and Techniques,* Marcel Dekker, New York (1984).

Florkin, M., *A History of Biochemistry. Parts I and II: Protochemistry to Biochemistry,* Comprehensive Biochemistry, *Vol. 30,* Elsevier/North Holland, Amsterdam (1972).

Herriot, J., G. Jacobson, J. Marmur, and W. Parson, *Papers in Biochemistry,* Addison-Wesley, Reading, MA (1984).

Jakubke, H.-D., and H. Jeschkeit, *Amino Acids, Peptides, and Proteins: An Introduction,* Wiley, New York (1977).

Kyte, J., and R. Doolittle, "A Simple Method for Displaying the Hydropathic Character of a Protein", *J. Mol. Biol.* **157**: 105–132 (1982).

Liu, P.-Y., ed., *Chemical Synthesis and Sequencing of Peptides and Proteins: Proceedings of an International Conference,* Elsevier/North Holland, Amsterdam (1981).

Margulis, L., *Early Life,* Science Books, Boston, MA (1982).

Meister, A., *Biochemistry of the Amino Acids,* Second Edition, Vol. 1, Academic, New York (1965).

Needleman, S. B., ed., *Advanced Methods of Protein Sequence Determination,* Springer-Verlag, Berlin (1977).

Nyhan, W. L., *Abnormalities in Amino Acid Metabolism in Clinical Medicine,* Appleton-Century-Crofts, Norwalk, CT (1984).

Rees, A. R., and M. J. E. Sternberg, *From Cells to Atoms: An Illustrated Introduction to Molecular Biology,* Blackwell Scientific Publications, Palo Alto, CA (1984).

Sulfur Amino Acids, Biochemical and Clinical Aspects: Proceedings of an International Symposium and the Fifth Annual Meeting of the Japanese Research Society on Sulfur Amino Acids (JRSSA), Alan R. Liss, New York (1983).

Wold, F., *Macromolecules: Structure and Function,* Prentice-Hall, Englewood Cliffs, NJ (1971).

Chapter 2

Structures and Functions of Proteins

> *The Infinity of various beings is abiding in the one, and is an evolution from the one.*
>
> —BHAGAVAD GITA

Enzymes catalyze virtually all of the biologically important reactions in a living cell. Rate enhancement depends on the highly specific three-dimensional arrangements of amino acyl residues in these proteins as well as on the interactions between protomeric (monomeric) species within a multicomponent enzyme complex. In this chapter we shall see how the primary structure of a protein (its amino acyl sequence) dictates its three-dimensional structure as well as its interactions with other cellular constituents. Thus, from simplicity we generate complexity and infinite variety. It is important to remember that in biology, the whole is usually greater than the sum of its parts.

2.1 PRIMARY STRUCTURES OF PEPTIDES AND PROTEINS

Amino acids are linked to one another in peptides via secondary amide bonds. If these bonds result from the condensation of the α-carboxyl group of one amino acid with the α-amino group of a second acid, we refer to this bond as a *peptide bond.* It is this bond that links all amino acyl residues in proteins.

Peptides found in nature may exhibit quite variable structures and functions. Some are cyclic and contain D-amino acids, hydroxy acids, and strangely derivatized residues. They may function as antibiotics, components of bacterial cell walls, biological reducing agents, substrates of enzyme-catalyzed reactions, pheromones, morphogens, or hormones. Those peptides that contain D-amino acids or unusual constituents which differ markedly in structure from those of the common amino acids listed in Table 1.2, and those that contain residues not linked by peptide bonds, are generally synthesized by highly specific enzymes, each of which functions solely in the synthesis of a specific bond. By contrast, those peptides that contain only the 20 common L-amino acids linked by peptide bonds are synthesized by a uniform process which involves a template mechanism. The genetic material of the cell, the deoxyribonucleic acid (DNA) is first transcribed to ribonucleic acid (RNA), and the RNA is translated into protein. As a consequence of this biosynthetic mechanism, the nucleotide sequence of the genetic material dictates the amino acid sequence of the protein. The way in which this complex process evolved is one of the major enigmas in biology.

The structure of a typical tripeptide is illustrated in Figure 2.1. By convention, peptides and proteins are always named from the N-terminus to the C-terminus as illustrated in the figure. The peptide bond that connects the two amino acyl residues is actually a resonating structure

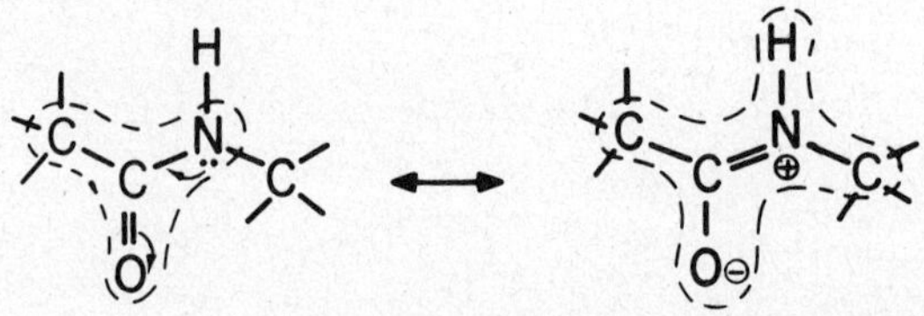

(2.1)

The second, less important resonance structure results from displacement of an electron pair on nitrogen to the more electronegative oxygen, giving rise to charge separation. Surprisingly, the C—N bond exhibits 40% double-bond character. Since all atoms associated with or bonded directly to a π double-bonded structure are coplanar, as illustrated by the dashed lines in equation 2.1 and Figure 2.1, free rotation of the backbone atoms in a peptide or protein can occur only about the α-carbon. A peptide can therefore be thought of as a linear array of overlapping, planar molecular groupings. Any model for protein secondary structure must accommodate this important fact.

2.2 SECONDARY STRUCTURAL FEATURES OF PROTEINS

Four secondary structural elements are commonly associated with proteins: (a) right-handed α-helices; (b) parallel and antiparallel β-strands; (c) β-turns; and (d) random

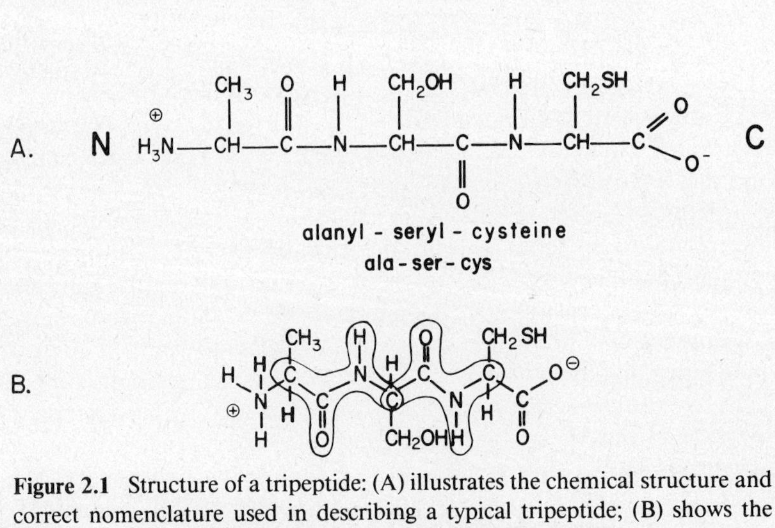

Figure 2.1 Structure of a tripeptide: (A) illustrates the chemical structure and correct nomenclature used in describing a typical tripeptide; (B) shows the regions of coplanarity that result from peptide bond resonance.

coils. The structures of the α-helix and antiparallel β-strands are illustrated in Figures 2.2(a) and (b), respectively, while the two types of β-turns are shown in Figures 2.3(a) and (b). The characteristics of these structures are summarized in Table 2.1 and discussed systematically below.

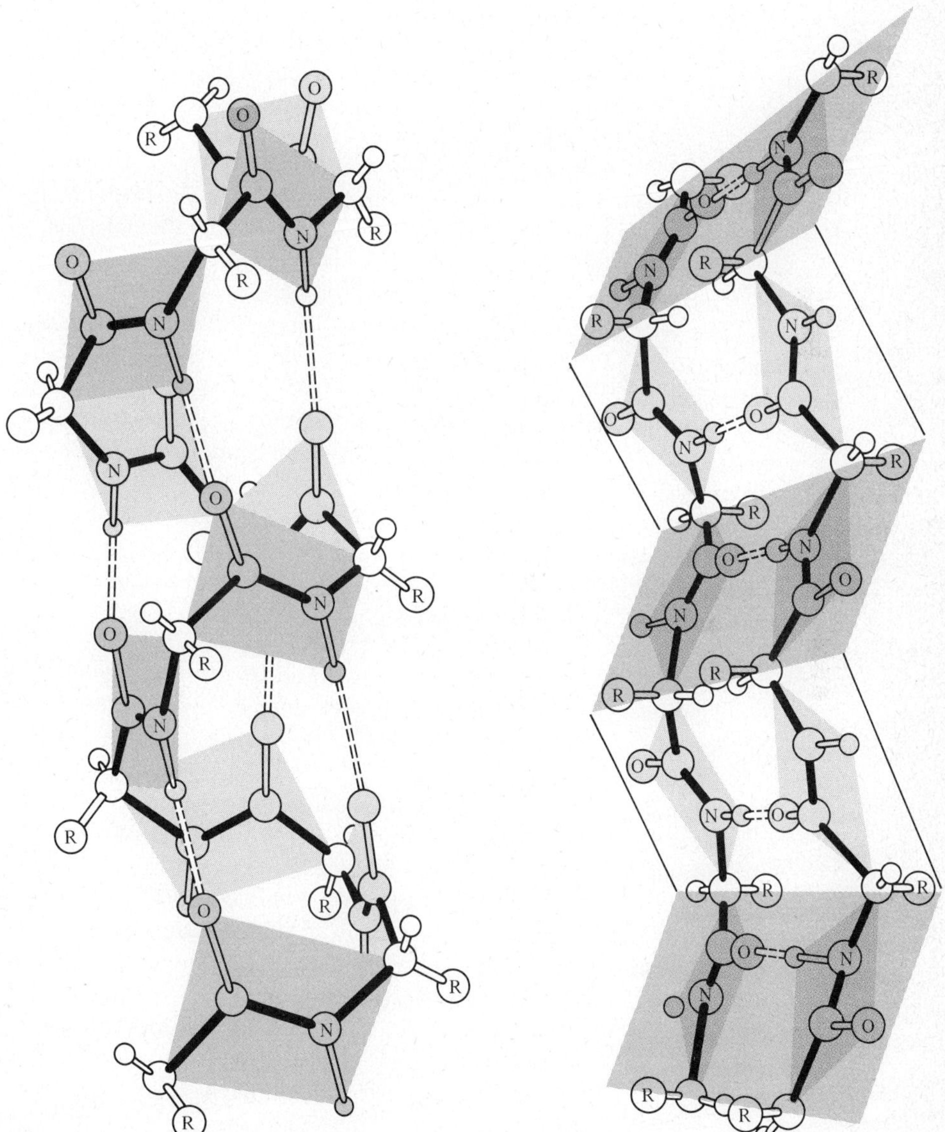

Figure 2.2 (A) The α-helix with 3.6 residues per turn has intrastrand hydrogen bonds which stabilize its structure. (B) Antiparallel β-strands have interstrand hydrogen bonds stabilizing the structure. Hydrogen bonds are shown as dashed lines. Regions of coplanarity are clearly indicated. (Reproduced by courtesy of Dr. I. Geis, Department of Biophysics and Theoretical Biology, University of Chicago, Chicago, IL 60637)

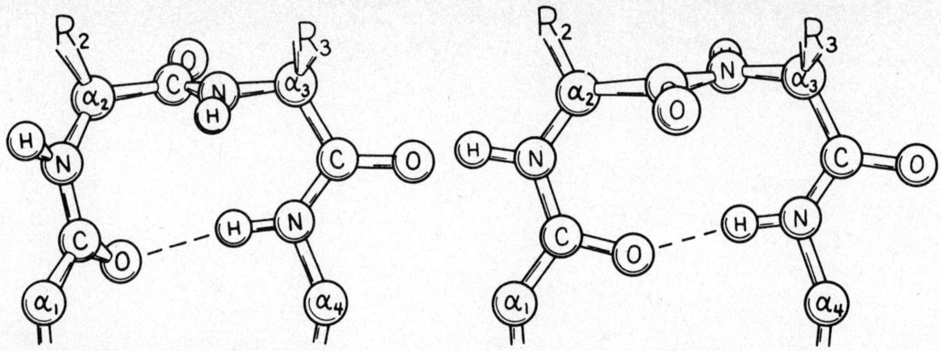

Figure 2.3 The two major types of β-turns found in proteins. (Reproduced with permission from F. R. Salemme and G. Zubay, "Anatomy of Protein Structure," in *Biochemistry,* G. Zubay, ed., Addison-Wesley, Reading, MA, 1983.)

The α-helix possesses a number of characteristic features as shown in Figure 2.2(a).

1. Intrachain hydrogen bonds are formed between the backbone amide hydrogen and the backbone carbonyl oxygens of residues which are four amino acids further along the chain.
2. The hydrogen bonds are nearly parallel to the axis of the helix.
3. The spacing between turns is 5.6 Å along the helix axis, and each turn incorporates 3.6 residues. Therefore, the advance per amino acyl residue is about 1.5 Å along the helical axis.
4. The amino acyl side chains all lie outside the coil of the α-helix.
5. Glutamyl, methionyl, and alanyl residues form particularly stable α-helices, while prolyl, glycyl, and disulfide-bonded cysteyl residues are frequent α-helix breakers.

The relative probabilities that different residues will occur in an α-helical configuration are listed in the first column of Table 2.2.

Although alternative hydrogen-bonded helical arrangements have been proposed, the right-handed α-helix is by far the most common helix found in native proteins. Both the tight packing resulting in part from the exclusion of amino acyl side chains from the center of the helix and the regular hydrogen bonding between all backbone carbonyl and amide groups, appear to account for its exceptional stability. Short (but not extended) left-handed helical structures, usually incorporating glycyl residues, are found in proteins, frequently as β-turns (see p. 20).

Like the α-helix, β-strands possess a number of characteristic features as illustrated in Figure 2.2(b) and summarized in Table 2.1.

1. Interchain hydrogen bonds are formed between the peptide backbone carbonyl groups and amide hydrogens of adjacent, parallel (or antiparallel) chains.
2. The hydrogen bonds are nearly perpendicular to the axis of the two extended strands.

TABLE 2.1 THE CHARACTERISTICS OF PRINCIPAL SECONDARY STRUCTURAL ELEMENTS IN PROTEINS: α-HELICES, β-STRANDS AND β-TURNS

Type of structure	The hydrogen bonds formed between the backbone C=O and N−H moieties are:	The orientation of the hydrogen bond(s) is (are):	Each residue advances:	Residue side chains project:	Residues that contribute greatest stability to the structure	Residues that usually are not accommodated
α-helix (Fig. 2.2a)	Intrastrand, involving every fourth residue	Parallel to the axis of the helix	1.5 Å along the helical axis	Outward, away from the axis of the helix	*glu* *met* *ala*	*pro* *gly* *cys*—S | *cys*—S
β-strand (Fig. 2.2b)	Interstrand, involving adjacent groups	Perpendicular to the axes of the two strands	6.5 Å (parallel) or 7.0 Å (antiparallel) along the backbone strand	Alternately on opposite sides of the sheet plane	Hydrophobic residues	*glu* *asp* *pro*
β-turn (Fig. 2.3)	Intrastrand, involving residues 1 and 4	Perpendicular to the axes of the two polypeptide chains entering the turn	About 45° through the turn	Outward from the loop (residues 2 and 3), or perpendicular to the axes of the strands (residues 1 and 4)	*gly* *asn* *pro*	Hydrophobic residues

TABLE 2.2 CONFORMATIONAL PARAMETERS OF SECONDARY STRUCTURAL ELEMENTS IN PROTEINS, BASED ON DATA AVERAGED FROM 29 PROTEINS.[a]

P_α		P_β		P_t	
glu	1.51	*val*	1.70	*asn*	1.56
met	1.45	*ile*	1.60	*gly*	1.56
ala	1.42	*tyr*	1.47	*pro*	1.52
leu	1.21	*phe*	1.38	*asp*	1.46
lys	1.16	*trp*	1.37	*ser*	1.43
phe	1.13	*leu*	1.30	*cys*	1.19
gln	1.11	*cys*	1.19	*tyr*	1.14
trp	1.08	*thr*	1.19	*lys*	1.01
ile	1.08	*gln*	1.10	*gln*	0.98
val	1.06	*met*	1.05	*thr*	0.96
asp	1.01	*arg*	0.93	*trp*	0.96
his	1.00	*asn*	0.89	*arg*	0.95
arg	0.98	*his*	0.87	*his*	0.95
thr	0.83	*ala*	0.83	*glu*	0.74
ser	0.77	*ser*	0.75	*ala*	0.66
cys	0.70	*gly*	0.75	*met*	0.60
tyr	0.69	*lys*	0.74	*phe*	0.60
asn	0.67	*pro*	0.55	*leu*	0.59
pro	0.57	*asp*	0.54	*val*	0.50
gly	0.57	*glu*	0.37	*ile*	0.47

[a] *P* values represent relative probabilities that a particular internal amino acyl residue in a protein will reside within an α-helix (P_α), a β-strand (P_β), or a β-turn (P_t).

3. *Parallel* β-sheets are arranged with the same N to C polypeptide sense with a repeat period of 6.5 Å per residue pair, while *antiparallel* β-sheets are arranged with alternately opposite N to C polypeptide senses with a repeat period of 7.0 Å.
4. The alternate amino acyl side chains point to opposite sides of the sheet, but have their peptide planes nearly in the sheet plane to insure good interchain hydrogen bonding.
5. Hydrophobic residues form β-strands with greatest stability, while glutamyl, aspartyl, and prolyl residues occur in β-strands with low probability.

The relative probabilities for the participation of the different residues in a β-stranded configuration are listed in the second column of Table 2.2.

Like the α-helix and β-strands, β-turns possess a number of characteristic features (Table 2.1).

1. β-turns [types I and II, Figures 2.3(a) and (b)] form tight loops which change the strand direction by 180° in a 4 residue turn. The first residue carbonyl group forms a hydrogen bond with the amide hydrogen of the residue in position 4 of the turn.
2. This hydrogen bond is nearly perpendicular to the axis of the two connected strands.
3. Each residue turns about 45° so that the 4 residue turn reverses the direction of the polypeptide chain.
4. The amino acyl side chains of residues 2 and 3 project outward, away from the center of the turn. Those of residues 1 and 4 project up or down, perpendicular to the strand axis.
5. Glycyl, prolyl, and asparaginyl residues occur in β-turns with highest frequency, while hydrophobic residues occur in these structures with low frequency (see the third column of Table 2.2). The flexibility of glycyl residues and the restricted conformation of prolyl residues, both of which are frequent α-helix breakers, may help to explain their high frequency in β-turns.

Some sections of the polypeptide chains in proteins do not form any one of the three common structural elements discussed above, and they do not form any sort of regular repeating unit. These portions of the chain are said to form a "random coil." The term "random coil" therefore refers to a part of a polypeptide chain that lacks organized secondary structure. It should be noted, however, that in any one protein, an amino acyl residue in a region of random coil is likely to assume one preferable, thermodynamically most stable position.

2.3 TERTIARY STRUCTURES OF WATER-SOLUBLE PROTEINS

As summarized in Table 2.2, different amino acyl residues form each of the three principal secondary structural elements found in proteins with differing facilities. It is evident that primary structure determines secondary structure. In most enzymes, tertiary structure, also determined by the amino acyl sequence, results from close packing of the secondary structural elements as they fold back on themselves. Forces that contribute to the stability of the folded coil include charge neutralization (electrostatic interactions), hydrophobic forces, and hydrogen bonds.

Generally, proteins cannot exist as single-layered structures in aqueous solution because at least two layers are required to bury the hydrophobic core residues. A general principle of protein folding requires that entropy be maximized by minimizing interaction between water and nonpolar residue side chains. Hydrophilic residues generally appear on the surface; hydrophobic residues comprise the core. Application of this principle requires efficient packing between extended structural elements such as α-helices, parallel β-sheets, and antiparallel β-sheets.

Proteins possess a diversity of structures that accommodate their multiplicity of functions (Table 2.3). Most water-soluble proteins are either compact globular structures as in the case of enzymes, or extended, multistranded fibrous structures as in the case of many structural and contractile proteins (Table 2.3). The latter may consist of extended but intertwined α-helices as in α-keratin, or they may consist of β-pleated sheets as in β-keratin. Globular proteins usually contain a variety of structural elements. For example, the small enzyme, lysozyme, contains six antiparallel β-strands arranged in two β-pleated sheets, six short α-helical segments and connecting stretches including six β-turns, and several regions of random coil. Small proteins such as lysozyme usually consist of single, tightly packed, globular structures. However, large proteins more often fold into two (or more) locally compact structural units called *domains.* The most common domain size is between 100 and 200 residues, but domains varying in

TABLE 2.3 FUNCTIONAL DIVERSITY OF PROTEINS

Classification	Representative examples	Function
1. Enzymes	Lysozyme	Hydrolysis of bacterial cell walls
	Trypsin	Hydrolysis of proteins
2. Storage proteins	Ovalbumin	Amino acid storage in egg white
	Ferritin	Iron storage in spleen
3. Transport proteins		
A. in blood	Hemoglobin	Oxygen transport
B. transmembrane solute carriers	Glucose permease	Transports glucose in and out of cells
C. electron carriers	Cytochrome *c*	Carries electrons from cytochrome *b* to cytochrome *c* oxidase
4. Protective proteins	Fibrinogen	Blood clotting
	Antibodies	Neutralization of foreign objects and cells
5. Contractile proteins	Actin and myosin	Cell and organismal motility
6. Toxins	Cholera toxin	Animal toxin produced by bacteria
	Melitin	Animal toxin produced by bees
7. Peptide hormones	Insulin	Intercellular communication: regulation of metabolism
	Growth hormone	Intercellular communication: regulation of bone growth
8. Structural proteins	α-keratin	In skin, hair, nails, etc.
	β-keratin	In silk and spiders' webs

size between 40 and 400 residues have been observed to exist in proteins. Sometimes two domains resemble each other to a striking degree, suggesting that they probably arose during evolutionary history from a single smaller unit as a result of the duplication of genetic material. In other cases, the two domains exhibit little or no structural similarity, suggesting independent origins.

Two-domain proteins consisting of a single polypeptide chain may possess independent globular domains, loosely connected by a flexible polypeptide chain, or the two domains may be in close proximity with many hydrophobic contacts preventing entry of water into the intervening space. The majority of two-domain proteins, however, exhibit an intermediate level of domain separation. In these proteins, a fair degree of contact occurs within the cleft between the domains, but the distinction between other portions of the two elongated globular structures clearly delineates them as separate. An example of an enzyme with such a structure is phosphoglycerate kinase, found in the glycolytic cycle.

Just as different enzymes exhibit domains with varying degrees of structural autonomy, they also exhibit varying degrees of functional autonomy. In the case of two-substrate enzymes consisting of two relatively independent domains, the binding site for one substrate may be associated with one domain, while that for the other substrate is associated with the other domain. In other cases one domain may function catalytically, while the other serves the purpose of allosteric regulation. Enzymes consisting of closely interacting domains frequently bind their substrates in a cleft between the two domains, which therefore serve a single catalytic function.

The structure of one overlapping, two-domain protein (the arabinose binding protein from *Escherichia coli*) is shown in Figure 2.4. This protein, which binds arabinose with high affinity and functions in the transmembrane transport of this sugar into bacterial cells, consists of two similarly structured domains. The sugar binds in the cleft between the two domains, and substrate binding induces a conformational change which partially closes the cleft, thereby locking the sugar into its binding site. This "breathing" motion is required not only for the reversible high-affinity binding of the sugar in the cleft region, it also functions secondarily to couple sugar binding to the transmembrane translocation step which is catalyzed by integral membrane protein constituents of the transport system with which the binding protein interacts. Conformational changes of this type usually accompany substrate binding and catalytic turnover of enzymes and transport systems.

2.4 TERTIARY STRUCTURES OF INTEGRAL MEMBRANE PROTEINS

About half of the proteins in a cell are associated with membranous structures. Many of these proteins are partly embedded within the hydrophobic matrix of the phospholipid bilayer which serves as the structural element of all biological membranes. The structures of several of these integral membrane proteins have been elucidated. Some such proteins consist of two domains which are linearly polarized. One end of the polypeptide chain forms a globular domain which extends from the membrane surface into the aqueous medium. The other end is more hydrophobic in nature and forms a small domain which is largely embedded in the phospholipid bilayer of the membrane.

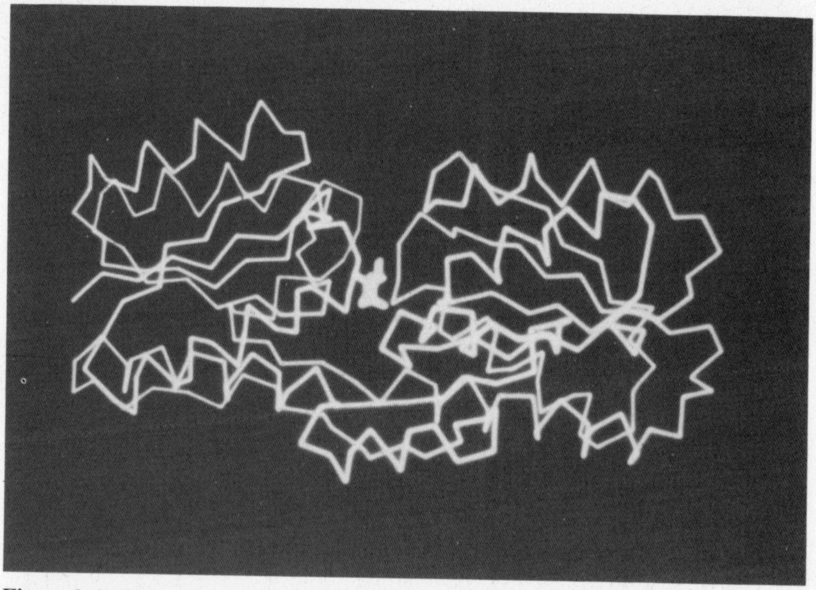

Figure 2.4 Schematic depiction of the L-arabinose binding protein, a constituent of the L-arabinose transport system in *E. coli.* The protein is shown binding its ligand, L-arabinose, in the cleft between the two domains of the protein. (Courtesy of Dr. F. A. Quiocho.)

Two protein components of a fatty acid reductase system found in the endoplasmic reticulum of animal cells possess such a structure. These proteins function as parts of an electron transport chain. Electrons are transferred from NADH to the first of these enzymes, called NADH:cytochrome b_5 reductase, then to a smaller protein of fundamentally similar structure called cytochrome b_5, and, finally, to the desaturase that is responsible for introduction of a carbon–carbon double bond into a previously saturated fatty acid. In both cytochrome b_5 and its reductase, the water-soluble moiety serves a catalytic role while the hydrophobic domain serves to anchor the molecule to the membrane.

A second integral membrane protein whose structure is known is called *glycophorin.* It is the glycoprotein in the human red blood cell that carries the MN blood group specificity and serves as the receptor for influenza virus. This protein is known to consist of three domains. The C-terminal part of the protein forms a water-soluble, globular structure on the cytoplasmic side of the membrane. The central portion of the protein, a very hydrophobic segment of the polypeptide chain which is about 20 amino acyl residues in length, passes through the membrane as an α-helix. Since α-helices form completely hydrogen-bonded backbone structures, they can be stably inserted into the hydrophobic matrix of a membrane provided that the amino acyl side chains are predominantly hydrophobic in nature. The larger N-terminal domain, the receptor domain of the protein, is water-soluble and extends into the aqueous medium on the external surface of the membrane. Thus, only the central portion of this protein resides in the lipid bilayer.

A third class of integral membrane proteins having structural features in common—possibly as a consequence of their common function—is represented by the transmembrane transport proteins. The polypeptide chains of all structurally well-characterized integral membrane proteins which catalyze the transport of solute molecules across biological membranes have been found to span the membrane several times. Two of the best characterized transport proteins are the mannitol and lactose permeases in *E. coli.* These two proteins transport their sugar substrates by different mechanisms: the mannitol permease is a component of the bacterial phosphotransferase system which catalyzes the phosphorylation of its sugar substrate as it passes through the membrane. Thus, the sugar substrate of this enzyme is extracellular mannitol, while the product of the reaction catalyzed by it is cytoplasmic mannitol-1-phosphate. On the other hand, the lactose permease does not modify its sugar substrate, but it can accumulate the substrate a thousandfold against a concentration gradient in energy-proficient cells because lactose uptake is coupled to the uptake of a proton which flows down its electrochemical gradient into the cell. This type of *chemiosmotic coupling* will be discussed in Chapters 5 and 7.

Elucidation of the nucleotide sequence of the gene which encodes the mannitol permease in *E. coli* allowed the amino acid sequence of the protein to be deduced. Computer analyses of the hydropathy indices of amino acyl residues along the polypeptide chain (as summarized in Figure 1.1) gave the hydropathy plot shown in Figure 2.5. In such a plot, a water-soluble, globular protein normally possesses an average hydropathy value of zero. Portions of the chain that are strongly hydrophilic fall below the midline, while those that are hydrophobic project above the midline. Careful scrutiny of Figure 2.5 reveals that the N-terminal half of the protein is strongly hydrophobic, while the C-terminal half of the molecule exhibits the characteristics of a typical water-soluble protein. Moreover, within the *N*-terminal half, there are seven stretches, each at least 20 amino acyl residues in length, which are of sufficient hydrophobicity to

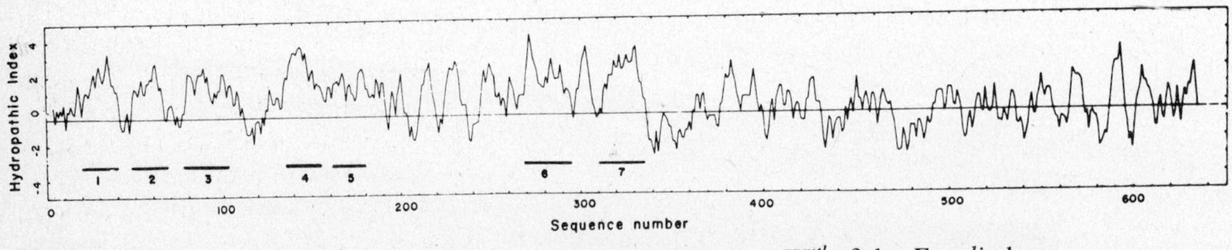

Figure 2.5 Hydropathic profile of the mannitol permease (Enzyme II^{mtl} of the *E. coli* phosphotransferase system) amino acid sequence. The hydropathy analysis was conducted employing a computer program which assigns values to each amino acid based on its hydropathic character (Figure 1.1). Using a moving-segment approach that continuously determines the average hydropathy of a segment of seven residues as it advances through the sequence, consecutive scores are plotted at the middle of each segment from the amino terminus to the carboxy terminus. As shown, seven hydrophobic regions of 19 residues or greater are indicated by the numbered lines below the graph. These regions are of sufficient length to pass through the membrane as α-helices. (Reproduced with permission from C. A. Lee and M. H. Saier, Jr., "Mannitol-specific Enzyme II of the Bacterial Phosphotransferase System III. The Nucleotide Sequence of the Permease Gene," *Journal of Biological Chemistry,* **258:** 10761–10767, 1983.)

allow the chains to enter into and pass through the phospholipid bilayer as α-helices. The axes of these helices are thought to be nearly perpendicular to the plane of the membrane. Each helix, with one exception, is flanked by an amino acyl sequence which may well form a β-turn. It therefore appears that the N-terminal domain passes through the membrane at least seven times, while the C-terminal domain is localized to the inner cytoplasmic surface of the membrane. The latter domain may consist largely of short α-helical segments which fold back on themselves. The proposed structure of the protein is shown in Figure 2.6.

Similar analyses conducted with the lactose permease of *E. coli* have led to the proposal that this protein, which is largely hydrophobic, consists of twelve transmembrane α-helices. Comparable studies with other integral membrane transport proteins from both bacterial and animal sources have revealed structures that probably traverse the membrane several times. Such structures therefore appear to be characteristic of this fundamental class of proteins.

2.5 QUATERNARY STRUCTURES OF PROTEINS

Many proteins exist in cells as oligomers of a single polypeptide chain and/or in complexation with other proteins. For example, yeast hexokinase is a dimer of two identical subunits, muscle phosphofructokinase is a tetrameric protein of four identical subunits, and glutamine synthase from *E. coli* contains twelve identical subunits (Table 2.4). *E. coli* aspartate transcarbamoylase also consists of twelve protein subunits, but these are of two types: six catalytic subunits that function to catalyze a chemical reaction, and six regulatory subunits that function solely to control the activities of the catalytic subunits. The pyruvate dehydrogenase complex of bovine heart mitochondria is one of the largest enzyme complexes known. It consists of 160 separate polypeptide chains of seven distinct types and has a molecular weight of about 7

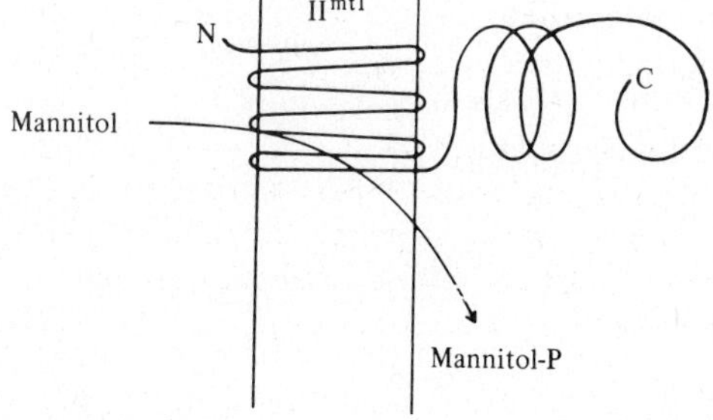

Figure 2.6 Possible disposition of the mannitol permease (Enzyme II^{mtl} of the *E. coli* phosphotransferase system) in the membrane. The model shows seven transmembrane segments within the hydrophobic amino terminal half of the enzyme. The hydrophilic carboxy terminal half of the protein is known to be a globular structure localized to the cytoplasmic surface of the membrane. The amino- and carboxy-termini are indicated by N and C, respectively. The figure also depicts the transport of extracellular mannitol across the membrane with the release of mannitol-1-phosphate in the cytoplasm. The phosphoryl donor for this process is phosphoenolpyruvate, and the permease is transiently phosphorylated before translocation of the sugar across the membrane can occur.

TABLE 2.4 MOLECULAR WEIGHTS AND SUBUNIT COMPOSITIONS OF ENZYMES AND TRANSPORT PROTEINS

Protein	Source	Molecular weight	Number of subunits
Enzymes			
Lysozyme	Egg white	14,000	1
Hexokinase	Yeast	102,000	2
Phosphofructokinase	Muscle	340,000	4
Glutamine synthase	*E. coli*	600,000	12
Aspartate transcarbamoylase	*E. coli*	310,000	12 (2 types)
Pyruvate dehydrogenase complex	Beef heart mitochondria	7,000,000	160 (6 types)
Transport proteins			
Cytochrome *c*	Beef heart mitochondria	13,000	1
Lactose permease	*E. coli*	45,000	1
Mannitol permease	*E. coli*	136,000	2
Cytochrome oxidase	Beef heart mitochondria	340,000	24 (12 types)

million. This large protein assembly actually catalyzes five primary reactions and is subject to multiple forms of control. The product of each primary reaction is passed directly on to the next enzyme where it serves as substrate for the next chemical conversion. Regulatory enzymes within the complex catalyze its covalent modification.

Finally, integral membrane proteins can exist either in the monomeric state within the phospholipid bilayer or they can associate to form oligomers. While the lactose permease in *E. coli* appears capable of functioning as a monomer, the monomeric form of the mannitol permease appears to self-associate to give a catalytically active dimer. Mammalian cytochrome oxidase, the terminal component of the mitochondrial electron transport chain, has a molecular weight of 340,000 and consists of up to twelve dissimilar polypeptide chains, all tightly associated with the matrix of the membrane.

From the preceding discussion, it should be clear that many proteins have evolved as oligomeric structures. This higher degree of complexity presumably serves to enhance reaction rates, to coordinate separate reactions in a single metabolic pathway, to allow allosteric regulation of enzyme activities, and to coordinate regulatory interactions with enzymes that control the activities of other enzymes. Many enzymes are undoubtedly integrated in the cell architecture. It is also possible, however, that the oligomeric structures of some enzymes reflect the evolutionary histories of these proteins and no longer serve a useful function.

Regardless of function, the structural basis of molecular association is fairly well understood. Protein oligomers generally are symmetrical, geometric structures, owing to the occurrence of repeated nearest-neighbor interactions between subunits which stabilize a closed structure. In cases where open structures are generated, fibers or helical arrays of subunits result from the continuous addition of protein monomers to the growing chain.

While symmetry is a characteristic feature of many enzyme complexes, it should not be assumed that symmetry is a requirement for self-association. X-ray crystallographic analyses have revealed several quaternary interactions that are not symmetrical, even between identical subunits. Moreover, structural asymmetry may be of functional significance. In an asymmetrical dimeric structure, one subunit may catalyze one reaction while the other functions in another capacity. For example, if the overall reaction catalyzed by a dimer consists of two sequential reactions, $A \xrightarrow{a} B \xrightarrow{b} C$, one subunit might catalyze reaction *a* while the second simultaneously catalyzes reaction *b* (Figure 2.7). Then, in the next catalytic event, the first subunit would catalyze reaction *b* while the second subunit catalyzes reaction *a*. Such alternating functions have been termed "half-of-sites" reactivity. Alternative designations include "alternating sites reactivity," "anticooperativity," "reciprocal interaction," and "flip flop." Some evidence suggests that such processes may be important to vectorial as well as chemical catalytic processes mediated by proteins. Examples of proteins that are thought to function by half-of-sites mechanisms will be discussed in Chapters 5, 6, and 7.

2.6 EVOLUTION OF PROTEIN STRUCTURE AND FUNCTION

As a consequence of the preceding discussion, it should be apparent to the reader that the structures of proteins are exceptionally diverse, accounting for the variety of catalytic functions required by living organisms. If the gene sequence dictates the primary amino acyl sequence of a protein, and the latter determines its structure and function, then analysis of the primary nucleotide sequence of a gene should potentially reveal

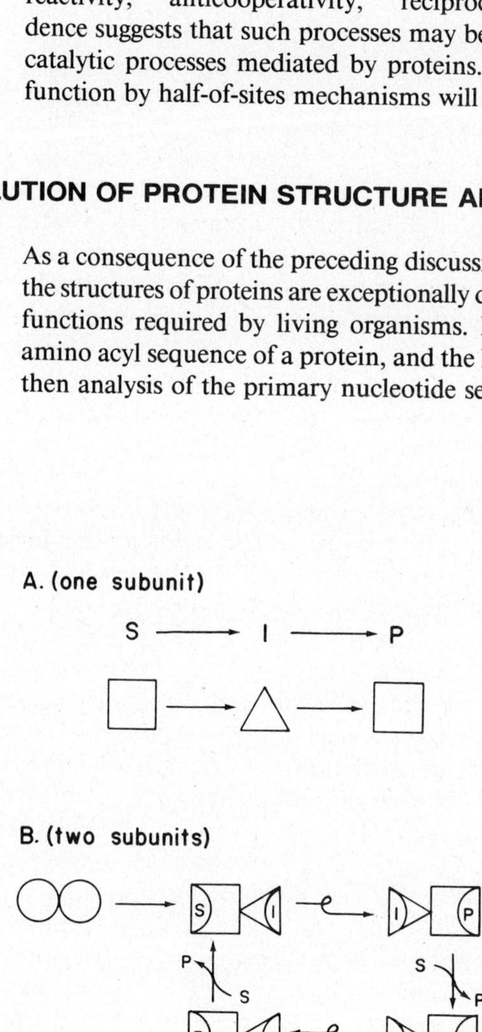

Figure 2.7 Schematic depiction of the process termed *half-of-sites* reactivity, or *flip-flop*, in which the structural asymmetry of an enzyme assumes functional significance. The dimeric enzyme depicted consists of two identical subunits, which can assume two ligand-induced conformational states (triangle and square). One conformation of the subunit (square) possesses affinity for the substrate S and the product P, but not for the intermediate I. The other conformation of the subunit possesses high affinity for I, but does not bind S or P. One conformational transition (square to triangle) is induced by the chemical interconversion S → I. I is a tightly bound intermediate which does not dissociate from the enzyme surface. The reverse conformational transition (triangle to square) is induced by the chemical interconversion I → P. As a consequence, the conformational change (square to triangle) of one subunit is tightly coupled to the reverse transition (triangle to square) of the other subunit, as shown. Although single-headed arrows have been drawn to indicate directionality, all reactions may occur reversibly.

every three-dimensional detail of the protein it encodes as well as the mechanism of its action. This theoretical possibility is far from being realized. Our predictive methods are too crude, and even when the tertiary structure of an enzyme is revealed by x-ray crystallographic techniques, much effort is required to establish its mechanism of action. Primary amino acyl sequence analyses do, however, tell us a great deal about the relatedness of different proteins which reflect their evolutionary origins. For example, cytochrome *c* is a class of small electron transport carriers present in mitochondria and aerobic bacteria. All such proteins isolated from different organisms exhibit similar amino acyl sequences and tertiary structures and are functionally interchangeable in *in vitro* assays regardless of their biological origin. The degree to which these proteins differ is a reflection of their evolutionary distance. In fact, one can estimate the time of evolutionary divergence of two or more different species by analyzing the amino acyl sequences of related proteins within these organisms. By carrying out such analyses in closely related present-day species, the sequences of proteins in extinct ancestral organisms can be accurately determined. By performing similar analyses on proteins from evolutionarily divergent species, the primary structures of proteins within primordial organisms that lived over a billion years ago can be predicted. In this way the evolutionary history of a protein can be traced. Such studies have led to a tentative understanding of the branching pathways that have led to protein diversification.

We can now state with fair certainty that all living organisms share a tremendous amount of related genetic material. This fact presumably reflects their common ancestry and leads to the suggestion that all present-day organisms, from bacteria to man, arose from a single cell.

Not only is it probable that homologous proteins in different organisms share a common evolutionary origin, but proteins of related structures and functions within a single organism probably also share a common evolutionary history. The bacterium, *E. coli,* contains about a dozen solute binding proteins which function in the transmembrane transport of sugars, amino acids, and salts. These proteins differ from one another with respect to their ligand specificities, but they contain the same general three-dimensional structural features as shown in Figure 2.4 for the L-arabinose binding protein. Most of these proteins exhibit a similar size, and the most closely related of these proteins show over 80% sequence homology. Others lack clearly identifiable sequence homologies, but they all show the same two-domain structure with the ligand binding site in the cleft between the two domains. It is therefore postulated that repeated duplication of the primordial binding protein gene followed by evolutionary divergence must have given rise to all of the binding proteins of differing specificities.

Further examination of the structure shown in Figure 2.4 reveals that the two domains within the L-arabinose binding protein exhibit structural similarities. In this protein both domains contain a six-stranded parallel β-sheet flanked by two α-helices on either side. This fact suggests that the two domains of the protein may have arisen by duplication of genetic material within a single primordial gene of about half of its present-day size prior to the duplication and divergence of the ancestral binding protein gene. Extensive sequence analyses conducted with many proteins have revealed that such occurrences must have been frequent throughout evolutionary history.

In subsequent chapters, many other examples of proteins exhibiting common structural features and evolutionary origins will be discussed. Proteins of very different functions have been shown to share a common ancestry. Some of these are multifunctional proteins which show sequence homology with proteins with only one or two of the multiple functions of the first protein. It seems that proteins gain and lose catalytic activities as mutations in their structural genes alter their structures. It is clear that the notion of one gene/one protein/one function is inadequate to account for the wide diversity of catalytic activities found in nature.

> *The truth is not a citadel of certainty to be defended against error: It is a shady spot where one eats lunch before tramping on.*
>
> —LYNN WHITE, *Machina ex Deo*

BIBLIOGRAPHY

Blake, C. C. F., and L. N. Johnson, "Protein Structure", *Trends Biochem Sci.*, **9:** 147–151 (1984).

Cheng, T. C., ed., *Structure of Membranes and Receptors,* Plenum, New York (1984).

Chothia, C., "Principles that Determine the Structure of Proteins," *Ann. Rev. Biochem.*, **53:** 537–572 (1984).

Doolittle, R. F., "Fibrinogen and Fibrin," *Scientific American,* **245:** 126–135 (1981).

Doolittle, R. F., "Similar Amino Acid Sequences: Chance or Common Ancestry?" *Science,* **214:** 149–159 (1981).

Doolittle, R. F., "Protein Evolution," in *The Proteins,* H. Neurath and R. L. Hill, eds., Volume IV, Academic, New York (1979).

Eisenberg, D., "Three-Dimensional Structure of Membrane and Surface Proteins," *Ann. Rev. Biochem.*, **53:** 595–623 (1984).

Gilliland, G. L., and F. A. Quiocho, "Structure of the L-Arabinose-Binding Protein from *Escherichia coli* at 2.4 Å Resolution," *J. Mol. Biol.*, **146:** 341–362 (1981).

Karplus, M., and J. A. McCammon, "Dynamics of Proteins: Elements and Function," *Ann. Rev. Biochem.*, **53:** 263–300 (1983).

Kim, P. S., and R. L. Baldwin, "Specific Intermediates in the Folding Reactions of Small Proteins and the Mechanism of Protein Folding," *Ann. Rev. Biochem.*, **51:** 459–489 (1982).

Kyte, J., and R. F. Doolittle, "A Simple Method for Displaying the Hydropathic Character of a Protein," *J. Mol. Biol.*, **157:** 105–132 (1982).

Lerner, R. A., "Synthetic Vaccines," *Scientific American,* **248:** 66–74 (1983).

Pestka, S., "The Purification and Manufacture of Human Interferons," *Scientific American,* **249:** 37–43 (1983).

Quagliariello, E., and F. Palmieri, eds., "Structure and Function of Membrane Proteins," in *Proceedings of the International Symposium on Structure and Function of Membrane Proteins,* Elsevier/North Holland, Amsterdam (1983).

Saier, M. H., Jr., *Mechanisms and Regulation of Carbohydrate Transport in Bacteria,* Academic, New York (1985).

Saier, M. H., Jr., and G. R. Jacobson, *The Molecular Basis of Sex and Differentiation,* Springer-Verlag, New York (1984).

Saier, M. H., Jr., and C. D. Stiles, *Molecular Dynamics in Membrane Biology,* Springer-Verlag, New York (1975).

Salemme, F. R., "Anatomy of Protein Structure," in *Biochemistry,* G. Zubay, ed., pp. 69–129, Addison-Wesley, Reading, MA (1983).

Schulz, G. E., and R. H. Schirmer, *Principles of Protein Structure,* Springer-Verlag, New York (1979).

Unwin, N., and R. Henderson, "The Structure of Proteins in Biological Membranes," *Scientific American,* **250:** 78–94 (1984).

Chapter 3

Enzyme Catalysis

> *In the center there is a narrow path that leads to the top of the mountain. That path suggests a harmony in life. It is the path of perfection.*
>
> —JUAN MASCARO

Among the most remarkable features of a living organism are the processes by which metabolic reactions are catalyzed and coordinated. Virtually every reaction in every cellular metabolic pathway is catalyzed by an enzyme regardless of whether it plays an anabolic (biosynthetic), catabolic (degradative), or amphibolic (both biosynthetic and degradative) role. As a consequence, a living cell contains thousands of enzymes which confer upon this minimal unit of life its vital characteristics.

In order to understand the ways in which proteins with the structural features described in the preceding chapter can enhance reaction rates up to 10^{20}-fold, enzyme catalysis must be dissected into its constituent rate-enhancement factors. These factors are discussed in Sections 3.2 and 3.3. One of the principal approaches to the study of enzymes involves the kinetic analysis of the reactions they catalyze. This subject is presented briefly in Sections 3.4 and 3.5, while parameters influencing reaction rates are considered in Sections 3.6 and 3.7.

The mechanisms by which the activities of enzymes are regulated are discussed in the last three sections of this chapter. It will be seen that enzymes have evolved increasing degrees of complexity in order to allow them to gain sensitivity to control by a variety of stimuli. Responsiveness to such stimuli allows each cell to precisely coordinate the multifaceted components of its catalytic machinery.

3.1 ENZYME CLASSIFICATION

As discussed in Chapter 2, thousands of enzymes have been characterized, and thousands more have yet to be discovered. Some estimates suggest that the genome of *E. coli* encodes about 5,000 enzymes, over half of which are currently known. Enzymes are classified into six major groups according to directives dictated by the International

Union of Biochemists. Each enzyme receives an Enzyme Commission (E.C.) number, which has four components indicating respectively the class, subclass, sub-subclass and the enzyme itself. This approach to enzyme classification is exemplified in Table 3.1 and briefly discussed below.

The six major enzyme classes include:

1. *Oxidoreductases,* which catalyze oxidation–reduction reactions;
2. *Transferases,* which transfer a chemical group from one molecule to another (intermolecular transfer) or within a single molecule (intramolecular transfer);
3. *Hydrolases,* which use water to cleave a single molecule into two distinct molecules;
4. *Lyases,* which split a molecule in two by a nonhydrolytic process;
5. *Isomerases,* which interconvert isomeric structures by intramolecular rearrangements; and
6. *Ligases* or *synthases,* which create a new chemical bond, usually coupled to nucleoside triphosphate hydrolysis, thereby joining two separate molecules into one.

Each of these classes is divided into subclasses, determined by the nature of the bond or molecular substituent that is acted on. Each subclass is further subdivided based on a variety of criteria. It should be pointed out that this classification system is somewhat arbitrary, frequently based more on biological function than on reaction mechanism. The examples provided in Table 3.1 were taken from a 200-page table which is constantly being revised and extended as more enzymes are discovered and characterized. As illustrated in Table 3.1, each enzyme is assigned a systematic name based on the substrates it acts upon, the class within which it falls, and sometimes on the bond or molecular group which is acted upon. Each enzyme also possesses a shorter, "trivial" name which is more commonly used by biochemists. As indicated in the table, many enzymes require a metal ion and/or some other cofactor for biological activity.

3.2 THE NATURE OF ENZYME CATALYSIS

Enzymes usually increase reaction rates between 10^{10}- and 10^{20}-fold over the uncatalyzed rate. They are frequently in excess of 10^{10}-fold more efficient than man-made catalysts and are always more specific with respect to the substrates acted on. For example, virtually all enzymes except racemases which act on optically active compounds exhibit absolute specificity for just one of the D- and L-isomers of an enantiomer pair. This fact dictates that each enzyme must interact with at least three of the four molecular groupings about the chiral center in question.

There are eight general processes or methods by which enzymes enhance reaction rates. These are listed in Table 3.2 and are discussed briefly below:

1. *Specific acid or base catalysis.* Like many organic chemical reactions, enzymes can utilize H^+ or OH^- from the solvent to protonate or deprotonate a substrate moiety.

TABLE 3.1 REPRESENTATIVE ENZYMES ILLUSTRATING A SYSTEMATIC APPROACH TO ENZYME CLASSIFICATION[a]

E.C. #	Systematic name	Trivial name	Active groups and cofactors	Reaction
1.	*Oxidoreductases*			
1.1.1.1	Alcohol:NAD$^+$ oxidoreductase	Alcohol dehydrogenase	Zn^{++}	Alcohol + NAD$^+$ → aldehyde or ketone + NADH
1.1.2.3	L-lactate:cytochrome *c* oxidoreductase	Lactate dehydrogenase	Flavin, heme	L-lactate + 2 cytochrome *c* (ox) → pyruvate + 2 cytochrome *c* (red)
2.	*Transferases*			
2.4.1.11	UDP glucose:glycogen α1,4-glucosyl transferase	Glycogen synthase	Mg^{++}	UDP glucose + $(glucose)_n$ → UDP + $(glucose)_{n+1}$
2.6.1.2	L-alanine:2-oxoglutarate amino transferase	Alanine aminotransferase	PLP	L-alanine + α-ketoglutarate → pyruvate + L-glutamate
2.7.1.1	ATP:D-glucose 6-phosphotransferase	Glucokinase	Mg^{++}	ATD + D-glucose → ADP + glucose-6-P
3.	*Hydrolases*			
3.1.3.1	Phosphoric monoester phosphohydrolase	Alkaline phosphatase	M^{++}	Phosphate ester + H_2O → an alcohol + H_3PO_4
3.4.4.4	Peptide peptidohydrolase	Trypsin		Peptide (or ester) hydrolysis
4.	*Lyases*			
4.1.1.15	L-glutamate 1-carboxy-lyase	Glutamate decarboxylase	PLP	L-glutamate → 4-aminobutyrate + CO_2
4.1.2.7	Ketone-1-phosphate: aldehyde lyase	Aldolase		A ketone-1-P → dihydroxyacetone-P + an aldehyde
5.	*Isomerases*			
5.1.1.1	L-alanine:D-alanine isomerase	Alanine racemase	PLP	L-alanine → D-alanine
5.3.1.1	D-glyceraldehyde-3-P keto-isomerase	Triose-P isomerase		D-glyceraldehyde 3-P → dihydroxyacetone-P
6.	*Ligases*			
6.1.1.1	L-tyrosine:tRNA ligase (AMP)	Tyrosyl-tRNA synthase	Mg^{++}, K^+	ATP + L-tyrosine + tRNA → AMP + P_2 + L-tyrosyl-tRNA
6.3.1.2	L-glutamate:ammonia ligase (ADP)	Glutamine synthase	Mg^{++}	ATP + L-glutamate + NH_3 → ADP + P_i + L-glutamine

[a] Abbreviations include: NAD$^+$: nicotinamide adenine dinucleotide; PLP: pyridoxal phosphate; CO_2: carbon dioxide; P_2: pyrophosphate; M^{++}: a divalent cation.

2. *General acid or base catalysis.* The reaction rate is accelerated by addition or removal of a proton, employing an amino acyl residue side chain in the enzyme.

3. *Charge neutralization.* In cases where a charged substrate is bound to the enzyme, electrostatic interactions with residues of opposite charge can facilitate binding. Similarly, when the energy level of a transition state is high because of the development

TABLE 3.2 MECHANISMS UTILIZED BY ENZYMES TO ENHANCE REACTION RATES

Process	Description	Amino acyl residues most frequently involved in this type of catalysis
1. Specific acid and base catalysis	Protons are added to or removed from the substrate employing OH^- or H^+ from the solvent	
2. General acid and base catalysis	Protons are added to or removed from the substrate employing weak bases or acids	*asp, glu, his, tyr, lys*
3. Charge neutralization	A formal or developing charge is neutralized by the proximity of a charged amino acyl residue	*asp, glu, his, lys, arg*
4. Nucleophilic catalysis	A nucleophilic group in the enzyme transiently forms a covalent bond with the substrate	*cys, ser, his, asp, glu*
5. Electrophilic catalysis	Electrons are withdrawn from the reaction center by protonation, a neighboring positive charge, or an electron sink	*lys, his, arg*
6. Bond angle strain	The substrate is bound to the enzyme in a configuration which more closely approximates the transition state	All hydrophobic and hydrophilic residues
7. Proximity effects [residue and substrate orientation] (anchimeric assistance)	The participating enzyme residue side chains and substrate moieties must be properly aligned for maximal reaction rate	Usually hydrophilic residues
8. Environmental effects (solvation)	Environmental substituents (water, salts, etc.) can be utilized for dipole stabilization, charge neutralization, etc.	

of a formal charge on the substrate, the proximity of a charged residue of opposite sign can reduce the activation energy.

4. *Nucleophilic catalysis.* Many enzymes form covalent bonds with their substrates, and in virtually all such cases the enzyme functions as a nucleophile, attacking an electropositive center in the substrate. The covalent enzyme–substrate bond is formed and broken at rates that are much more rapid than the overall conversion of substrate to products in the absence of enzymatic nucleophilic participation.

5. *Electrophilic catalysis.* Rates of enzyme-catalyzed reactions are sometimes accelerated by the withdrawal of electron density from the reaction center. This process may occur by (a) transfer of a proton to a substrate moiety from a general acid, (b) the presence of a metal ion or positively charged amino acyl side chain, or (c) the presence of an electron-withdrawing electron sink, usually in the form of a cationic nitrogen.

Nucleophilic and electrophilic catalysis are in a sense directly opposite means of catalysis (one involving attack by an electron-rich moiety on a positive center, and the other involving the withdrawal of electrons from a reaction center), but the division between the two is not sharp. Often, nucleophilic attack and electron withdrawal occur as a consequence of a single reaction. In other reactions, a step which is electrophilically catalyzed might involve nucleophilic catalysis in the reverse direction, and vice versa. Whether such ambiguous reactions are defined as examples of electrophilic or nucleophilic catalysis depends somewhat arbitrarily on which steps seem most important in the facilitation of the reactions in the direction in which they are normally written.

6. *Bond strain.* Enzymes do not usually bind their substrates in the configuration normally observed when that substrate is free in aqueous solution. Instead, they undergo conformational rearrangements which induce bond strain, causing the substrate to assume bond angles and lengths that more closely approximate those of the transition state. Therefore, in these enzymes the active site cannot be visualized as a perfect fit for its substrates and products, but rather for molecules sharing a blend of the characteristics of these molecules and the transition state(s). Hydrogen bonds, hydrophobic (entropy) interactions, electrostatic interactions, π stacking, etc., contribute to the energy of binding. Induced approximation of the transition state upon substrate binding lowers the activation energy essentially by increasing the ground-state energy level of the substrate(s). Because the binding site is not designed for the substrate but is designed for something approaching the transition state, molecules that possess structures resembling the transition state may bind more tightly to the enzyme surface than does the substrate itself. Such compounds are called *transition-state inhibitors.* It should be pointed out that the active site need not retain a single conformation but can undergo reversible and cyclic conformational transitions as the reaction sequence progresses. Enzyme conformational changes almost always accompany substrate binding.

7. *Proximity effects.* In order for rapid catalysis to occur, all participating amino acyl residue side chains and substrate moieties must be aligned in proper orientation relative to one another. Only a single orientation of all participating molecular groupings gives rise to the maximal reaction rate. Misalignment by a fraction of an angstrom, introduced by the wrong substrate or by a defect in the enzyme, can reduce the reaction rate by several orders of magnitude. Sometimes the substrate is held in a cyclic conformation so that a molecular grouping on one part of the molecule can facilitate the reaction that occurs at another part of the same molecule. Such a mechanism in which different parts of the same substrate participate both in catalysis and in reaction is called *anchimeric assistance.*

8. *Environmental effects.* Finally, the solvent (water) or elements from the environment (salts, amino acids, lipids, other macromolecules) can enhance reaction rates by providing dipole stabilization for, by neutralizing developing charges in, and by providing hydrogen bonds to, a transition state. Any such mechanism stabilizes the transition state and consequently reduces the activation energy for the overall reaction.

3.3 GENERALIZED MECHANISMS OF ENZYME CATALYSIS

All enzymes use the same principles to accelerate reaction rates as discussed in the previous section. This statement is based on the results of studies conducted with thousands of enzymes over the past 50 years. It is therefore possible to take a particular enzyme, any enzyme catalyzing any reaction, and propose a reaction mechanism based on the principles of the organic chemist, the guidelines outlined in the previous section, and any information available concerning the enzyme of interest. In doing so, we can propose a *plausible* reaction mechanism which may or may not approximate the *correct* mechanism for that particular enzyme. Alternatively, if nothing is known about the enzyme that catalyzes a reaction of interest, one can always propose a reaction mechanism, or more than one mechanism, by which the enzyme may function. In any case, such procedures are useful not only for instructional purposes, they also allow the biochemist to propose alternatives which can be compared and tested experimentally. This procedure is illustrated in Figures 3.1 and 3.2 for a hypothetical enzyme catalyzing peptide bond hydrolysis.

$$R-\overset{\overset{\displaystyle O}{\|}}{C}-NH-R' \xrightarrow{H_2O} R-CO_2^- + R'-NH_3^+ \qquad (3.1)$$

Our hypothetical enzyme, designated peptidase H, initiates its reaction sequence by binding its substrate, a peptide, to the active site which lies in a cleft between the two domains of the enzyme. The enzyme has a molecular weight of about 40,000, and each domain contains about 200 amino acyl residues. Binding of substrate, which occurs with a rate that is diffusion-limited, can occur in many different ways and with different orientations of substrate relative to the enzyme. Since the polypeptide chain of the substrate is long, many different portions of the chain can bind to the active site. In any binding orientation, however, two residues fit snugly into the catalytic groove, with the remaining residues projecting outward from the enzyme surface. Upon binding, the interaction of enzyme with substrate induces a conformational change in the enzyme so that one enzyme domain rotates several degrees relative to the other, and partial cleft closure occurs, locking the substrate into the active site.

Any two amino acyl residues along the chain of the substrate can bind within the cleft, but not all bind with equal affinity or induce the conformational change that orients catalytic residues properly for catalysis of the reaction. For this particular enzyme, high affinity binding and proper rotation of the two domains only occurs if R in equation (3.1) is a lysyl residue and R' is an isoleucyl residue. Binding of the side chain of the lysyl residue occurs in a fashion that brings the positively charged ϵ-amino group of the substrate lysyl residue ($S_3-NH_3^+$ in Figure 3.1) adjacent to its own carbonyl oxygen, the carbonyl of the secondary amide bond which will be hydrolyzed. This positively charged ϵ-amino group will function catalytically to neutralize the developing negative charge on oxygen, which will become a formal negative charge in two of the reaction intermediates (I_1 and I_4 in Figure 3.1). Because the substrate is held in a cyclic configuration which allows it to participate catalytically in the reaction, anchimeric assistance is exemplified.

Binding of the peptide backbone, of the lysyl side chain (R), and of the hydrocarbon side chain of the isoleucyl residue (R') is effected by the proximity of *complementary* enzyme residues. For example, the positioning of the peptide backbone is stabilized by hydrogen bonds to hydrophilic groups in the enzyme; the isoleucyl side chain must fit into a hydrophobic pocket of the protein consisting of hydrophobic residue side chains; and the positioning of the ϵ-amino group of residue R in equation (3.1) is established in part by the proximity of a side-chain carboxyl group (the β- or

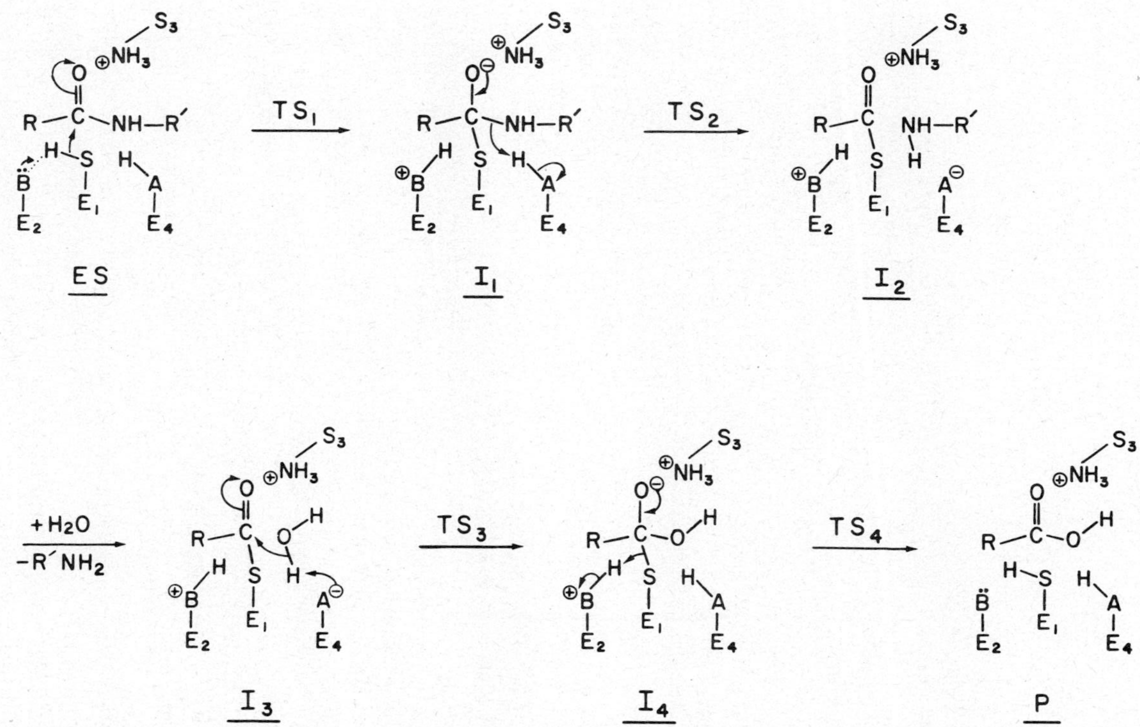

Figure 3.1 Proposed reaction mechanism for a hypothetical protease, peptidase H. Three enzymic groups (E_1, E_2, and E_4) and one moiety of the substrate (S_3) participate in catalysis. E_1–SH is a nucleophilic catalyst; E_2–B: is a general base catalyst; S_3–NH_3^+ functions in charge neutralization (anchimeric assistance), and E_4–AH is a general acid catalyst. The reaction proceeds in several steps: the enzyme–substrate complex (ES) first forms, and then passes through the first transition state (TS_1) to the first metastable intermediate (I_1). The secondary amide bond of the substrate is hydrolyzed (TS_2) to give a stable acylated enzyme (I_2). Water displaces the hydrolyzed peptide fragment (R′–NH_2) at the active site (I_3). Attack by water on the carbonyl group of the acylated enzyme (TS_3) generates another metastable intermediate (I_4) which spontaneously hydrolyzes to regenerate the native form of the enzyme (E) to which the product (P) is bound. The product finally dissociates from the active site, and the enzyme is ready to bind another substrate molecule and repeat the cycle.

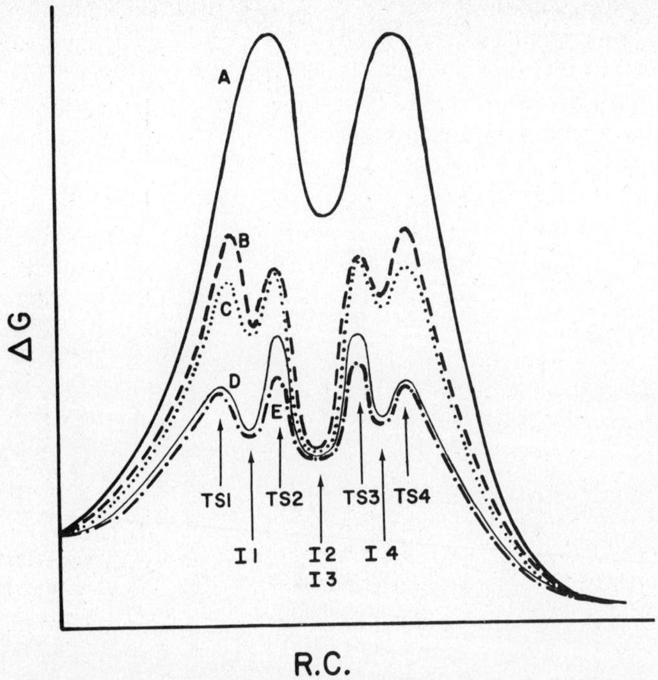

Figure 3.2 Free energy (ΔG)-reaction coordinate (R.C.) diagram for the hydrolysis of a peptide bond. The five different curves (A–E) show the expected free energy–reaction coordinate profiles for catalysis involving an increasing number of catalytic factors (1–4): (A) the uncatalyzed hydrolytic reaction (——); (B) the hydrolytic reaction facilitated *only* by nucleophilic catalysis (1) (---); (C) the same reaction in which both nucleophilic catalysis (1) and general base catalysis (2) facilitate the reaction (· · ·); (D) the same reaction involving nucleophilic catalysis (1), general base catalysis (2) and charge neutralization (3) (——), and (E) the same reaction in which nucleophilic catalysis (1), general base catalysis (2), charge neutralization (3), and general acid catalysis (4) all accelerate the reaction rate (-·-·-). I_1, I_2 (or I_3), and I_4 correspond to the intermediates shown in Figure 3.1. Transition states TS_1, TS_2, TS_3, and TS_4 correspond to those indicated in Figure 3.1.

γ-carboxyl group of an *asp* or *glu,* respectively) on the far side of the substrate carbonyl. Thus, the position of the positively charged ϵ-amino group is stabilized by a hydrogen bond to the carbonyl oxygen in the substrate on one side and by an enzymic carboxyl group on the opposite side. The formation of an ion pair functions to facilitate orientation of the substrate.

Binding of the polypeptide to the enzyme surface effects bond strain in the substrate. The trigonal symmetry of the carbonyl group in equation (3.1) is altered, causing bond angles to decrease and assume an orientation more closely approximating tetrahedral symmetry. As a result of bond strain, the energy level of the bound substrate increases, and this increase is compensated for by a decrease in the energy level of the enzyme when it assumes the more stable configuration induced by substrate binding. The enhanced energy level of the bound substrate raises the ground state of the molecule and thereby lowers the activation energy required for hydrolysis of the peptide bond. The reaction rate consequently increases.

Peptidase H uses a *cys* residue as a nucleophilic catalyst (Figure 3.1). Because of the diffuse electron cloud around sulfur, the sulfhydryl group ($E_1{-}SH$) is both a good nucleophile and a good leaving group. The energy of the transition state that gives rise to a tetrahedral carbon atom from the trigonal carbonyl is therefore decreased, lowering the activation energy for formation of intermediate I_1 in Figure 3.1 as shown by the dashed line (b) in Figure 3.2.

In order to increase the nucleophilicity of the sulfhydryl group (TS_1) and to facilitate its subsequent displacement by water, the sulfhydryl group ($E_1{-}SH$) is weakly hydrogen-bonded to an electronegative atom, a basic residue in the enzyme, ($E_2{-}B$:). This association increases the negative character of the sulfur atom because of the tendency of the proton to be lost to $E_2{-}B$:. $E_2{-}B$: therefore functions as a general base. The sulfhydryl group loses its proton, and $E_1{-}S^-$, a very potent nucleophile, becomes the agent that attacks the substrate carbonyl. The effect of base catalysis on the free energy–reaction coordinate diagram is shown by the dotted line (c) in Figure 3.2.

As stated above, the ϵ-amino group of the substrate lysyl residue [side chain R in equation (3.1) or $S_3{-}NH_3^+$ in Figure 3.1] functions to neutralize the negative charge which develops on the carbonyl oxygen when the π electron pair is transferred to oxygen and tetrahedral symmetry is established. Charge neutralization lowers the energies of the two intermediates, I_1 and I_4, as well as that of each transition state that bears a partial negative charge. The free energy–reaction coordinate diagram that takes charge neutralization into account is depicted by the thin solid line (d) in Figure 3.2. By use of an acidic residue ($E_4{-}AH$) as a general acid, a proton is transferred to the leaving amino group, giving that group a formal positive charge. $E_4{-}A^-$, the basic form of the enzymic weak acid utilized in the previous step as a general acid catalyst, subsequently accepts a proton from a hydrogen-bonded water molecule, thereby rendering the oxygen atom of the water molecule a more potent nucleophile which attacks the carbonyl group of the substrate (TS_3). General acid catalysis therefore increases the reaction rate by lowering the activation energies of TS_2 and TS_3 [dashed–dotted line (e) in Figure 3.2]. Assuming that one or both of these reactions is rate-limiting for the overall reaction, the rate will increase.

Finally, the reaction rate is further increased by insuring that all catalytic residues are maintained at distances from the substrate that are optimal for catalysis. That is, each of the catalytic groups ($E_1{-}SH$, $E_2{-}B$:, $S_3{-}NH_3^+$, and $E_4{-}AH$) are positioned for catalysis by enzyme conformational changes which are induced by substrate binding. Solvation of developing dipoles in the substrate molecule or the catalytic residues can further stabilize transition states and intermediates. The net result of these effects is an increase in the rate of peptide hydrolysis about 10^{15}-fold over that observed in the absence of a catalyst [Line (a) in Figure 3.2].

3.4 ENZYME KINETICS: MICHAELIS–MENTEN TREATMENT FOR ONE-SUBSTRATE REACTIONS

The mechanisms of enzyme-catalyzed reactions cannot be visualized directly, and the biochemist must therefore rely on indirect methods to gain information about these processes. One of the most informative approaches is to study the kinetic characteristics of the reaction; that is, to characterize the rate of the reaction as a function of various parameters such as substrate concentration, enzyme concentration, temperature, pH, etc. Such studies can provide valuable information concerning the mechanism utilized by a particular enzyme.

Frequently, when the rate of an enzyme-catalyzed reaction v is plotted versus substrate concentration $[S]$, a hyperbolic curve is observed as shown in Figure 3.3(a). Initially, at low $[S]$, the reaction rate increases linearly with increasing $[S]$. At higher $[S]$ the rate tapers off until, at saturating concentrations, no further increase in rate is observed.

In order to explain this behavior it is assumed that the substrate binds to the active site of the enzyme E at a rate determined by an "on" kinetic constant k_1 to form an enzyme–substrate complex ES. Subsequently, the substrate can either dissociate from the enzyme surface at a rate determined by the "off" kinetic constant k_{-1}, or it can react to give the product of the reaction P and free enzyme. The kinetic constant for the interconversion process k_2 is usually much smaller than k_1 *or* k_{-1}.

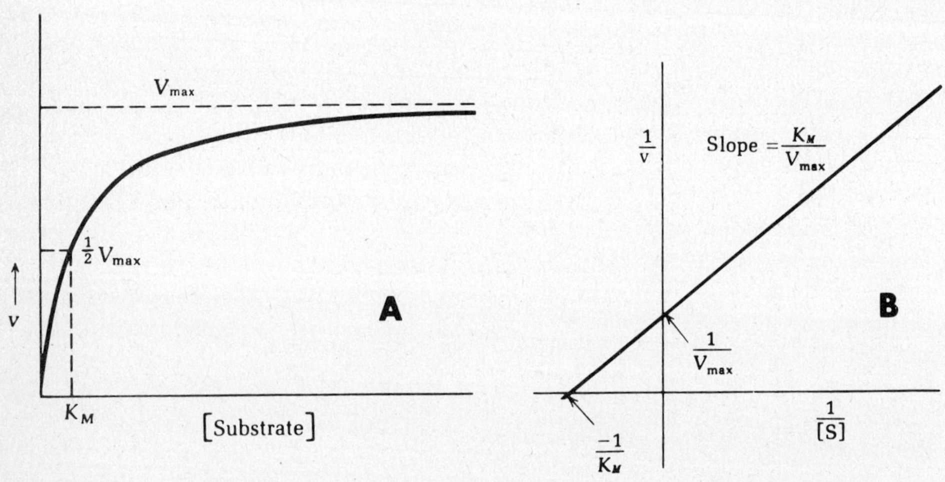

Figure 3.3 Michaelis–Menten kinetics for a simple, single-substrate, enzyme-catalyzed reaction. (A) Effect of substrate concentration ($[S]$) on the rate (v) of an enzyme-catalyzed reaction. The maximal rate of reaction corresponds to the V_{max} value. When the velocity (v) equals 1/2 V_{max}, the substrate concentration equals the Michaelis–Menten constant K_M. Reaction rate follows saturation or hyperbolic kinetics. (B) A double reciprocal (Lineweaver–Burk) plot of the curve shown in (A). A plot of $1/v$ versus $1/[S]$ gives a straight line for any enzyme which exhibits simple saturation kinetics. The line intersects the ordinate at infinite substrate concentration ($1/[S] = 0$). This value corresponds to the reciprocal of the maximal reaction rate ($1/V_{max}$). The curve intersects the abscissa at $1/[S] = -1/K_M$. The slope of the curve is equal to K_m/V_{max}.

That is, the activation energy for chemical reactivity is usually much greater than the activation energy for binding or dissociation of the substrate from the enzyme surface.

The overall reaction can thus be described:

$$E + S \underset{k_{-1}}{\overset{k_1}{\rightleftharpoons}} ES \overset{k_2}{\rightarrow} E + P \tag{3.2}$$

If we define $[S]$ as the concentration of substrate, $[E_T]$ as the total concentration of enzyme, and $[ES]$ as the concentration of the enzyme–substrate complex, then the net rate of formation of the enzyme–substrate complex as a function of time will be equal to the rate of its formation (determined by k_1 times the concentrations of E and S) minus the rate of its disappearance (determined by the rate of its dissociation to E and S which equals $k_{-1}[ES]$) together with the rate at which substrate is converted to product ($k_2[ES]$). In other words,

$$\frac{d[ES]}{dt} = k_1([E_T] - [ES])[S] - (k_{-1} + k_2)[ES] \tag{3.3}$$

If we assume steady-state conditions, ($d[ES]/dt = 0$), which is justified if $[S]$ is much greater than $[E]$, then

$$\frac{([E_T] - [ES])[S]}{[ES]} = \frac{k_{-1} + k_2}{k_1} \equiv K_M \tag{3.4}$$

The new constant K_M is the Michaelis–Menten constant which equals the dissociation constant, defining the affinity of the enzyme for the substrate ($K_d = k_{-1}/k_1$) if k_2 is much less than k_{-1}.

The reaction rate is defined as the rate of product formation as a function of time ($v = dP/dt$). Therefore,

$$v = \frac{dP}{dt} = k_2[ES] \tag{3.5}$$

Solving equation (3.4) for $[ES]$ and eliminating this term from equation (3.5) gives

$$v = \frac{k_2(E_T)}{K_M/[S] + 1} = \frac{V_{\max}}{K_M/[S] + 1} \tag{3.6}$$

where $V_{\max}$ is defined as the maximal velocity, or maximal reaction rate, which is observed when all of the enzyme is present as the enzyme–substrate complex ES. This condition applies at infinite or very large substrate concentrations, as shown in Figure 3.3(a). The concentration of S at which $v = \frac{1}{2}V_{\max}$ is equal to the K_M value. Rearrangement of equation (3.6) gives

$$\frac{V_{\max}}{v} = \frac{K_M}{[S]} + 1 \tag{3.7}$$

which is the Michaelis–Menten equation.

From this equation it can be seen that a plot of $1/v$ versus $1/[S]$ should give a straight line as shown in Figure 3.3(b). If we set $1/v = 0$, then equation (3.7) reduces to $K_M = -[S]$. The Michaelis–Menten constant K_M can therefore be calculated from the point at which the plot of $1/v$ versus $1/[S]$ crosses the abscissa. If we set $1/[S]$

equal to zero in equation (3.7), $1/v = 1/V_{max}$. Therefore, V_{max} is the value of v (extrapolated to infinite substrate concentration) where the line in Figure 3.3(b) crosses the ordinate. The slope of the line is equal to K_M/V_{max}.

From these considerations, it can be seen that whenever an enzyme exhibits Michaelis–Menten kinetics (also called hyperbolic or saturation kinetics), a plot of $1/v$ versus $1/[S]$ gives a straight line. In Section 3.9 we shall see that this result implies that all of the substrate binding sites within the population of enzyme molecules exhibit the same affinity for the substrate and that the enzyme does not exhibit the property of *cooperativity*. It behaves like a simple, monomeric protein.

3.5 ENZYME KINETICS: TWO-SUBSTRATE REACTIONS

While many enzymes such as peptidase H discussed in Section 3.3 act on a single substrate (other than the solvent), the reactions of many more enzymes require the participation of at least two substrates in order for reaction to occur. For example, oxidoreductases (class I enzymes) cannot function without an electron donor and acceptor; transferases (class II enzymes) must function with group transfer donors as well as acceptors. Hydrolases, lyases, and isomerases (classes III–V) frequently act on a single substrate, but ligases (class VI enzymes) require the participation of two or more substrates. Enzymes that act on more than one substrate and still exhibit Michaelis–Menten kinetics usually fall within two classes with respect to kinetic behavior and mechanism of action.

In the first class, both substrates must bind *simultaneously* to the active site of the enzyme. These enzymes therefore possess distinct, nonoverlapping binding sites for the two substrates at the active site. Double reciprocal plots ($1/v$ versus $1/[S_1]$) at constant but different concentrations of S_2 give intersecting straight lines as shown in Figure 3.4(a). This sort of kinetic behavior implies that both substrates must bind to the enzyme surface before reaction can occur. The enzyme is usually not modified as an obligatory part of the catalytic cycle. This type of kinetic behavior is called *sequential.*

In the second class of two-substrate enzymes, the two substrates never bind simultaneously, usually because a single binding site accommodates both substrates. The two substrates frequently share certain structural features. Double reciprocal plots ($1/v$ versus $1/[S_1]$) at three different but constant concentrations of S_2 give parallel straight lines that never intersect, as shown in Figure 3.4(b). The enzyme E is covalently modified to E' as a result of the reaction which converts S_1 to P_1. It is then the conversion of S_2 to P_2 that restores the enzyme to the original E form. This type of reaction mechanism is referred to as *ping–pong.*

Sometimes it is possible to predict which of these two mechanisms is operative for a particular enzyme. For example, if an oxidoreductase such as alcohol dehydrogenase (E.C.1.1.1.1; Table 3.1) does not contain a prosthetic group which can serve as an electron acceptor, then the electron pair must be transferred directly from the electron donor (ethanol) to a free electron acceptor (NAD^+). A sequential mechanism should be anticipated. On the other hand, alanine aminotransferase (E.C.2.6.1.2; Table 3.1) contains tightly bound pyridoxal phosphate, a coenzyme which can accept an amino group from a substrate such as alanine and transfer it to a keto acid such as

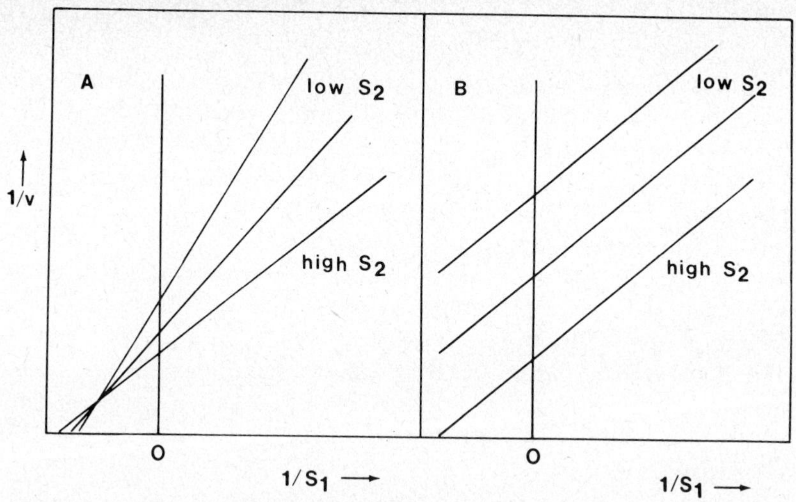

Figure 3.4 Kinetic analysis of two-substrate reactions. Double reciprocal plots ($1/v$ versus $1/[S_1]$) at three different (but constant) concentrations of S_2 give two types of kinetic behavior. (A) Intersecting straight lines are observed for the "sequential" reaction mechanism which occurs if both S_1 and S_2 bind *simultaneously* to the enzyme surface before reaction can occur. (B) Parallel straight lines for the "ping pong" reaction mechanism are observed when only one of the two substrates binds to the enzyme at any one time. S_1 modifies the original enzyme E to give the first product P_1 and an altered enzyme E'. E' then binds the second substrate S_2, and the second reaction in which S_2 is converted to P_2 restores the original form of the enzyme (E).

α-ketoglutarate. The prosthetic group in the enzyme is aminated so that the pyridoxal phosphate form of the enzyme is temporarily converted to the pyridoxamine form. A ping–pong mechanism can be anticipated in this case.

3.6 PARAMETERS INFLUENCING REACTION RATES

A multitude of external conditions influence the rates of enzyme-catalyzed reactions, and the study of these dependencies can provide information concerning the mechanism of an affected reaction. The turnover number, pH dependency, metal ion and cofactor requirements, temperature dependency, and substrate and inhibitor specificities of an enzyme are all normally studied when it is first characterized. These parameters will be discussed in this section.

3.6.1 Turnover Number

Each enzyme catalyzes a chemical reaction at a certain maximal rate, termed the maximal velocity or V_{max}, which is attained at saturating substrate concentrations. Each enzyme preparation is characterized by a *specific activity* value which tells how many molecules of substrate can be converted to product per second per milligram of protein at a particular temperature and under a given set of conditions. If the enzyme has been purified to homogeneity and its molecular weight has been determined, its *turnover number,* the number of substrate molecules converted to product per second per enzyme molecule present, can be calculated. Measurements of turnover numbers reveal that some enzymes are highly efficient, converting up to 10^6 substrate molecules to product per second per molecule of enzyme under optimal conditions. Other enzymes are relatively inefficient, having turnover numbers a billionfold smaller. For example, the turnover numbers for lysozyme, which hydrolyzes the bacterial cell wall, lactate dehydrogenase, which oxidizes lactate to pyruvate, and carbonic anhydrase, which hydrates carbon dioxide to give bicarbonate, are 1, 10^3, and 10^6, respectively. Some enzymes are clearly far more efficient than others, but the latter enzymes may perform much more difficult tasks.

3.6.2 Temperature

All enzymes exhibit reaction rates that are dependent on temperature. The degree to which a reaction rate increases with temperature is related to the activation energy of the reaction. If the activation energy is small, the reaction rate will be very fast, and the rate will not increase markedly when the temperature is increased. Slow reactions, characterized by high activation energies, show more pronounced dependencies on temperature. Most enzymes show a 50% to 300% increase in reaction rate when the temperature is increased 10°C. The ratio of rate constants at two temperatures 10°C apart therefore varies between about 1.5 and 4.0 for most enzymes. This value is termed the Q_{10}.

When the logarithm of the reaction rate is plotted versus the reciprocal of the absolute temperature, a straight line is frequently observed for soluble enzymes within a restricted range of temperatures (Figure 3.5; solid line). The enzyme is said to follow a linear *Arrhenius plot.* At high temperatures (usually between 40°C and 90°C depending on the enzyme) almost all enzymes are denatured and lose their activities.

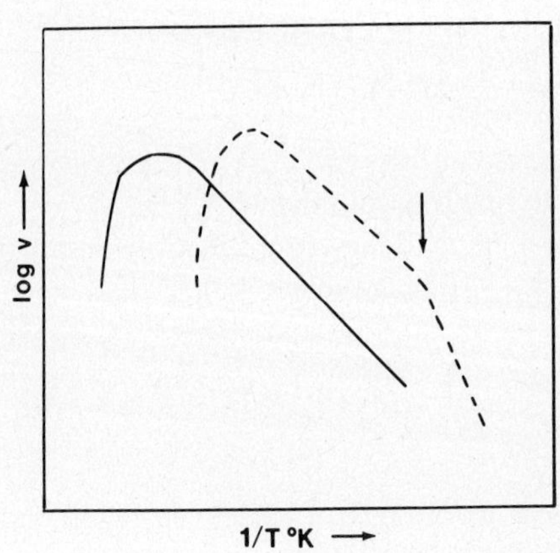

Figure 3.5 Temperature dependencies of two different enzymes revealed when the logarithm of the reaction rate (v) is plotted versus the reciprocal of the absolute temperature (K = °C + 273°). The plot on the left (solid line) shows the Arrhenius plot of a typical soluble enzyme. The plot on the right (dashed line) may represent a soluble enzyme which undergoes a conformational transition at the temperature corresponding to the discontinuity (arrow), or it may be an integral membrane enzyme which senses the lipid environment of the membrane. In this case the membrane undergoes a thermal phase transition at the temperature of the discontinuity. Denaturation and loss of activity occur at high temperature.

Catalytic function is rapidly lost above an enzyme's denaturation temperature because catalysis depends on the specific conformation of the native protein. Some enzymes exhibit nonlinear Arrhenius plots as shown for the enzyme represented by the dashed line to the right in Figure 3.5. This enzyme may be a cytoplasmic enzyme which undergoes a conformational transition at the temperature of the discontinuity. If so, the two conformations of the enzyme must catalyze the reaction with different activation energies. Alternatively, if the enzyme is embedded within the phospholipid matrix of a cellular membrane, nonlinear kinetics may reflect the sensitivity of the enzyme to the viscosity of the hydrophobic matrix of the membrane which is highly temperature-dependent. It should be noted that the enzyme on the left (solid line) denatures at a higher temperature than the enzyme on the right (dashed line). The denaturation temperature of an enzyme is a highly characteristic attribute under well-defined conditions.

While most enzymes denature with increasing temperature and are said to be heat sensitive, others denature at low temperature and are termed cold sensitive. This distinction has been attributed to the nature of the forces holding the enzyme in its native state. Bonds stabilized by enthalpy are disrupted with increasing temperature while bonds stabilized by entropy are weakened by lowering the temperature. The hydrophobic associations, attributed in part to the presence of structured water molecules around the hydrocarbon chains of the amino acyl residues serve as the principal type of entropy bond. As the temperature is lowered, the degree of water structuring increases, thereby decreasing the significance of the entropy term. A number of membrane-associated enzymes have been found to be cold sensitive.

3.6.3 pH

Virtually all enzymes catalyze reactions that exhibit pH dependencies. The pH dependencies of different enzymes vary widely. Some show a bell-shaped curve as reproduced in Figure 3.6. Frequently such curves reflect the deprotonation of an ionizable substrate or amino acyl side chain in the enzyme. For example, for the enzyme depicted in Figure 3.6, half maximal activity is observed at pH 4.5 and pH 7.0. As revealed in Table 1.2 (Chapter 1), the pKa value of the side-chain carboxyl group of an *asp* or *glu* residue in a protein is about 4.5 while that of *his* residues in proteins is 7.0.

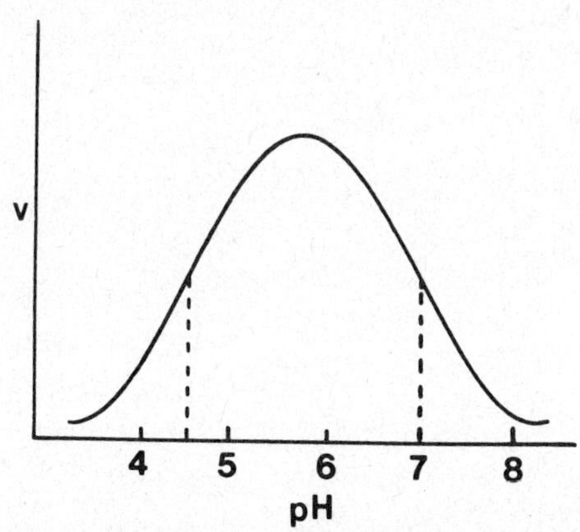

Figure 3.6 The pH dependency of an enzyme-catalyzed reaction. The reaction rate v is plotted versus pH. A bell-shaped curve with half maximal activity at pH 4.5 and 7.0 suggests the possible participation of a side-chain carboxyl group and the imidazole ring of a histidyl residue. Note, however, that the pKa values of active-site amino acyl side chains frequently differ markedly from those in peptides because of the proximity of other polar amino acyl residues or local, environmental effects.

Assuming that the pH curve of the enzyme reflects the ionization state of *glu* and *his* residues, it is apparent that the *glu* residue must be in its anionic form while the *his* residue must be protonated (positively charged) in order for reaction to occur. Both the K_M and V_{max} values may vary as a function of pH.

All enzymes denature at extremes of pH (e.g., <3 and >10). If an enzyme shows an abrupt loss of activity as the pH is brought to a more extreme value, denaturation and irreversible loss of activity may be the explanation. If the loss of activity occurs more gradually as a function of pH, it may reflect side-chain deprotonation or a reversible conformational change. Restoration of the optimal pH would then be expected to restore full enzymatic activity.

3.6.4 Metal Ions

Many enzymes depend on the presence of a divalent cation for activity; fewer enzymes are activated by the presence of monovalent cations, anions, or salts. Some enzymes are activated specifically by a monovalent cation such as K^+, others by an anion such as chloride or HPO_4^{2-}, and still others by ionic strength. These effects are frequently attributed to conformational influences or to the control of subunit interactions. Divalent cations may also interact with a protein to influence its conformation or its interactions with other proteins, for example, by forming salt bridges between ionic residue side chains. On the other hand, divalent cations frequently participate directly in the reaction sequence of an enzyme. They may function to polarize a functional group by complexation with lone electron pairs, such as those of a carbonyl group or an alcoholic oxygen. The ionic requirement of a particular enzyme may be highly specific. Divalent cations required by different enzymes include Mg^{++}, Mn^{++}, Co^{++}, Zn^{++}, Ca^{++}, Ni^{++}, and Fe^{++}. If a divalent metal ion is required for activity, the enzyme is frequently inhibited by divalent cation-chelating reagents such as EDTA. Inhibition by metal ion chelators is highly suggestive of a dependency on one of these ions. However, insensitivity to them may merely suggest that the metal ion is very tightly bound to the enzyme and therefore difficult to remove. The enzyme may be a more efficient chelator than the chelating reagent added.

Other cofactors may be required for enzyme activity. Among these are the coenzymes and prosthetic groups to be discussed in Chapter 4 and subsequent chapters. These cofactors invariably participate directly in the reaction, and a knowledge of their presence greatly facilitates deduction of the reaction mechanism.

3.7 INHIBITOR SPECIFICITIES

Inhibitors of enzyme functions fall into two major categories: reversible and irreversible inhibitors. Irreversible inhibitory agents may either covalently modify specific amino acyl residue side chains or coenzymes, or they may denature the protein to an inactive state. Among the former agents are *N*-ethylmaleimide, which reacts with the sulfhydryl groups of *cys* residues; diethylpyrocarbonate, which specifically derivatizes the imidazole ring of *his* residues; and phenylmethylsulfonyl fluoride, which specifically inactivates serine proteases by covalent reaction with the activated hydroxyl groups of the active-site *ser* residues. Reagents that exhibit specificity toward each of the charged hydrophilic residues in proteins are available. The careful use of these reagents can provide evidence for the involvement of a particular residue side chain in the mechanism of an enzyme-catalyzed reaction.

Denaturing agents include organic solvents, acids, bases, heavy metals, and anionic and cationic detergents. The last-mentioned agents bind to a protein via hydrophobic interactions, enhancing the net charge associated with the molecule and causing it to expand. Chaotropic agents such as urea, guanidinium–hydrochloride, and thiocyanate also denature proteins. In the case of these agents, the mechanism is quite different. Chaotropes (chaos-inducing agents) appear to disrupt water structure, thereby weakening hydrophobic interactions. Protein denaturation is an essentially irreversible process unless the protein is small and great care is taken in the renaturation process.

Reversible inhibitors usually do not covalently modify or denature their target enzymes. Instead, they interact noncovalently, usually at specific sites on the enzyme surface. These agents fall within three classes: competitive, noncompetitive, and uncompetitive inhibitors. While competitive inhibitors alter the apparent affinity of the enzyme for its substrate without affecting the maximal reaction velocity, noncompetitive inhibitors depress the V_{max} without changing the K_M. Uncompetitive inhibitors alter both the K_M and V_{max} of the enzyme-catalyzed reaction. As a result, competitive inhibition can be fully reversed by adding excess substrate; uncompetitive inhibition can be *partially* overcome by substrate addition; but noncompetitive inhibition is characterized by the same inhibitory effects at both high and low substrate concentrations. These three types of inhibitory behavior are illustrated in the Lineweaver–Burk plots shown in Figure 3.7.

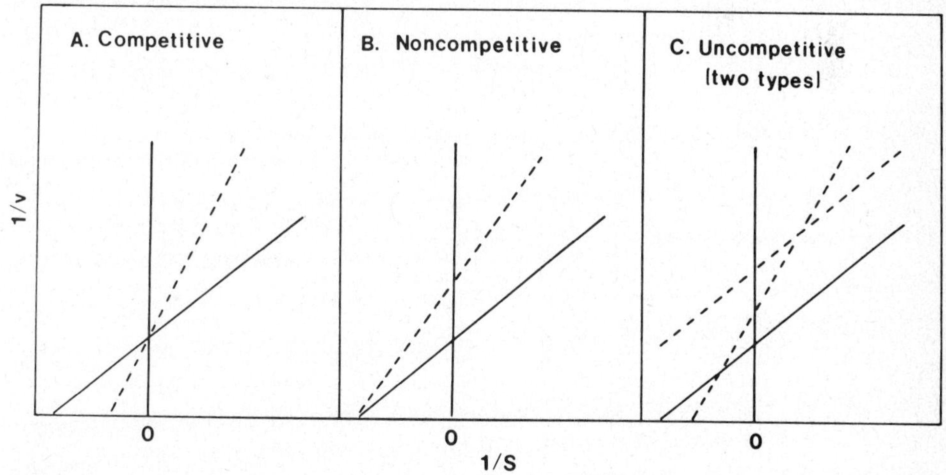

Figure 3.7 Lineweaver–Burk (double reciprocal) plots revealing the effects of the three types of reversible enzyme inhibitory agents on reaction rates. Each curve shows expected behavior for an enzyme in the absence (——) or the presence (---) of the following type of inhibitor: (A) competitive, (B) noncompetitive, (C) uncompetitive. NOTE: Two types of uncompetitive inhibitors are depicted. Both influence the apparent V_{max} value as well as the apparent K_M value.

Competitive inhibitors are usually structural analogues of the substrate, the molecule with which they are competing. They bind to the active site but either do not possess a structure which is conducive to chemical modification or do not induce the proper orientation of catalytic amino acyl residues required to effect catalysis. Consequently, they displace the substrate from the active site and thereby depress the rate of reaction, but they are not themselves acted on.

Noncompetitive inhibitors, on the other hand, bind elsewhere on the surface of the enzyme, altering the conformation of the enzyme so that it no longer functions with maximal efficiency. Presumably they alter the positional orientations of catalytic residues without influencing the positions of residues which function in substrate binding.

Uncompetitive inhibitors may bind to a site either distant from the active site or different from but overlapping with it. In either case, the consequence of uncompetitive inhibitor binding is to lower both the catalytic efficiency of the enzyme and its apparent affinity for the substrate.

Frequently an enzyme can bind several structural analogues at the active site. If these analogues are acted on to undergo chemical transformation, we refer to the array of substrates acted on by the enzyme as its *substrate specificity.* When two different substrates are compared, it is found that they are generally acted on at different maximal rates, and they bind with differing affinities. In some cases, high-affinity substrates are only slowly transformed into products. Such compounds may be poor substrates, but they are potent competitive inhibitors of the reaction that occurs with a preferred substrate.

Usually the natural substrate of an enzyme binds to the active site with higher affinity than a structural analogue of the substrate. Occasionally, however, one of these analogues binds with higher affinity than does the natural substrate. Careful examination of the possible structures of reaction intermediates or transition states reveals that the high-affinity inhibitor frequently possesses a structure that closely resembles that of an intermediate or transition state. Because the enzyme is designed to introduce bond strain, causing the natural substrate to more closely resemble the transition state, the inhibitor fits more easily into the active site than does the substrate. Such inhibitors are termed *transition state inhibitors,* as mentioned in Section 3.2. Their identification can provide confirmatory evidence for a possible reaction pathway.

Some modulators of enzyme activity control the conformations of multisubunit enzymes in a complex but physiologically meaningful way: they indirectly modulate the conformations of the active sites of all subunits, either to enhance or depress reaction rates by altering either the apparent K_M and/or V_{max} values. Moreover, in such an enzyme, the binding of substrate to one subunit can alter the affinity of a neighboring subunit for the same substrate. If the binding of substrate to the first subunit enhances binding to the remaining subunits, we refer to the phenomenon as *positive cooperativity.* When the binding of substrate to the first subunit lowers the affinity of the other subunits for substrate, the phenomenon is referred to as *negative cooperativity.* In complex enzyme systems, a substrate of one catalytic center may function as an allosteric regulatory agent, controlling the reaction rate at another reaction center. Such interactions will be the subject of the last three sections in this chapter.

3.8 A DIVERSITY OF REGULATORY MECHANISMS CONTROLLING ENZYME ACTIVITY

The activities of enzymes are controlled by several different mechanisms. Some enzymes are synthesized in an inactive or less-active precursor form called a proenzyme (or pre-proenzyme), and these precursor forms are converted to the active, mature enzymes by proteolytic cleavage of specific peptide bonds in the protein. These inactive precursor forms of enzymes are sometimes referred to as *zymogens.* Enzymes that are synthesized as inactive precursors frequently are digestive enzymes, destined to be released to an extracellular site. They would be highly deleterious to the cell if activated prior to export.

In other cases, catalytic function is regulated by covalent modification. Although many examples of physiologically relevant covalent enzyme modification reactions have been documented, enzyme phosphorylation reactions are by far the most important. Regulatory phosphorylations of enzymes, transport proteins, structural proteins and contractile proteins are well-documented. ATP-dependent protein kinases catalyze the phosphorylation of seryl, threonyl, and tyrosyl residues in these proteins. Some of the protein kinases are regulated by cytoplasmic molecules including cyclic AMP, cyclic GMP, Ca^{++}, and other second messengers which function to relay messages from hormone and neurotransmitter receptors on the cell surface to the kinases. Phosphorylation converts the target protein to a form that exhibits either greater or lesser activity depending on the system under study. The phosphorylated protein is hydrolyzed to the free protein and inorganic phosphate by a protein–phosphate phosphatase. Regulatory mechanisms involving covalent modification appear to be ubiquitous, having been described in animals, plants, fungi, eukaryotic protists, and bacteria.

Although covalent modification of enzymes is a common mechanism for regulating the activities of enzymes, noncovalent regulation by both macromolecules and small ligands is more common. As an example of a noncovalent regulatory system involving direct protein–protein interactions, dozens of enzymes in eukaryotic cells are regulated by a Ca^{++}-binding protein that modulates the effects of cytoplasmic Ca^{++}. This protein, aptly called *calmodulin,* has a molecular weight of 16,800, and is highly conserved throughout the four major eukaryotic kingdoms. The structure of the protein with its four Ca^{++}-binding domains (I–IV) is shown in Figure 3.8. Darkened circles represent residues included within α-helical segments of the protein. Analyses of internal sequence homology suggest that the protein may have arisen from a smaller protein of about half its present size with only two Ca^{++} binding sites. When Ca^{++} binds to calmodulin, the divalent ion induces a conformational change that causes the protein to bind to and alter the activities of many of its target enzymes. Because the Ca^{++}-calmodulin complex regulates the cyclic AMP biosynthetic and degradative enzymes, called adenylate cyclase and cyclic AMP phosphodiesterase, respectively, regulatory mechanisms involving covalent and noncovalent modifications overlap. Regulation of an enzyme system by multiple mechanisms will be observed repeatedly in the metabolic examples to be considered in later chapters.

A second somewhat different example of a macromolecular, allosteric, regulatory mechanism involves direct protein–protein interactions in bacteria. Adenylate cyclase (which catalyzes cyclic AMP synthesis), various permeases which transport carbohy-

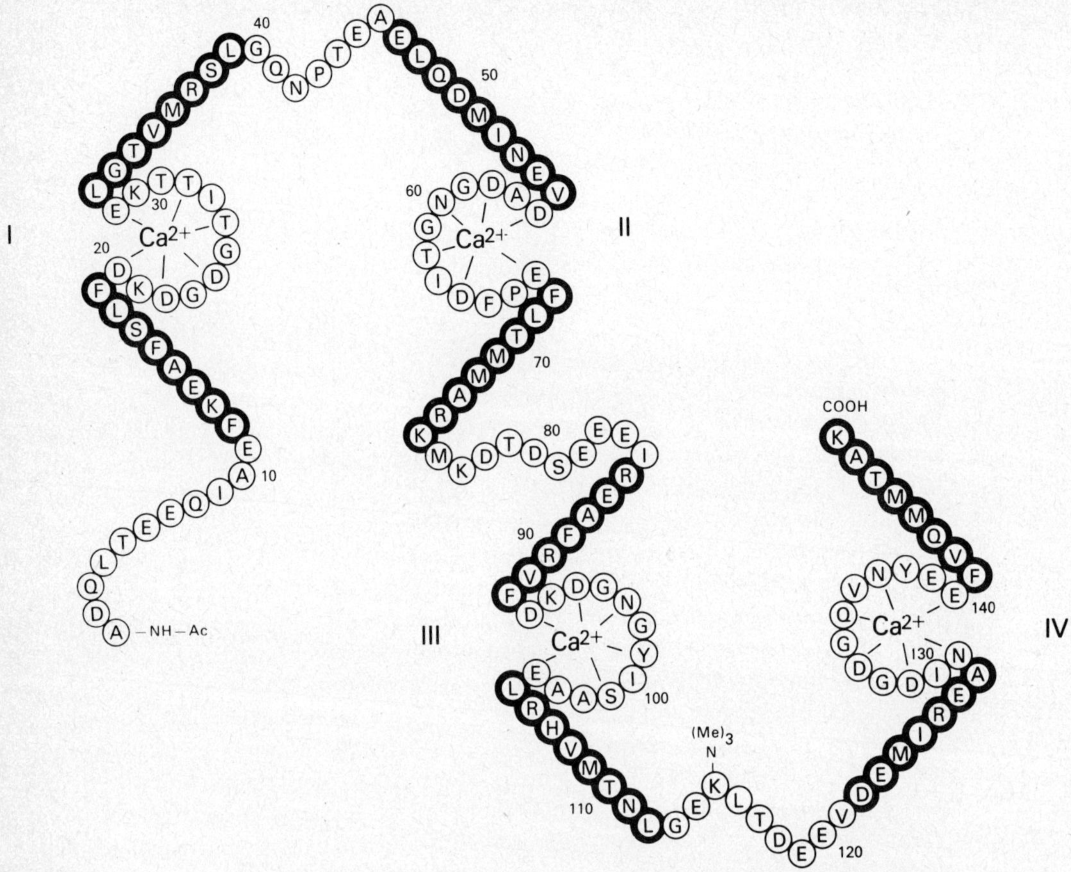

Figure 3.8 Primary structure of bovine brain calmodulin. The sequence is shown with one-letter abbreviations for the amino acyl residues listed in Table 1.2. These residues are (in alphabetical order): A, Ala; C, Cys; D, Asp; E, Glu; F, Phe; G, Gly; H, His; I, Ile; K, Lys; L, Leu; M, Met; N, Asn; P, Pro; Q, Gln; R, Arg; S, Ser; T, Thr; V, Val; W, Trp; Y, Tyr. The four Ca^{++}-binding domains are indicated. Dark circles are regions of α-helix. There is considerable sequence homology between domains I and III and between domains II and IV. Note that the N-terminus is acetylated, that lysyl residue-115 is N-methylated, and that the protein lacks cysteine and tryptophan. [From C. B. Klee, T. H. Crouch, and P. G. Richman, *Annual Review of Biochemistry,* **49,** 496 (1980). The corrected structure was reproduced, courtesy of Dr. Claude B. Klee, Laboratory of Biochemistry National Cancer Institute, National Institutes of Health, Bethesda, MD. 20205.]

drates into the bacterial cell, and certain enzymes which initiate carbohydrate utilization, are allosterically controlled by a regulatory protein termed RPr. Like calmodulin, this protein is small and heat stable, but unlike calmodulin, its regulatory activity is controlled not by Ca^{++} but by the phosphorylation of a histidyl residue in the protein. The phosphorylation of RPr is catalyzed by a phosphotransferase system. Both the lactose permease and glycerol kinase are allosterically inhibited by direct interaction with RPr. The phosphorylated form of RPr does not bind to the target proteins. Because cyclic AMP and carbohydrate inducers in bacteria regulate transcription of operons which synthesize the carbohydrate catabolic enzyme systems, RPr actually regulates the syntheses as well as the activities of the carbohydrate permeases and metabolic enzymes. The regulation of glycerol kinase by RPr will be discussed in the next section.

3.9 ENZYME COOPERATIVITY AND THE ALLOSTERIC CONTROL OF CATALYTIC FUNCTION

As pointed out in Chapter 2, many cellular proteins exist as oligomers. In addition to catalytic subunits or domains, these enzyme complexes may contain subunits or domains which function exclusively in the allosteric regulation of the catalytic active site. In more complex cases, the binding of a substrate to one catalytic subunit may alter the catalytic potential of another nearby subunit regardless of whether it catalyzes the same reaction as, or a different reaction from, the first subunit. The transmission of conformational information from one subunit to another depends on a close, tightly binding interaction of the subunits. When the subunit associations are loosened or dissolved, cooperative or antagonistic regulatory interactions are lost. We shall first consider the phenomenon of enzyme cooperativity in general terms and subsequently discuss some representative examples.

Consider the tetrameric enzyme E_4, each subunit of which possesses a single homogeneous substrate binding site which is identical to the other three. If the four subunits function independently of one another, a plot of reaction velocity versus substrate concentration will give a hyperbolic curve [Figure 3.9(a), solid line] because the enzyme follows simple saturation kinetics. The double reciprocal plot gives a straight line [Figure 3.9(b), solid line]. The assumptions made in deriving the Michaelis–Menten equation are apparently valid (Section 3.4). However, if the subunits strongly interact, and the binding of S to the first subunit of E_4 induces the remaining three subunits to assume altered conformations which differ in their catalytic properties from the unliganded enzyme, hyperbolic kinetics will not be observed.

The binding of S to the first subunit of E_4 can alter the V_{max} and/or the K_M of the other subunits, and can increase or decrease either parameter. If initial substrate binding *increases* the affinity of the other enzyme subunits for S, we refer to the phenomenon as *positive cooperativity.* Positive cooperativity gives a sigmoidal curve when v is plotted versus $[S]$ [Figure 3.9(a), dashed line]. A double reciprocal plot of such a curve gives obvious deviation from a straight line, the plot being sigmoidal [Figure 3.9(b), dashed line]. Extrapolation of the data to the two concentration extremes gives two different K_M values, a high value at low concentrations of S (low affinity) and a low value at high concentrations of S (high affinity).

If initial substrate binding *decreases* the affinity of the other subunits for S, we refer to the phenomenon as *negative cooperativity.* When an enzyme shows negatively cooperative behavior, the plot of reaction rate versus substrate concentration gives a curve as shown by the dotted line in Figure 3.9(a). The double reciprocal plot [Figure 3.9(b), dotted line] shows nonlinearity but extrapolates to two different K_M values at low and high substrate concentrations as observed for positive cooperativity. This

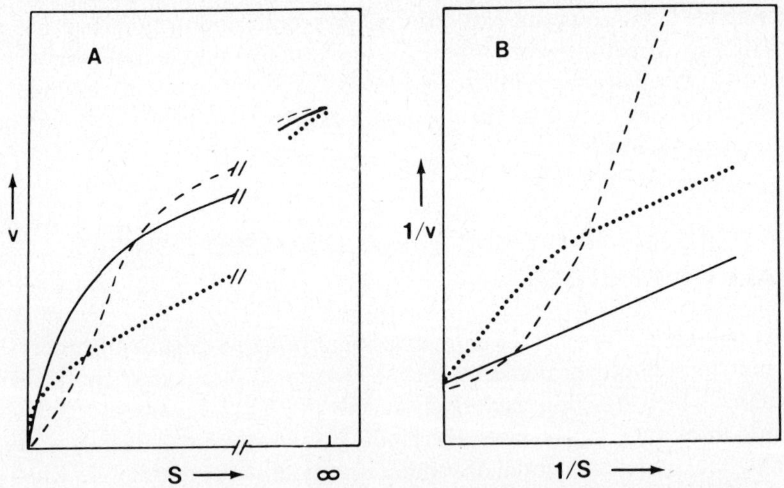

Figure 3.9 Illustration of kinetic behavior observed for three enzymes that exhibit hyperbolic or Michaelis–Menten kinetics (solid line), positive cooperativity (dashed line), or negative cooperativity (dotted line). (A) Reaction rate is plotted versus substrate concentration. (B) Double reciprocal (Lineweaver–Burk) plots of the data in (A).

time, however, the K_M is smaller at low concentrations of substrate than at high concentrations because substrate binding decreases the affinity of the enzyme for S.

X-ray diffraction analyses of multisubunit enzymes have revealed that while some such enzymes show asymmetry, others are symmetrical about a point, line, or plane. In these latter enzymes, symmetry is maintained regardless of the number of substrate molecules bound. However, each subunit in the oligomeric enzyme can exist in two or more conformations, and the substrate preferentially binds to one of these conformations. Addition of substrate to a solution of the enzyme consequently shifts the equilibrium toward the form which has highest affinity for it. If symmetry is to be maintained, all subunits must have the same conformation at any one time. This situation is likely to exist whenever the coupling between subunits is tight as depicted in Figure 3.10(c).

If the subunits are relatively loosely coupled, a conformational change in one, promoted by substrate binding, may induce less drastic conformational shifts in the adjacent subunits. Under such conditions, if the subunits differ in conformation from one another, the oligomeric enzyme will not maintain symmetry [Figure 3.10(b)]. An enzyme with loose subunit conformational coupling [Figure 3.10(b)] is intermediate in behavior between one that exhibits tight coupling and always maintains symmetry [Figure 3.10(c)] and one that shows no conformation coupling and is therefore never symmetrical unless all or none of the subunits have substrate bound to them [Figure 3.10(a)]. Tightly coupled oligomeric enzymes represent one limiting case or extreme in which the allosteric effector, here a substrate molecule, exerts a maximal effect. Oligomeric enzymes that show no conformational coupling and exhibit Michaelis–Menten kinetics represent the other limiting case or extreme. In this case, substrate binding to one subunit exerts no effect on the catalytic functioning of the others. Thus,

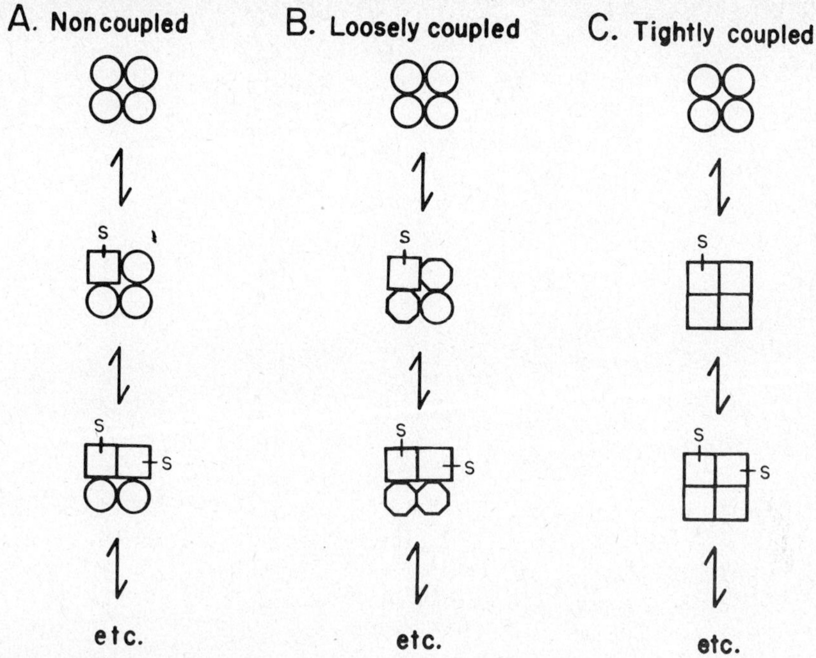

Figure 3.10 Schematic diagram of three tetrameric enzymes which exhibit differing degrees of conformational coupling. (A) The conformational states of the subunits in this first enzyme are not coupled. Consequently, the enzyme exhibits Michaelis–Menten (hyperbolic) kinetics. This situation represents one limiting case. (B) The conformations of the subunits in this second tetrameric enzyme are loosely coupled so that an asymmetric enzyme is observed when one, two, or three substrates are bound to the enzyme. This enzyme exhibits cooperative behavior and represents the general case. (C) The conformations of the four subunits in this third enzyme are tightly coupled so that the enzyme always exhibits a symmetrical structure. The subunits of this enzyme exhibit a maximal degree of cooperativity with respect to substrate binding. This situation represents the other limiting case.

a single mathematical treatment, based on the assumption of varying degrees of coupling between the subunits of an oligomeric enzyme, can account for the kinetic response of virtually any multisubunit enzyme to substrate.

Some enzymes are subject to allosteric regulation by cellular metabolites that are structurally unrelated to the substrates. These enzymes usually occur at critical branch points in metabolic pathways [Figure 3.11(a)] and catalyze reactions which are essentially irreversible. An example is the enzyme aspartate transcarbamoyltransferase (aspartate transcarbamoylase or ATCase) of *E. coli* [Figure 3.11(b)]. This enzyme condenses carbamoyl-P with L-aspartate to give *N*-carbamoyl-L-aspartate and inorganic phosphate. This reaction is the first unique step in the synthesis of the nucleoside triphosphate, cystidine triphosphate (CTP). ATCase is subject to feed-back inhibition by the end product of the biosynthetic pathway, CTP, as well as to feed-forward activation by an initial reactant involved in the synthesis of carbamoyl-P, ATP.

Kinetic analyses revealed that the allosteric effectors of aspartate transcarbamo-

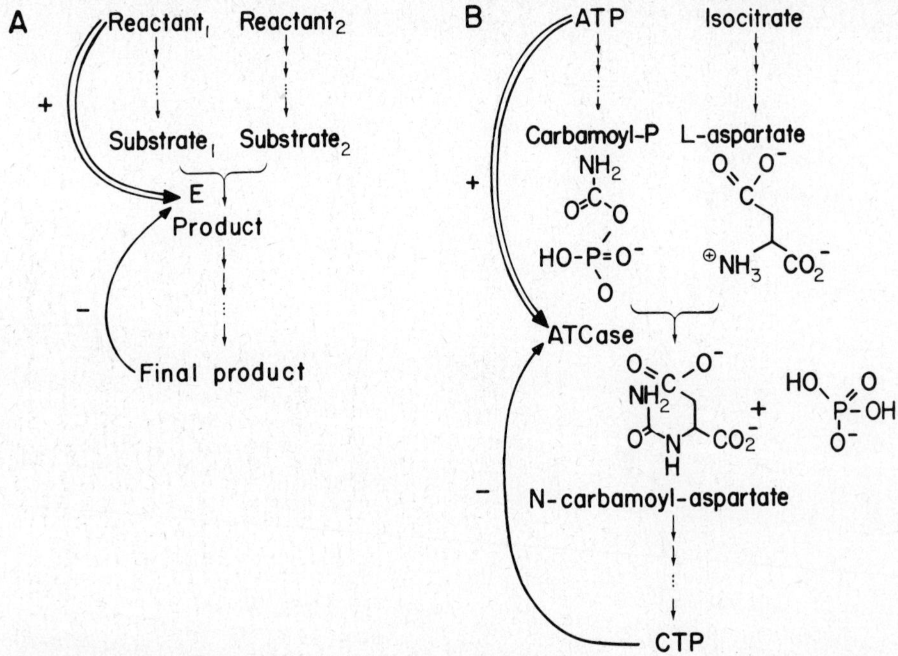

Figure 3.11 Schematic depiction of a converging biosynthetic pathway illustrating feed-forward activation (⟹) as well as feed-back inhibition (⟶). (A) A central enzyme E is subject to feed-forward activation (positive control) by an early metabolite (reactant 1) as well as feed-back inhibition (negative control) by the final product. (B) The process is exemplified by the biosynthetic pathway for the synthesis of cytidine triphosphate (CTP). Aspartate transcarbamoylase (ATCase) condenses carbamoyl phosphate and L-aspartate in the first unique step toward the synthesis of CTP. The enzyme is feed-forward activated by ATP and feed-back inhibited by the end product CTP.

ylase alter the apparent affinity of this enzyme for its amino acid substrate, L-aspartate (Figure 3.12). Thus, in the absence of an effector molecule, a plot of reaction rate versus L-aspartate concentration gives a slightly sigmoidal curve. Addition of CTP, the feed-back inhibitor, to the reaction mixture shifts the curve to the right, rendering it more sigmoidal (greater cooperativity with respect to substrate binding). By contrast, addition of ATP, the feed-forward activator, to the reaction mixture, shifts the curve to the left, rendering it more hyperbolic (little or no cooperativity with respect to substrate binding).

Treatment of this enzyme with the sulfhydryl reagent, *p*-chloromercuribenzoate (*p*CMB) abolishes all allosteric effects. The enzyme retains full catalytic function, but it is no longer sensitive to regulation by ATP or CTP, and this "desensitized" enzyme now exhibits normal Michaelis–Menten kinetics. Native ATCase exhibits a molecular weight of 300,000. Its structure is shown in Figure 3.13 (left). Analyses have revealed that treatment with *p*CMB causes dissociation of the enzyme into two constituent proteins. One, which retains full catalytic activity, is designated C and was found to be a trimer with a monomer molecular weight of 33,000 (Figure 3.13, right). The

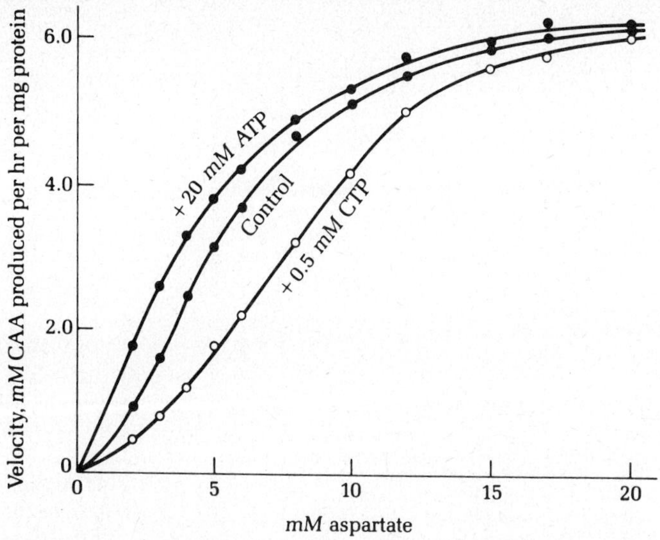

Figure 3.12 Response of aspartate transcarbamoyltransferase (ATCase) to the allosteric effectors CTP and ATP. CTP is a negative effector because it effectively decreases the apparent affinity of the enzyme for L-aspartate (i.e., shifts the curve to the right, making it more sigmoidal), while ATP is a positive effector because it increases the apparent affinity of the enzyme (i.e., it shifts the curve to the left, rendering it more hyperbolic).

other constituent protein exhibits no catalytic activity but has a binding site for nucleoside triphosphates. This second protein, the regulatory constituent of ATCase, is designated R and was found to be a dimer with a subunit molecular weight of 17,000.

Two moles of the catalytic trimer and three moles of the regulatory dimer are recovered per mole of ATCase exposed to the reagent (Figure 3.13). It is therefore clear that the holoenzyme consists of six identical catalytic subunits and six identical regulatory subunits. The three-dimensional structure of this regulatory protein was revealed by x-ray crystallography.

These observations provide a structural basis for the regulatory interactions that control the activity of aspartate transcarbamoyltransferase. It should not be assumed, however, that all allosteric enzymes are regulated by the same mechanism. Glycerol kinase from *E. coli,* for example, is a tetrameric enzyme (MW = 220,000) which consists of four identical subunits of 55,000-dalton molecular weight. This enzyme phosphorylates glycerol with ATP as the phosphoryl donor, yielding α-glycerol phosphate and ADP as products. It binds ATP and glycerol at the active site and is allosterically inhibited both by fructose-1,6-diphosphate (FDP) and by the regulatory protein of the bacterial phosphotransferase system, RPr, discussed in Section 3.8. FDP can be thought of as a feed-back inhibitor of the enzyme which senses the intracellular metabolite levels of the cell, while RPr senses the availability of extracellular carbohydrates which serve as better carbon and energy sources for growth than does glycerol. RPr is normally phosphorylated in the bacterial cytoplasm, and phospho-RPr neither

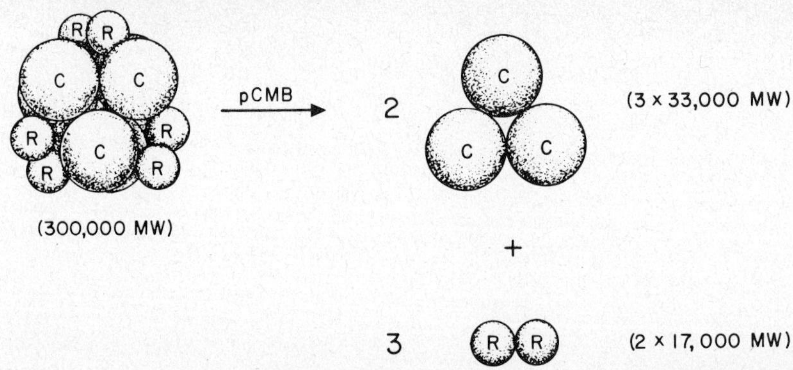

Figure 3.13 Illustration of the structure of native aspartate transcarbamoylase (left) and the dissociated catalytic (C) and regulatory (R) subunit constituents (right). While the catalytic trimers possess full enzyme activity and exhibit Michaelis–Menten kinetics, the regulatory dimers possess two nucleoside triphosphate binding sites per dimer. Dissociation of the regulatory subunits from the catalytic subunits is effected by treating the enzyme with the sulfhydryl reagent *p*-chloromercuribenzoate (*p*CMB).

binds to nor inhibits glycerol kinase. When glucose or another sugar substrate of the phosphotransferase system is added to the medium, RPr is rapidly dephosphorylated and thereby converted to the free form of the protein which inhibits glycerol kinase. This mechanism allows the preferential utilization of glucose and certain other carbohydrates over glycerol.

Genetic analyses have shown that the binding sites on glycerol kinase specific for RPr and FDP are distinct. Mutant enzymes that no longer bind RPr are still sensitive to inhibition by FDP, while mutant enzymes that no longer bind FDP retain full sensitivity to RPr. Each subunit apparently contains separate binding sites for FDP and RPr, and these are distinct from the active site. The binding of either FDP or RPr to the native tetramer decreases the maximal rate of glycerol phosphorylation without changing the affinity of the enzyme for either substrate. However, when both FDP and RPr are present, the inhibitory effects of these two allosteric effectors are frequently less than additive. Although the two allosteric binding sites are distinct, they interact functionally, presumably because the binding of either ligand induces the same, inhibitory, conformational change at the active site of the kinase. The presence of two separate allosteric regulatory sites associated with the same polypeptide chain that bears the catalytic substrate binding cleft suggests that each subunit may possess two or more domains, one or two of which are responsible for regulation with a third functioning in catalysis. Glycerol kinase therefore differs from aspartate transcarbamoylase in having its regulatory domain(s) "fused" to its catalytic domain and in exhibiting V_{max} rather than K_M responses to allosteric effectors. A schematic model illustrating the presumed structure of glycerol kinase is shown in Figure 3.14. The exact structure–function correlates for this enzyme must await x-ray crystallographic analyses of the enzyme and its complexes with substrates and allosteric effectors.

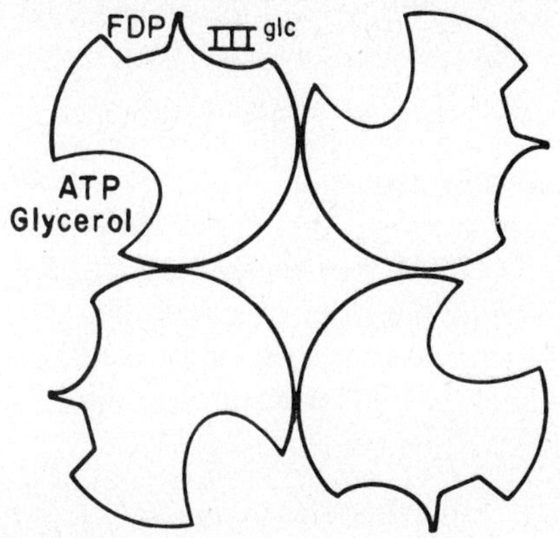

Figure 3.14 Schematic model illustrating presumed structural features of glycerol kinase from *E. coli.* Each subunit of the tetrameric enzyme possesses an active site which binds ATP and glycerol as well as two distinct allosteric regulatory sites, one of which binds fructose-1,6-diphosphate (FDP), the other which binds the regulatory protein (RPr) of the phosphoenolpyruvate: sugar phosphotransferase system. RPr has been shown to be the glucose Enzyme III (III^{glc}) discussed in Section 5.4 of Chapter 5. The symmetrical arrangement of the four identical subunits in the enzyme has not been established.

3.10 CLASSIFICATION OF ALLOSTERIC INTERACTIONS

In the previous section it was seen that a single enzyme may be subject to simultaneous feed-back inhibition and feed-forward activation by an indirect, allosteric mechanism. It was further seen that not all enzymes in a metabolic pathway are subject to this type of control. Rather, one or a few key, rate-limiting enzymes that usually catalyze essentially irreversible reactions act as the target of regulatory control. These enzymes may be regulated not only by cellular metabolites but also by chemical energy sources, by chemiosmotic energy sources, and by macromolecular sensors of the various metabolic states of the cell.

Many pathways serve multiple functions, leading to the production of several key biosynthetic precursors and/or energy sources. This fact is particularly true of amphibolic pathways such as those of glycolysis, gluconeogenesis, and the Krebs cycle. It also applies to branched, diverging, biosynthetic pathways as well as to forked, converging, degradative pathways. In order to satisfy the multiplicity of regulatory needs that are based on the ultimate functions of the pathways, a variety of allosteric control mechanisms have evolved. These mechanisms will be briefly summarized in this section.

3.10.1 Metabolite-Sensitive Allosteric Regulation

a. Simple One-Effector Feed-Back or Feed-Forward Regulation A single metabolic product inhibits or a single precursor activates the enzyme, signaling a sufficiency of the product or an excess of the precursor. Aspartate transcarbamoylase, discussed in the previous section, is a prime example of this type of regulation.

b. Cumulative Feed-Back Inhibition In cases where the activity of a key enzyme leads to the synthesis of several metabolites, each such end-product may only partially inhibit the activity of the enzyme, and each may inhibit independently of the others due to the presence of multiple binding sites for the different end-products on the surface of the enzyme. The effects of any two, three, or more inhibitors are roughly *additive.*

Only when all such inhibitors are present is inhibition maximal. Glutamine synthase of *E. coli,* discussed in Chapter 9, is an example of an enzyme sensitive to cumulative inhibition.

c. Synergistic or Antagonistic Feed-Back Inhibition When two end-products feed-back inhibit an enzyme simultaneously, they may inhibit more strongly or less strongly than the sum of their independent effects. The former effect is referred to as *synergistic* or *cooperative* feed-back inhibition while the latter effect is called *antagonistic* feed-back inhibition. Because of the cooperative properties of allosterically regulated enzymes, these phenomena may be reflective of either single or multiple conformational transitions.

3.10.2 Sensitivity of Enzymes to Cellular Energy States

a. Chemical Energy Many enzymes are regulated by metabolites that serve as sensors of the energy state of the cell. For example, an enzyme that regulates a pathway that generates ATP may be inhibited by ATP but activated by AMP and inorganic phosphate. Phosphofructokinase from *E. coli,* discussed in Chapter 5, is an example of such an enzyme. The opposite may be true of an enzyme in a pathway that utilizes ATP for biosynthetic purposes.

b. Chemiosmotic Energy Other enzymes, particularly those embedded within the membrane of a cell or organelle, may be sensitive to control by chemiosmotic energy. These enzymes sense the electrochemical gradient of an ion such as H^+ or K^+ across the membrane. While the mechanism by which the activity of such an enzyme is regulated is not well understood, interactions between an electric field and the electric dipole moment of the protein may bring about a conformational change in the protein which alters its activity. Alternatively, it has been suggested that the electrochemical potential may regulate enzyme activity by controlling cysteyl oxidation ($2\ SH \rightleftharpoons S{-}S$). Transport systems such as the mannitol and lactose permeases in *E. coli* may be subject to this type of control.

c. Macromolecular Control Studies over the past few years have revealed that macromolecules, usually but not always proteins, can sense the energy state of a cell and thereby regulate the activities of enzymes. They may also sense the concentrations of cytoplasmic "second messengers" such as Ca^{++} and cyclic nucleotides, which in turn are responsive to energy sources, metabolite concentrations, or extracellular stimuli such as hormones and neurotransmitters. Regardless of the agent sensed, two very different mechanisms of macromolecular control appear to be emerging: structural and catalytic. Structural control requires direct macromolecular interactions to effect a change in functional state, while catalytic control depends on the catalytic activity of the macromolecular effector to bring about a covalent modification of the target enzyme. Calmodulin in eukaryotic cells and the regulatory protein RPr of the phosphotransferase system in prokaryotic cells (discussed in the preceding two sections) are examples of structural macromolecular effectors. Protein kinases and protein methylases are examples of catalytic macromolecular effectors.

It is clear from this discussion that several independent regulatory mechanisms involve covalent and noncovalent interactions. These mechanisms allow enzymes to sense metabolite concentrations, chemiosmotic sources of energy, and macromolecular sensors of second messengers. In fact, a single enzyme may be responsive to many such mechanisms. In *E. coli,* aspartate transcarbamoylase is regulated by both feed-back inhibition and feed-forward activation (Section 3.9); glycerol kinase is regulated by both metabolite and structural macromolecular allosteric control (Section 3.9); phosphofructokinase is regulated allosterically by both metabolite concentrations and the adenylate energy charge (Chapter 5); glutamine synthase is regulated by both cumulative feed-back inhibition and covalent adenylylation (catalytic macromolecular control) (Chapter 9); isocitrate dehydrogenase is regulated by feed-back inhibition, feed-forward activation, and covalent phosphorylation (Chapter 6); and the pyruvate dehydrogenase complex is regulated by at least four distinct mechanisms which are still poorly understood (Chapter 6). It is clear that studies of the intricacies of metabolic regulation, including the control of these regulatory interactions, will provide biochemists with challenges and intellectual entertainment for years to come.

> *Abandon the search for God. Learn who is within you. Learn the source of sorrow, joy, love, hate. If you carefully investigate these matters, you will find Him in yourself.*
>
> —HIPPOLYTUS

BIBLIOGRAPHY

Blackburn, S., *Enzyme Structure and Function,* Marcel Dekker, New York (1976).

Breslow, R., and G. Zubay, "Enzyme Catalysis I and II," in *Biochemistry,* G. Zubay, ed., pp. 130–195, Addison-Wesley, Reading, MA (1983).

Clark, J. M., Jr., and R. L. Switzer, *Experimental Biochemistry,* W. H. Freeman, San Francisco, CA (1964).

Cornish-Bowden, A., *Fundamentals of Enzyme Kinetics,* Butterworth, London (1979).

De Bernard, B., et al., eds., "Calcium-Binding Proteins, 1983," in *Proceedings of the International Symposium on Calcium-Binding Proteins in Health and Disease,* Elsevier/North Holland, Amsterdam (1983).

Dixon, M., E. C. Webb, C. J. R. Thorne, and K. F. Tipton, *Enzymes,* Third Edition, Academic, New York (1979).

Ebner, K. E., ed., *Subunit Enzymes: Biochemistry and Function,* Marcel Dekker, New York (1975).

Enzyme Nomenclature, 1978: Recommendations of the Nomenclature Committee of the International Union of Biochemistry on the Nomenclature and Classification of Enzymes, Academic, New York (1979).

Freedman, R. B., and H. C. Hawkins, *The Enzymology of Posttranslational Modification of Proteins,* Academic, New York (1980).

Hammes, C. G., *Enzyme Catalysis and Regulation,* Academic, New York (1982).

Houghton, J. E., D. A. Bencini, G. A. O'Donovan, and J. R. Wild, "Protein Differentiation: A

Comparison of Aspartate Transcarbamoylase and Ornithine Transcarbamoylase from *Escherichia coli* K-12," *Proc. Nat. Acad. Sci. USA,* **81:** 4864–4868 (1984).

Huang, C. Y., S. G. Rhee, and P. B. Chock, "Subunit Cooperation and Enzymatic Catalysis," *Ann. Rev. Biochem.,* **51:** 935–971 (1982).

Hunter, T., "The Proteins of Oncogenes," *Scientific American,* **251:** 70–79 (1984).

Jacobson, G. R., and M. H. Saier, Jr., "Biological Membranes: Structure and Assembly," in *Biochemistry,* G. Zubay, ed., pp. 573–619, Addison-Wesley, Reading, MA (1983).

Johnson, B. C., ed., "Posttranslational Covalent Modifications of Proteins," in *International Conference on Posttranslational Covalent Modifications of Proteins for Function,* Oklahoma City, Oklahoma, 1982, Academic, New York (1983).

Kane, J. F., ed., *Multifunctional Proteins: Catalytic/Structural and Regulatory,* CRC Press, Boca Raton, FL (1983).

Ke, H., R. B. Honzatko, and W. N. Lipscomb, "Structure of Unligated Aspartate Carbamoyltransferase of *Escherichia coli* at 2.6-Å Resolution," *Proc. Natl. Acad. Sci. USA,* **81:** 4037–4040 (1984).

Lefkowitz, R. J., J. M. Stadel, and M. G. Caron, "Adenylate Cyclase-Coupled Beta-Adrenergic Receptors: Structure and Mechanisms of Activation and Desensitization," *Ann. Rev. Biochem.,* **52:** 159–186 (1983).

Lipscomb, W. N., "Structure and Catalysis of Enzymes," *Ann. Rev. Biochem.,* **52:** 17–34 (1983).

Novotny, M. J., W. L. Frederickson, E. B. Waygood, and M. H. Saier, Jr., "Allosteric Regulation of Glycerol Kinase by Enzyme III^{glc} of the Phosphotransferase System in *Escherichia coli* and *Salmonella typhimurium,*" *J. Bacteriol.,* **162:** 810–816 (1985).

Purich, D. L., ed., *Contemporary Enzyme Kinetics and Mechanism,* Academic, New York (1983).

Ricard, J., and A. Cornish-Rowden, eds., *Dynamics of Biochemical Systems,* Plenum, New York (1984).

Segel, I. H., *Enzyme Kinetics: Behavior and Analysis of Rapid Equilibrium and Steady-State Enzyme Systems,* Wiley, New York (1975).

Spector, L. B., *Covalent Catalysis by Enzymes,* Springer-Verlag, New York (1982).

Spiro, T. G., ed., *Calcium in Biology,* Wiley, New York (1983).

Srere, P. A., "Why are Enzymes So Big?," *Trends Biochem. Sci.,* **9:** 387–390 (1984).

Walker, R., *The Molecular Biology of Enzyme Synthesis: Regulatory Mechanisms of Enzyme Adaptation,* Wiley, New York (1983).

Walter, C., *Enzyme Reactions and Enzyme Systems,* Marcel Dekker, New York (1976).

Chapter 4

Cofactors of Enzyme-Catalyzed Reactions

> *Intellectual food is like any other; it is pleasanter and more beneficial to take it with a spoon than with a shovel.*
>
> —MARK TWAIN

The amino acyl side chains in proteins are not sufficiently diverse in structure to allow catalysis of all requisite chemical interconversions at rates which are sufficiently rapid to support life. As discussed in the preceding chapter, these residues function primarily in general acid and base catalysis, in nucleophilic and electrophilic catalysis, in charge neutralization, and in the formation of noncovalent enthalpy and entropy bonds (hydrogen and hydrophobic bonds, respectively). In order to increase the versatility of enzymes, a variety of cofactors have been incorporated into the majority of enzymes. These cofactors include molecules that, by virtue of their structures, readily undergo oxidation–reduction reactions, molecules that activate amino groups and allow resonance stabilization of reaction intermediates, and molecules that generate potent nucleophiles with unusual properties. Some of these cofactors are simple metal ions, but others are organic compounds which form either covalent or noncovalent linkages with enzymic side chains at or near the active sites of the proteins. In general, we can define an enzyme cofactor (a coenzyme) as a molecule that binds to an enzyme and acts cooperatively with it to accelerate the rate of a biochemical reaction. When the cofactor is tightly (even covalently) bound to the enzyme, it is frequently referred to as a *prosthetic group.* Some coenzymes such as the nicotinamide coenzymes bind relatively loosely, and really function as *cosubstrates.* The terms *coenzyme* and *enzyme cofactor* are universally applied to all of these agents.

4.1 RELATIONSHIPS OF VITAMINS TO COENZYMES

Table 4.1 lists the major water-soluble vitamins, the biologically active coenzymes derived from these vitamins, and the reactions in which these coenzymes participate. A vitamin is defined as a nutritional substance which an animal cannot synthesize but which is required for normal body function in small amounts. It will be noted that each vitamin generally has two designations, a nutritional and a biochemical

TABLE 4.1 WATER-SOLUBLE VITAMINS AND THEIR DERIVED COENZYMES

Vitamin designation		Coenzyme or prosthetic group (abbreviation)	Reactions catalyzed
Nutritional	Biochemical		
B_1	Thiamine	Thiamine pyrophosphate (TPP)	(a) Decarboxylation (b) Transketolation
B_2	Riboflavin	Flavin coenzymes (FMN, FAD)	Redox
B_3 (Niacin)	Nicotinate	Nicotinamide coenzymes (NAD^+, $NADP^+$)	Redox
B_6	Pyridoxine	Pyridoxal phosphate (PLP)	(a) Amino transferation (b) Decarboxylation (c) Racemization (d) α,β-elimination (e) Dealdolization
Folate	Folate	Tetrahydrofolate coenzymes (FH_4)	Transfer and interconversion of methyl, hydroxymethyl, methylene, formyl, formimino, and methenyl groups
B_{12}	Cobalamine	Coenzyme B_{12} or cobamide coenzymes (CoB_{12})	(a) Alkyl transfer (b) Dehydration (c) Redox
H	Biotin	Biocytyl–protein	Carboxylation
Pantothenate	Pantothenate	Coenzyme A (CoA) Acyl carrier protein (ACP)	Thioesterification and thioester modification
Lipoate	Lipoate	Lipoyl-proteins	Redox and acyl transfer
Metal ion	Metal ion	Mg^{++}, Fe^{++}, Cu^{++}, Zn^{++}, etc.	Redox; substrate activation and binding
Metal ion	Metal ion	Heme	O_2 and electron transfer
Metal ion	Metal ion	Iron–sulfur center	Electron transfer

designation. For example, the five major B-type vitamins (B_1, B_2, B_3, B_6, and B_{12}) are called by biochemists thiamine, riboflavin, nicotinate, pyridoxine, and cobalamin, respectively. Nicotinate was also given the nutritional designation of "niacin," solely because bread companies felt that the word "nicotinate" sounded too much like "nicotine." They wanted to be able to claim that their product was vitamin enriched without association with a harmful substance.

Vitamin H is termed "biotin" by the biochemist. Nutritional and biochemical designations for the remaining vitamins listed in Table 4.1—folate, pantothenate, and lipoate—are the same. Of the remaining well-known vitamins, vitamin C can be synthesized by most animals except humans, bats, guinea pigs, and certain birds and fish. It is required in relatively large amounts for normal bodily functions. Therefore its designation as a vitamin is sometimes considered to be a misnomer. Vitamins A, D, and E constitute lipid-soluble vitamins which do not function as classical enzyme cofactors.

Each of the water-soluble vitamins absorbed by intestinal epithelial cells can be transported through the plasma, transported into the cells of the body, and converted to the coenzyme form of the molecule which possesses inherent biological activity.

Thiamine is converted to thiamine pyrophosphate (Figure 4.2), which functions in decarboxylation, transketolation, and other reactions. Riboflavin serves as the precursor of the two flavin coenzymes, flavin mononucleotide (FMN) and flavin adenine dinucleotide (FAD) (Figure 4.5), which function as oxidation–reduction (redox) coenzymes. Nicotinate is converted to the two nicotinamide coenzymes, nicotinamide adenine dinucleotide (NAD^+) and nicotinamide adenine dinucleotide phosphate ($NADP^+$) (Figures 4.8 and 4.9), which function primarily in oxidation–reduction reactions. Pyridoxine is phosphorylated and oxidized to give pyridoxal phosphate (PLP) (Figure 4.13). This coenzyme functions as a cofactor for many enzymes which act on amino acids and other amines. Such enzymes include aminotransferases, decarboxylases, and racemases. The active forms of vitamin B_{12} (cobalamin) are called the cobamide coenzymes. They function in a diversity of mechanistically related reactions, including alkyl transfer, dehydration, and internal oxidation–reduction. 5′-Deoxyadenosyl cobalamin (coenzyme B_{12}) is the principal form of this coenzyme (Figure 4.18). Folate is reduced to tetrahydrofolate (Figure 4.16), which functions in the transfer and interconversion of various one-carbon substituents as indicated in Table 4.1. Finally, the last three vitamins listed in the table become covalently incorporated into specific proteins where they function as an enzyme-bound cosubstrate [lipoate; Figure 4.20(a)], as a coenzyme [biocytin; Figure 4.20(b)], or as a substrate–carrier (pantothenate; Figure 4.21).

4.2 AROMATIC NUCLEOPHILIC DISPLACEMENT (S_{N2}) REACTIONS

Numerous enzymes function by S_{N2} substitution reactions in which a nucleophile attacks an electrophilic center, displacing an electronegative atom. In biology, free radical mechanisms are less common than displacement reactions, presumably because of the potentially deleterious effects of free radicals to living organisms. In fact, except for certain redox (electron transfer) cofactors to be discussed in Chapter 7, the only two types of coenzymes known to sometimes function by free radical mechanisms are the flavin coenzymes (FMN and FAD) and coenzyme B_{12}. Because the simple

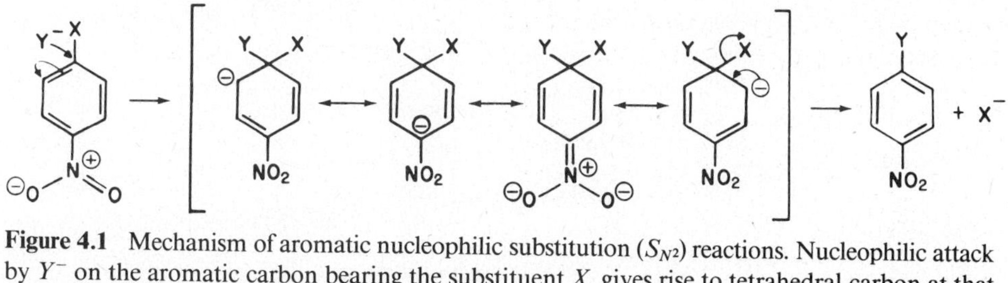

Figure 4.1 Mechanism of aromatic nucleophilic substitution (S_{N2}) reactions. Nucleophilic attack by Y^- on the aromatic carbon bearing the substituent X, gives rise to tetrahedral carbon at that position, destroying the aromatic character of the ring. This intermediate is extensively stabilized by resonance as shown within the brackets. The presence of a nitro group ortho or para to the position of substitution stabilizes the intermediate by permitting additional resonance structures. The presence of two nitro groups both ortho and para to the position of substitution stablizes the reaction intermediate further, thereby facilitating the reaction as discussed in the text. 2,4-Dinitrofluoro-benzene is an example of a protein reagent that is activated for nucleophilic attack by nitro groups.

principles of the organic chemist are applicable to so many coenzyme- and enzyme-catalyzed reactions, these principles will be reviewed here.

Figure 4.1 reviews the process and mechanism of aromatic nucleophilic substitution reactions. The lysyl-derivatizing reagent, 2,4-dinitrofluorobenzene, contains an electronegative fluorine atom as well as two electron-withdrawing nitro groups in the 2 (ortho) and the 4 (para) positions of the ring, relative to the fluorine atom. Attack at the ring carbon bearing the fluorine atom by the ϵ-amino group of a lysyl residue in a protein (*Y* in Figure 4.1) gives rise to an intermediate which is extensively stabilized by resonance. Figure 4.1 shows the resonance stabilization structures which can exist when the simpler but less reactive reagent, *p*-nitrofluorobenzene, is used. The subsequent elimination of the fluorine atom as a fluoride ion (*X* in Figure 4.1) regenerates the aromatic ring and gives as product the nitrophenylated lysyl side chain in the protein. Because proteins contain other effective nucleophiles (such as the sulfhydryl groups of cysteyl residues), dinitrofluorobenzene is not specific for lysyl residues.

As Figure 4.1 illustrates, the presence of a nitro group in the 2 or 4 (ortho or para) position of the ring greatly facilitates the substitution reaction because it stabilizes the tetrahedral intermediate by providing an additional resonance structure for the intermediate. Additionally, the ring is rendered a better electrophile for attack by the amine because of the electron-withdrawing effect of the nitro group. The nitro group facilitates attack by a nucleophile and at the same time inhibits attack by an electrophile. The extent of acceleration or inhibition per nitro group is actually about four orders of magnitude. Because the resonance structure with the ring electron pair residing on a nitro group can only be drawn when the attacking nucleophile is in an ortho or para position, relative to the nitro group, the nitro group is an *o,p*-director for aromatic nucleophilic substitution. In contrast, attack by an electrophile would be meta-directed (directed to the 3-position on the ring, relative to the nitro group). The resonance-stabilized structures for the intermediate following attack by an electrophile, exhibit resonance structures with a positive charge on the ortho and para positions relative to the position of substitution. The electron-withdrawing effect of a nitro group at either of these two positions therefore *destabilizes* the resonance structures more than if a nitro group was in the meta position.

Table 4.2 summarizes the effects of a variety of biologically relevant substituents on aromatic substitution reactions. Three generalizations can be made. First, it can be seen that any substituent which accelerates the rate of an electrophilic substitution

TABLE 4.2 EFFECTS OF VARIOUS BIOLOGICALLY IMPORTANT SUBSTITUENTS ON THE REACTIVITY OF AROMATIC RINGS WITH RESPECT TO ELECTROPHILIC AND NUCLEOPHILIC SUBSTITUTION REACTIONS

	Substitution			
	Electrophilic		Nucleophilic	
Group	Effect	Directing	Effect	Directing
$-NO_2$, $-C(=O)NH_2$, $-C{\equiv}N$, $-SO_3H$	↓	meta	↑	ortho, para
$-CH_3$, $-OH$, $-OCH_3$, $-NH_2$	↑	ortho, para	↓	meta

reaction will have the opposite effect on a nucleophilic substitution reaction. The converse also holds. Second, any substituent which directs electrophiles to the meta position, directs nucleophiles to the ortho and para positions. The converse of this generalization is also valid. Finally, for the substituents shown in Table 4.2, and for virtually all common biological substituents, activating substituents of aromatic S_{N2} reactions will be *o,p*-directors, while inhibitory substituents will be meta-directors. Of course, the converse is true for electrophilic substitution reactions. With these principles in mind, we will be able to more easily proceed to a consideration of the mechanisms of action of the aromatic coenzymes.

4.3 THIAMINE PYROPHOSPHATE (TPP)

Vitamin B_1, or thiamine, is the precursor of the coenzyme thiamine pyrophosphate (TPP). The effects of extreme thiamine deficiency include heart failure, mental disturbances, neuritis (the inflammation of nerves causing impaired reflexes or paralysis), and beriberi, a form of multiple neuritis characterized by loss of muscular power, emaciation, and exhaustion. Thiamine cannot be synthesized by most higher organisms including mammals and, therefore, is an essential dietary supplement. Intracellular thiamine is transformed into TPP in a reaction catalyzed by TPP synthase. A pyrophosphate group is transferred to the vitamin from ATP in the reaction shown in Figure 4.2. The by-product is AMP.

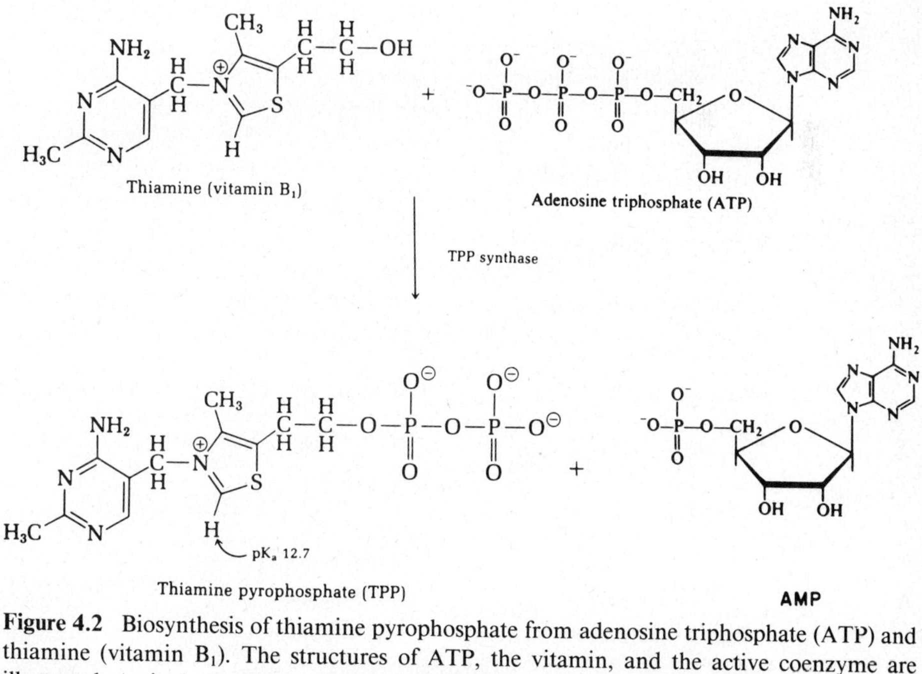

Figure 4.2 Biosynthesis of thiamine pyrophosphate from adenosine triphosphate (ATP) and thiamine (vitamin B_1). The structures of ATP, the vitamin, and the active coenzyme are illustrated. A single reaction converts thiamine to thiamine pyrophosphate as shown. The byproduct of the reaction is adenosine monophosphate (AMP). The enzyme catalyzing this reaction is called thiamine pyrophosphate synthase.

The thiazolium ring of TPP serves as the reactive center of the coenzyme. The ring substituents function only as handles for the enzyme and apparently do not provide direct catalytic assistance. However, the acidity of the proton at the C-2 position of the thiazolium ring (Figure 4.2) is enhanced by the presence of the adjacent quarternary nitrogen which acts as an *electron sink.* There are two important resonance structures of the carbanion. One is a dipolar ion (a ylid; structure 1 in Figure 4.3) and the other is a neutral carbene (structure 2 in Figure 4.3) which results from transfer of the π electron pair to nitrogen. The carbanion formed by loss of the proton at C-2 is stabilized not only by the electron-withdrawing capacities of the adjacent nitronium ion but also by the ring sulfur atom. It has been postulated that delocalization of the free electron pair of the carbanion into the vacant *d*-orbitals of the adjacent sulfur atom occurs. Because of these stabilizing effects, the proton at C-2 is quite acidic (pKa = 12.7), and the carbanion which results from dissociation of this proton is consequently available to function as a nucleophile, attacking the partially positive carbon in polar carbonyl groups.

The reactions catalyzed by TPP-dependent enzymes usually involve the synthesis or cleavage of a bond adjacent to a reactive carbonyl function. These processes can be either oxidative or nonoxidative. Generally, if an enzyme catalyzes decarboxylation of an α-keto acid, it probably requires TPP. Many TPP-dependent α-keto acid decarboxylases are known.

The nonoxidative decarboxylation of pyruvate as catalyzed by yeast pyruvate decarboxylase provides an excellent example of the mechanistic action of TPP. As shown in Figure 4.4(a), the TPP carbanion undergoes nucleophilic addition to the keto group of pyruvate, displacing the π-electrons to the carbonyl oxygen. CO_2 is lost in the next step (b), with the decarboxylation intermediate stabilized by resonance. Protonation of the decarboxylated substrate–enzyme adduct then gives hydroxyethyl-TPP. Finally, reformation of the carbonyl bond in the substrate provides the driving force for dissolution of the carbon–carbon bond between substrate and coenzyme (c). Acetaldehyde is produced, and the anionic form of TPP is regenerated.

An analogous process is responsible for the oxidative decarboxylation of pyruvate in *E. coli.* The enzyme responsible for this reaction is pyruvate oxidase, an enzyme which contains two cofactors, TPP and flavin adenine dinucleotide (FAD). Initially, hydroxyethyl-TPP is produced exactly as for the yeast pyruvate decarboxylase reaction. However, regeneration of the substrate carbonyl bond [as in Figure 4.4(c)] promotes

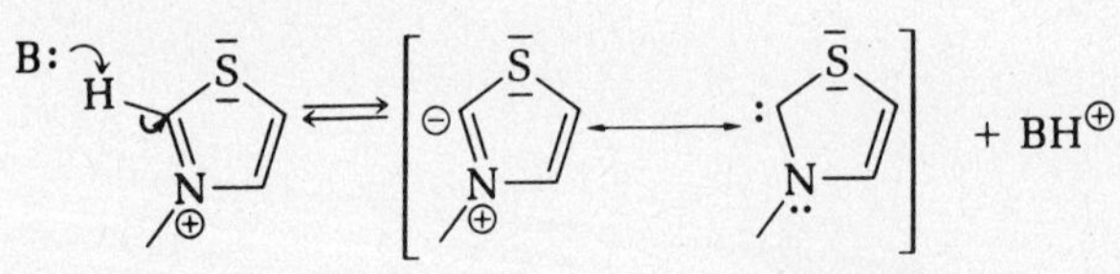

(1) Ylid (2) Nucleophilic carbene

Figure 4.3 Formation and resonance stabilization of the anionic form of thiamine pyrophosphate (TPP). These two resonance structures are: (1) the bipolar ionic form of TPP$^-$ called a ylid, and (2) the nucleophilic carbene. The proton is removed from the coenzyme employing a general base in the enzyme B.

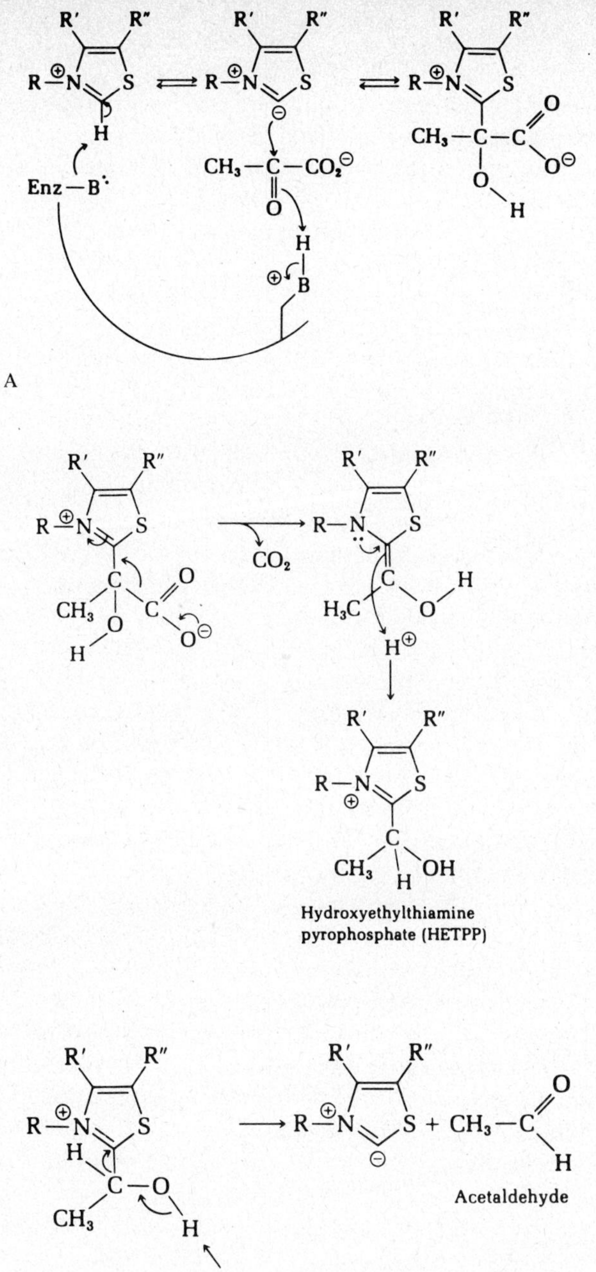

Figure 4.4 Mechanism of action of pyruvate decarboxylase from yeast. The reaction sequence is shown as occurring in three stages: step A, formation of a covalent coenzyme substrate complex; step B, decarboxylation; and step C, dissociation of the product from the coenzyme.

transfer of a hydride ion from C-1 in hydroxyethyl-TPP to FAD instead of breaking the carbon–carbon bond between the substrate and coenzyme, yielding acetyl-TPP and $FADH_2$. Hydrolysis of acetyl-TPP then gives acetate plus the free form of TPP. For illustration of this more complicated reaction sequence, see Figure 4.6 in the next section.

Of greatest importance with respect to the mechanism of action of TPP are the stability of the thiazolium ring carbanion, the facility with which it reacts with partially positive carbonyl carbons and the stability of the substrate carbanion due to delocalization of the electron pair into the thiazolium ring. These features are unique to TPP—no other coenzyme functions by an analogous mechanism.

4.4 THE FLAVIN COENZYMES (FMN AND FAD)

Flavin mononucleotide (FMN) and flavin adenine dinucleotide (FAD) are coenzyme derivatives of vitamin B_2, also called riboflavin. Although riboflavin can be synthesized by many microorganisms, it is an essential dietary supplement of higher organisms including mammals. The effects of riboflavin deficiency in humans include photophobia and fissuring of the skin. A single enzyme, flavokinase (ATP:riboflavin phosphotransferase), catalyzes the conversion of riboflavin to riboflavin-5′-phosphate (FMN). This enzyme is present in bacteria, yeast, plants, and many diverse animal tissues. FAD is synthesized reversibly from FMN by the action of flavin nucleotide pyrophosphorylase, another widely distributed enzyme. This enzyme catalyzes the transfer of the AMP portion of an ATP molecule to the 5′-phosphate group of FMN with concomitant release of pyrophosphate into the cytoplasm. The reaction is rendered irreversible by hydrolysis of the pyrophosphate bond catalyzed by a pyrophosphatase. Both the kinase and the pyrophosphorylase mentioned above require Mg^{++} for catalytic activity. Figure 4.5 outlines the biosynthesis of FAD and FMN from riboflavin and illustrates the structures of these three compounds. It should be noted that AMP is a constituent of three important coenzymes, FAD, $NAD(P)^+$, and coenzyme A.

The flavins were named after the Latin word *flavus* (yellow) because of the bright yellow color of the oxidized isoalloxazine ring. FMN and FAD are functionally equivalent cofactors, and the specificity of an enzyme for one or the other coenzyme depends entirely on its binding specificity. Most flavoproteins (which require a flavin coenzyme for activity) contain the coenzyme tightly but noncovalently bound at the active site. In only a few exceptional cases is the coenzyme covalently bound to the enzyme. One such enzyme, succinate dehydrogenase, will be discussed in Chapter 7.

Flavoproteins catalyze a wide variety of oxidation–reduction reactions. They can be grouped as dehydrogenases, which catalyze redox reactions without molecular oxygen; oxidases, which utilize molecular oxygen as the electron acceptor, generating hydrogen peroxide; and mono-oxygenases, also called hydroxylases, which introduce one atom of oxygen from O_2 into the substrate while reducing the other to H_2O. Some flavoproteins also require transition metals for activity, and these enzymes are called metalloflavoproteins. Because flavoproteins can function by hydride (H^-) transfer, by substrate carbanion additions, or by a free radical mechanism, they can link two-electron transfer processes (such as those involving NADH oxidation) to one-electron

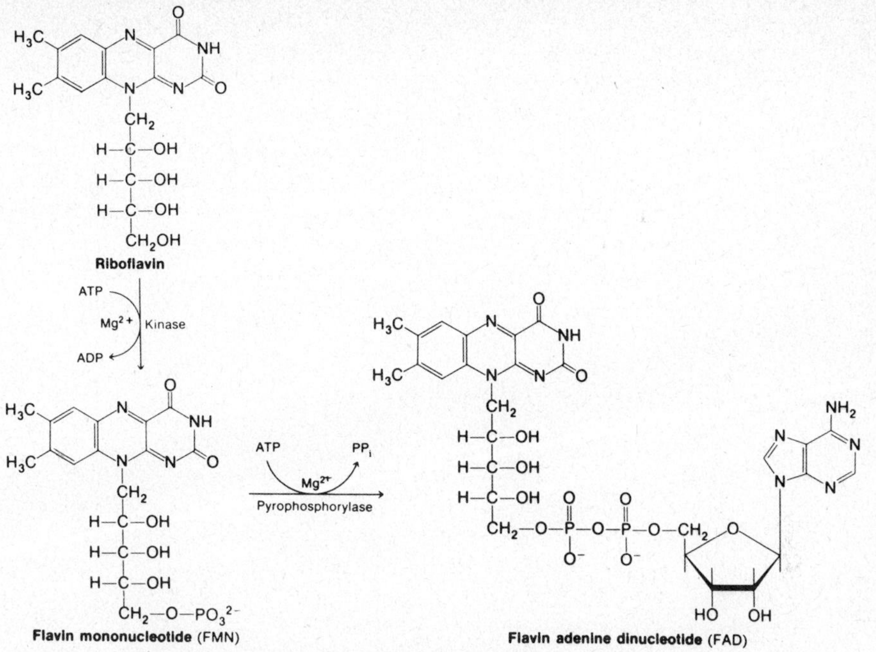

Figure 4.5 Biosynthesis of flavin mononucleotide (FMN) and flavin adenine dinucleotide (FAD) from riboflavin (vitamin B_2). This figure illustrates the structures of the vitamin and its two coenzyme forms as well as the biosynthetic pathway. (Reproduced with permission from P. A. Frey, "Structure and Function of Coenzymes" in *Biochemistry,* G. Zubay, ed., Addison-Wesley, Reading, MA, 1983.)

transfer processes (such as those catalyzed by iron-sulfur proteins, quinones, and cytochromes). This fact will be discussed in the following paragraphs and in Chapter 7.

Reduction of FMN or FAD disrupts the conjugated π system of the isoalloxazine ring, and as a result, the hydroquinones, $FMNH_2$ and $FADH_2$, are nearly colorless. As noted in the preceding paragraph, reduction of the flavin coenzymes can occur by direct hydride transfer, by carbanion additions, or by the stepwise transfer of single electrons (and protons) to the isoalloxazine ring with radical semiquinones as intermediates. Reduction of flavins by direct hydride transfer is exemplified by the plausible mechanism of action of pyruvate oxidase, discussed at the end of the preceding section on TPP, and is illustrated in Figure 4.6. FAD may be reduced by transfer of a hydride ion from hydroxyethyl-TPP to the central nitrogen atom in the isoalloxazine ring, but a carbanion addition reaction is equally probable.

Flavoenzymes which catalyze one-electron transfer reactions function in a more complex manner. In the unprotonated free radical form of the coenzyme (Figure 4.7; center, right) the isoalloxazine ring has a net charge of -1 and is bright red. Protonation gives a blue species which has a net neutral charge (Figure 4.7; center, left). The transfer of a second electron to the semiquinone radical produces an anion which quickly acquires a proton to give the fully reduced, neutral coenzyme as shown at the bottom of Figure 4.7. Because the fully reduced coenzyme lacks extended conjugation,

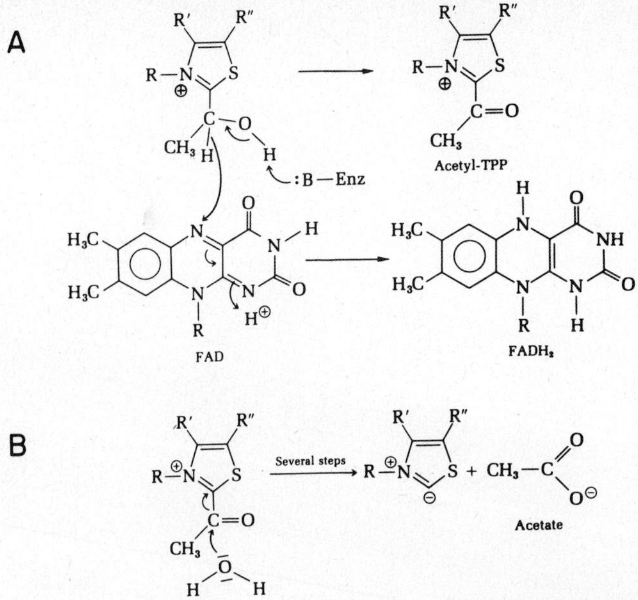

Figure 4.6 Illustration of the reduction of FAD to $FADH_2$ by a hydride shift-type mechanism. This figure shows the participation of FAD in the oxidation of hydroxyethyl-TPP to acetyl-TPP (A). Subsequently, acetyl-TPP hydrolyzes to give free acetate and TPP (B). The reaction is catalyzed by pyruvate oxidase from *E. coli.* While the mechanism shown involves hydride shift, the details of this process have not been elucidated. A carbanion addition reaction may occur.

it is colorless. The semiquinoid radical is relatively stable because its unpaired electron can resonate through the extended π-system of the isoalloxazine ring. It is as a result of this stability that flavin semiquinones are able to act as intermediates between one-electron and two-electron transfer systems. The substrates which accept electrons from $FADH_2$ and $FMNH_2$ can accept either two electrons, as do NAD^+ and $NADP^+$ (see the next section), or one electron, as do cytochromes, quinones, and iron–sulfur proteins. Molecular oxygen is also an acceptor of electrons from flavoproteins as well as a source of oxygen in oxygenation reactions.

4.5 THE NICOTINAMIDE COENZYMES (NAD^+ AND $NADP^+$)

The structures of nicotinamide adenine dinucleotide (NAD^+) and the 2′-phosphate ester of NAD^+, $NADP^+$, are indicated in Figure 4.8. The nicotinamide ring is derived from the vitamin nicotinate, which is a 3′-carboxyl-substituted pyridine ring. Nicotinate was originally so named because it was an acidic substance obtained by the chemical oxidation of the plant alkaloid, nicotine, according to the following reaction:

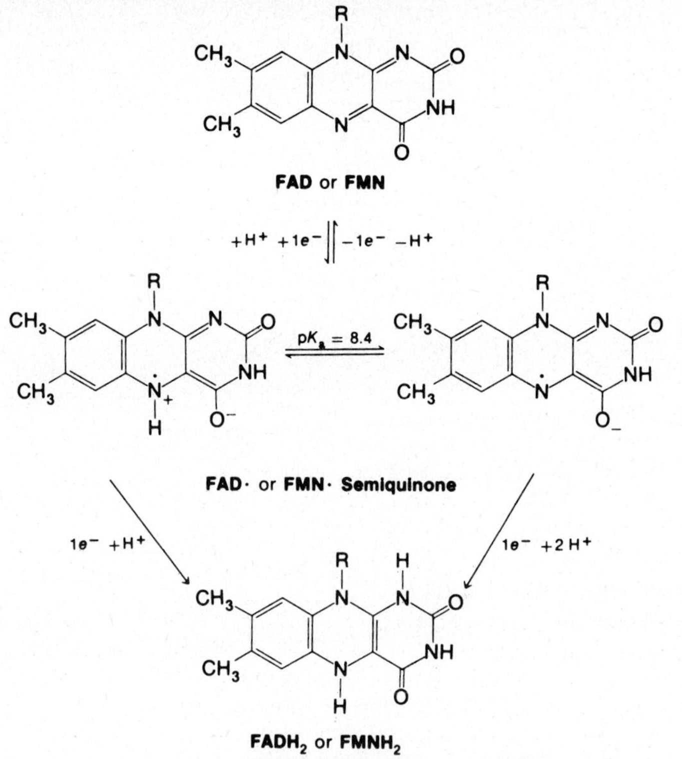

Figure 4.7 Illustration of the free radical mechanism for the reduction of FAD or FMN (top) to $FADH_2$ or $FMNH_2$ (bottom). The figure shows the two free radical forms of each coenzyme which result from the transfer of a single electron to the oxidized coenzyme: middle left, the zwitterionic semiquinone radical which predominates below pH 8.4, and middle right, the free radical anion which predominates above pH 8.4. (Reproduced with permission from P. A. Frey, "Structure and Function of Coenzymes" in *Biochemistry,* G. Zubay, ed., Addison-Wesley, Reading, MA, 1983.)

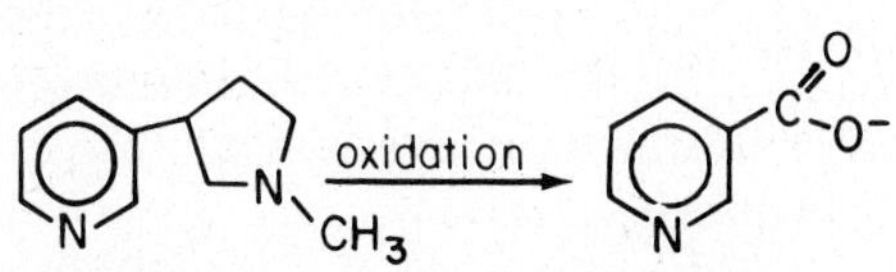

(4.1)

Nicotine Nicotinate

Nicotine, which represents 2 to 8% of the dry weight of tobacco leaves, is toxic to humans in milligram quantities when taken orally. Thus, the highly toxic alkaloid is a structural analogue of a biologically essential cofactor. Toxic effects of biologically inactive structural analogues of essential cellular constituents are frequently observed.

Vitamin deficiencies usually result in psychological and physiological disorders,

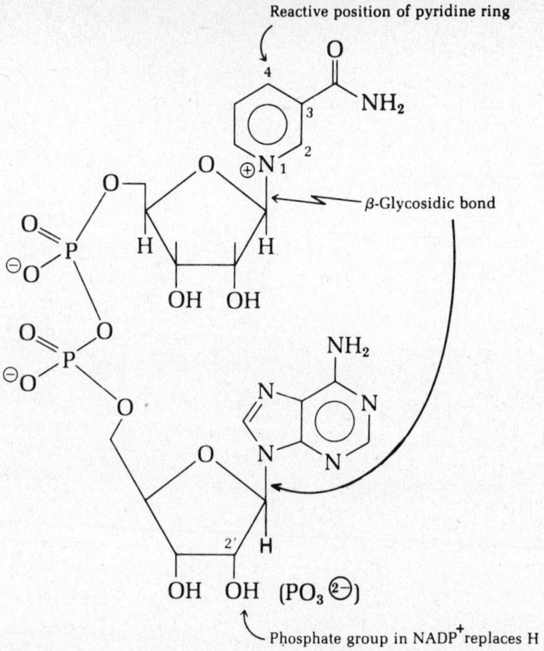

Figure 4.8 Structures of nicotinamide adenine dinucleotide (NAD^+) and its phosphorylated derivative ($NADP^+$). Reduction of these coenzymes results from hydride transfer to the 4 position in the pyridine ring (top). Both the nicotinamide and adenine bases are linked to the 1 position of the ribose rings via β-glycosidic linkages. The esterified phosphate group in $NADP^+$ is on the 2′ position of the ribosyl residue in the AMP moiety of the coenzyme. The AMP or 2′-phosphoryl AMP moiety of the coenzyme functions primarily in enzyme recognition rather than catalysis.

and nicotinate deficiency (pellagra) is no exception. People who suffer from mild nicotinate deficiency experience headaches, dizziness, and are frequently tired and apprehensive. As the condition becomes more severe, metabolic disorders (indigestion, diarrhea, etc.) as well as more severe neurological symptoms (hallucinations and insanity) are observed. In extreme cases, death can result from nicotinate deprivation.

The biosynthesis of NAD^+ and $NADP^+$ from nicotinate can occur by more than one pathway. These pathways are outlined in Figure 4.9. Starting with either nicotinate or nicotinamide, the ring nitrogen can function as a nucleophile to displace the pyrophosphate group of an intermediate of nucleotide synthesis, phosphoribosyl pyrophosphate (PRPP). When nicotinamide is the attacking nucleophile, the product of this reaction is nicotinamide mononucleotide (NMN^+). Although this molecule resembles the reactive portion of NAD^+, it is never used as an efficient substrate in biological redox reactions. The reaction that gives rise to NAD^+ from NMN^+ involves nucleophilic attack by a negatively charged oxygen of the phosphate moiety of NMN^+

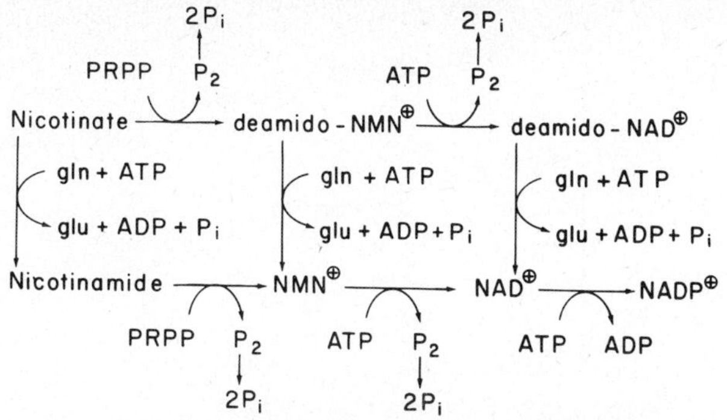

Figure 4.9 Biosynthetic pathways for the syntheses of NAD^+ and $NADP^+$ from nicotinate and nicotinamide. The vertical arrows indicate the amidation reactions while horizontal arrows illustrate all other biosynthetic interconversions. Abbreviations include: PRPP, phosphoribosyl pyrophosphate; P_2, pyrophosphate; NMN, nicotinamide mononucleotide; gln, glutamine; glu, glutamic acid.

on the electrophilic α-phosphorous atom of ATP (Figure 4.9). Pyrophosphate (P_2) is displaced, and this can be hydrolyzed to two molecules of inorganic phosphate ($2P_i$), rendering the reaction essentially irreversible. Finally, for the synthesis of $NADP^+$, NAD^+ is phosphorylated on the 2′ position of the ribosyl ring of the AMP moiety of the coenzyme (Figures 4.8 and 4.9). ADP is the by-product of this last reaction.

In order to understand the mechanism of action of NAD^+ and $NADP^+$ (which function identically although with different enzymes) the role that each part of the molecule plays in the reduction reaction must be realized. In the reduction of NAD^+, a hydride ion, H^-, is transferred from the substrate to the 4-carbon at the top of the pyridine ring (Figure 4.10), destroying the aromatic character of the ring and creating a quinoid structure. This reaction is facilitated by the ring amide which is an *o,p*-director for nucleophilic substitution as well as an electron-withdrawing substituent (see Table 4.2). However, the positively charged ring nitrogen serves the even more important function of electron sink. As a result, the reduced form of the molecule, termed NADH and having the structure shown in Figure 4.10, is a stable molecule which can be isolated and crystallized. While the positive charge of the nicotinamide ring renders the oxidized form of the enzyme stable to acid but labile to base, NADH is more stable in basic solutions and is labile in acidic solutions.

As noted previously, NMN^+ contains the reactive portions of NAD^+, but it is not readily utilized as a coenzyme by oxidoreductases. This fact implies that the adenosine monophosphate moiety of the coenzyme plays the role of "handle." Without this moiety the compound binds only weakly and with low specificity to the various nicotinamide coenzyme-dependent enzymes.

The nicotinamide ring in NAD^+ is planar due to its aromaticity. With the ring amide in front of the plane of the paper as shown in Figure 4.10, the hydride ion can be introduced either from above or below the plane of the ring. Because of the asymmetry of the ring, resulting from the presence of the amide group, the two hydrogens

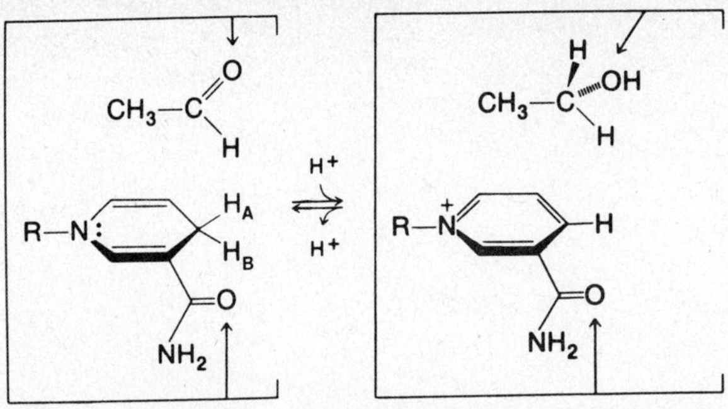

Figure 4.10 Schematic illustration of the enzyme-substrate and enzyme-product complexes for alcohol dehydrogenase with the two-carbon substrate acetaldehyde (left) or ethanol (right) above the coenzyme, NADH (left) or NAD^+ (right). This figure illustrates the stereospecific transfer of H^- from one of two possible positions at C-4 of the pyridine ring of the reduced coenzyme to a specific position in acetaldehyde, to give ethanol. If the atom transferred is deuterium, the monodeuterated ethanol produced is optically active by virtue of the new chiral center at C-1. Similarly, enzymatically produced monodeuterated NADH is optically active by virtue of the chiral center at C-4 of the pyridine ring of NADH. The subscripted stereochemical symbols A and B are explained in the text and are the same as the R and S designations, respectively. The arrows represent enzyme binding interactions. (Reproduced with permission from P. A. Frey, "Structure and Function of Coenzymes," in *Biochemistry,* G. Zubay, ed., Addison-Wesley, Reading, MA, 1983.)

bonded to the 4-carbon of NADH are not equivalent when bound to the enzyme surface.

Most oxidoreductases acting on NAD^+ or $NADP^+$ exhibit stereospecificity for both the substrate and the coenzyme. That is, the hydride ion removed from a specific position in the substrate is introduced into only one of the two possible positions of $NAD(P)^+$, the A (or R) position or the B (or S) position as shown in Figure 4.10. If the oxidized substrate is again reduced by NAD(P)H, the hydride ion returns to the same position it was removed from, even if the reactive carbon is not chiral (asymmetric), as in ethanol. These observations result from the fact that both the substrate and coenzyme in the ternary enzyme–substrate–coenzyme complex are bound at the active site, each in a highly specific configuration with only a single hydrogen atom positioned between the substrate and coenzyme in correct orientation for transfer.

Let us now elaborate on this point from the experimental standpoint. Suppose our substrate is deuterated ethanol, with two deuterium atoms bonded to carbon-1. Oxidation of the substrate reduces NAD^+ to deuterated NADH. If transfer were stereospecific, a chiral center would be generated at the 4-position of the pyridine ring because the four atomic groupings at C-4 would differ from one another. Optical activity results from the fact that ^1H is distinguishable from ^2H. Stereospecific transfer is in fact observed, with the deuterium appearing only on the A (or R) side of the ring. If alcohol dehydrogenase is subsequently allowed to reduce ordinary acetaldehyde with the deuterated NADH made from deuterated ethanol, 100% of the deuterium would be transferred from the deuterated NADH to acetaldehyde, releasing monodeuterated ethanol from the enzyme surface. The product would be optically active with a new chiral center at carbon-1. Since these results are in fact observed, the enzyme must recognize and specifically bind the carbonyl group of acetaldehyde and the amide group of the nicotinamide ring so that only one orientation of the substrate can be assumed relative to the coenzyme.

A diagrammatic representation of the active site of lactate dehydrogenase is shown in Figure 4.11. This enzyme, like alcohol dehydrogenase, exhibits A-stereospecificity. Several features of the active site of lactate dehydrogenase are worth noting. First, the two substrates fit into a pocket of the enzyme, and this pocket comprises the active site. Second, a variety of enzyme amino acyl side chains participate in hydrogen-bonding the NAD^+ stereospecifically at the active site. Other residues further insure that the configuration shown is maintained. *Lys*-250 is of particular importance in preventing rotation of the nicotinamide ring. Third, the substrate, L-lactate, which reduces NAD^+, or pyruvate, which oxidizes NADH, is bound adjacent to the C-4 atom of the nicotinamide aromatic ring so that direct hydride transfer from lactate to NAD^+ (or from NADH to pyruvate) can readily occur without altering the position of either substrate. *Arg*-171 neutralizes the charge of the carboxyl group. Fourth, the carbonyl group of pyruvate is hydrogen-bonded to the protonated imidazole ring of *his*-195. This group functions both in substrate binding and as a general acid catalyst. Upon reduction of pyruvate to lactate, the proton is transferred to lactate which then becomes hydrogen-bonded to the neutral imidazole ring of *his*-195. It should be noted that Figure 4.11 shows an "abortive complex" of the enzyme with its two oxidized substrates, NAD^+ and pyruvate.

The discussion of oxidoreductases acting on NAD^+ presented on the preceding pages can be applied to hundreds of enzymes, and comparative data have shown that several generalizations can be made. First, the stereospecificity of each dehydrogenase for its nicotinamide coenzyme is fixed and does not depend on the source of the enzyme. Thus, all alcohol dehydrogenases and all lactate dehydrogenases from various animal, plant, and microbial sources are of the A-type, while glyceraldehyde-3-phosphate dehydrogenases and glucose-6-phosphate dehydrogenases are of the B-type regardless of their biological source. This fact leads to the suggestion that the dehydrogenases specific for a given substrate are usually evolutionarily related and that the stereospecific recognition of the nicotinamide ring has been a highly conserved characteristic of an enzyme throughout its evolutionary history.

A second generalization which can be made states that most dehydrogenases that act on phosphorylated carbohydrates are of the B-type while the majority of A-type enzymes act on nonphosphorylated carbohydrates. For example, glycerol-3-phosphate dehydrogenases and mannitol-1-phosphate dehydrogenases are of the B-type although both the glycerol and mannitol dehydrogenases are of the A-type.

Still a third generalization notes that NAD^+ (or NADH) is usually involved in catabolic or degradative (energy-yielding) processes while $NADP^+$ or (NADPH) is

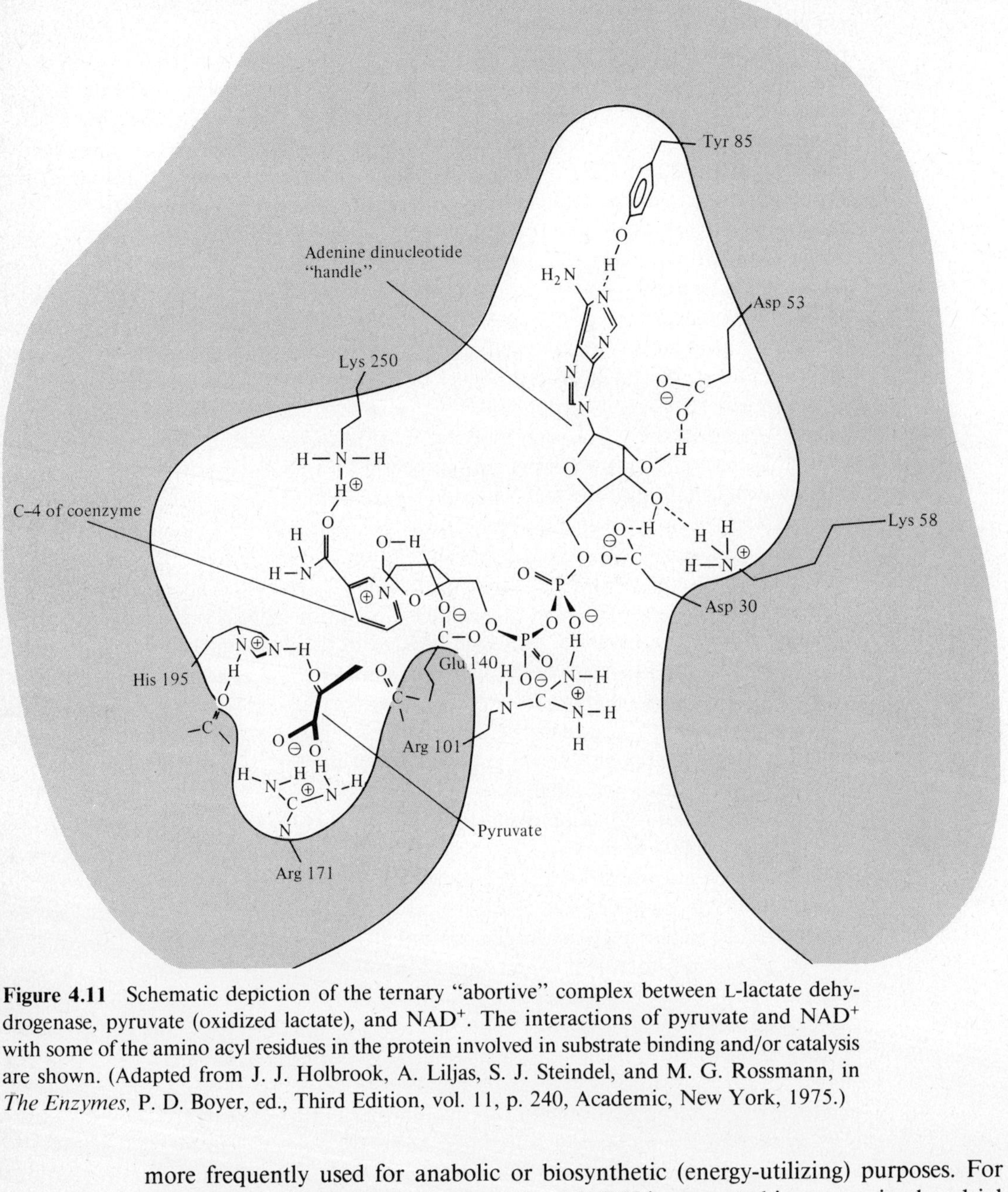

Figure 4.11 Schematic depiction of the ternary "abortive" complex between L-lactate dehydrogenase, pyruvate (oxidized lactate), and NAD$^+$. The interactions of pyruvate and NAD$^+$ with some of the amino acyl residues in the protein involved in substrate binding and/or catalysis are shown. (Adapted from J. J. Holbrook, A. Liljas, S. J. Steindel, and M. G. Rossmann, in *The Enzymes,* P. D. Boyer, ed., Third Edition, vol. 11, p. 240, Academic, New York, 1975.)

more frequently used for anabolic or biosynthetic (energy-utilizing) purposes. For example, it will be seen in Chapter 6 that NADH is generated in most mitochondrial redox reactions, and the reducing power so generated feeds into the electron transport chain. On the other hand, NADPH is synthesized by the oxidation of glucose-6-phosphate and 6-phosphogluconate via the pentose phosphate pathway in the cytoplasm of the cell where the reduced coenzyme is used primarily for biosynthetic purposes

(Chapter 6). Furthermore, in Chapter 8 we shall see that mitochondrial fatty acid oxidation generates NADH while cytoplasmic fatty acid biosynthesis utilizes NADPH. These distinctions cannot merely be attributed to compartmentalization, because the same specificities are observed in bacteria where the catabolic and anabolic processes occur within a single cytoplasmic compartment. Appreciation of this and other functional distinctions may provide an explanation as to why *two* nicotinamide coenzymes, differing only slightly in structure and exhibiting no mechanistic differences, may have universally evolved in biological systems.

In the preceding discussion, NAD^+ was shown to function as a redox cosubstrate, but this is not its sole function. NAD^+-dependent enzymes are known which catalyze epimerization, elimination, and aldolization reactions. The natural substrates of these enzymes always lack the intrinsic chemical properties necessary to facilitate the required reactions. In these cases, NAD^+ functions to *transiently* oxidize a hydroxyl group within the substrate to a more reactive carbonyl group so that this group or an adjacent group may be transformed as necessary. The tightly bound NAD^+ is simultaneously (and transiently) reduced. Thus, NAD^+ is a true coenzyme and *not* a cosubstrate in these reactions, and the last step in the reaction sequence is always to reduce the carbonyl back to a hydroxyl group before the product is released from the enzyme surface, generating a restored and reoxidized NAD^+ molecule in the process.

This catalytic function of NAD^+ is exemplified by UDP-galactose-4-epimerase which interconverts UDP-α-D-glucopyranoside and UDP-α-D-galactopyranoside. The two-step reaction mechanism is shown in Figure 4.12. The ability of this enzyme to reduce the oxidized substrate to either of the two possible products must result either because NADH can vacillate between two alternative positions on the enzyme surface with the reactive hydrogen at position 4 in the pyridine ring either above or below the plane of the carbonyl π system, or because both the A- and the B-hydrogens at the 4-position of NADH can serve as the hydride donor. If the latter situation is true, then this enzyme provides an example of one which, in contrast to alcohol dehydrogenase and most $NAD(P)^+$-dependent oxidoreductases, lacks stereospecificity both with respect to the substrate and to the coenzyme. This lack of stereospecificity would be the basis

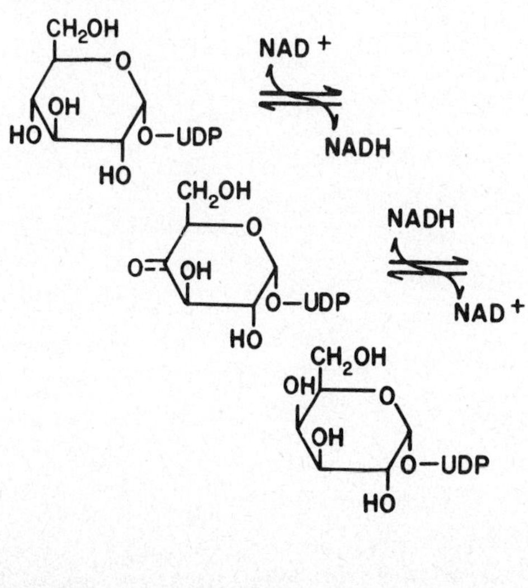

Figure 4.12 Mechanism of the epimerization reaction catalyzed by UDP-galactose 4-epimerase. UDP-α-D-glucopyranoside (top) is oxidized by NAD^+ to give an intermediate which can be reduced by NADH to UDP-α-D-galactopyranoside (bottom). No molecular grouping in the substrate activates C-4 for the epimerization reaction at this chiral center. Hence, the reversible oxidation process shown is required to effect the interconversion.

for the catalytic function of this enzyme. Although the question of this mechanistic feature has not yet been resolved, use of the deuterium isotope techniques discussed earlier in this section with respect to the alcohol dehydrogenase reaction should provide a definitive answer to this interesting question.

4.6 PYRIDOXAL-5-PHOSPHATE (PLP)

Pyridoxine, the most common form of vitamin B_6, is converted first via an ATP-dependent phosphorylation reaction to the phosphorylated form of the vitamin, pyridoxine phosphate, and then by oxidation to the principal coenzymic form of this vitamin, pyridoxal phosphate (PLP) (Figure 4.13). PLP can be further interconverted with pyridoxamine phosphate (PMP) by a transamination reaction. Vitamin B_6 deficiency sometimes manifests itself as anemia. The patient has a low red blood cell count and exhibits weakening of the blood vessels. Increased sensitivity to noise is common, and in severe cases epileptic seizures and death can result.

Like NAD^+, the aromatic ring of PLP contains several substituents which contribute to the catalytic efficiency of the coenzyme. First, the aldehydic function at the 4 position of the pyridinium ring condenses with an amino group in the substrate to form a secondary imine, an aldimine called a *Schiff's base.* Almost all substrates of

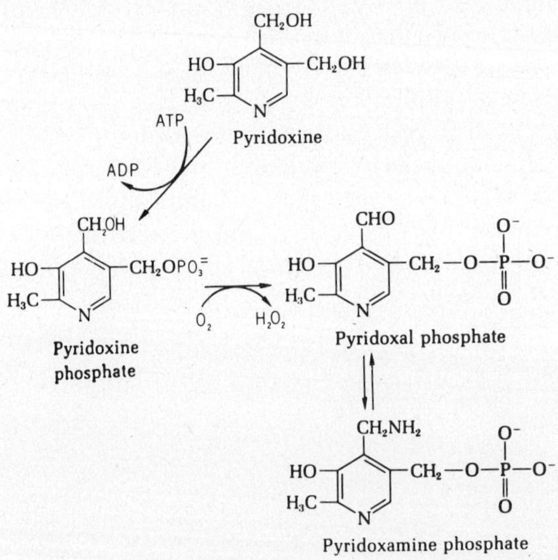

Figure 4.13 Biosynthetic pathways for the conversion of pyridoxine (top)—the most common form of vitamin B_6—first to pyridoxine phosphate (middle, left) and then to the principal coenzyme form, pyridoxal phosphate (PLP) (middle, right). PLP can secondarily be converted to the second coenzyme form of the vitamin, pyridoxamine phosphate (PMP) (bottom), which is a coenzyme of transamination (aminotransfer) reactions.

PLP-containing enzymes are amines, and the Schiff's base is a universal intermediate in PLP-catalyzed reactions involving these substrates. Second, the hydroxyl group in position 3 can stabilize the aldimine by forming an internal hydrogen bond, or it may function as a general acid or base. Third, as in the nicotinamide ring of NAD^+ and the thiazolium ring of TPP, the positively charged ring nitrogen atom serves as an electron sink, promoting the delocalization of electron density into the ring. Finally, the phosphomethylene group at the 5 position appears to function primarily as a handle, important only for enzyme recognition. In fact, pyridoxal binds weakly to many PLP-dependent enzymes, replacing the natural coenzyme. Further, free pyridoxal nonspecifically catalyzes virtually all of the reactions catalyzed by PLP-dependent enzymes by nonenzymatic means, provided that a metal ion is available and the reaction is allowed to proceed at higher temperatures. This fact is illustrated in Figure 4.15 and discussed below.

While the coenzyme alone will catalyze each of the reactions promoted by a specific PLP-dependent enzyme, the protein serves several essential functions. First, in almost all PLP-dependent enzymes, the ε-amino group of a lysyl residue in the protein first condenses with the coenzyme to form a Schiff's base as shown in Figure 4.14. This condensation reaction is of catalytic importance because the protonated aldimine is much more reactive in nucleophilic addition reactions than is the carbonyl group of the parental coenzyme. The enzyme-conjugated prosthetic group therefore undergoes *transimination,* forming a Schiff's base with the amino acid substrate at a much greater rate (with a lower activation energy) than does free PLP. Second, amino

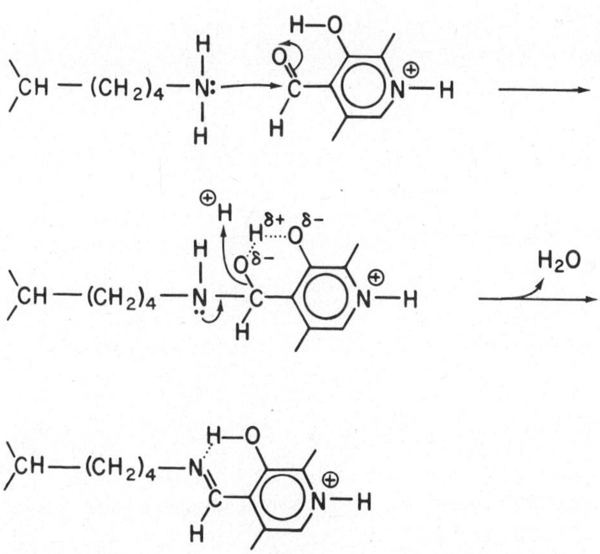

Figure 4.14 Stepwise condensation of an ε-amino group of a lysyl residue (top left) with pyridoxal phosphate (PLP) (top, right) at the active site of a PLP-dependent enzyme. The final product is an aldimine, or Schiff's base (bottom), which covalently links the coenzyme to the protein. This reaction is readily reversible in the presence of water or an amine.

A

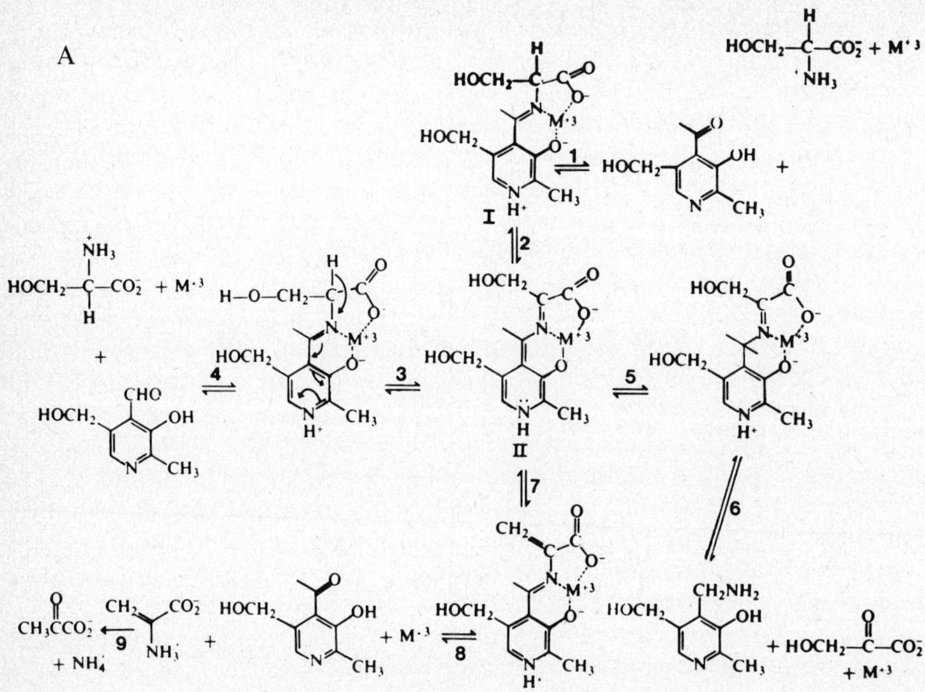

B

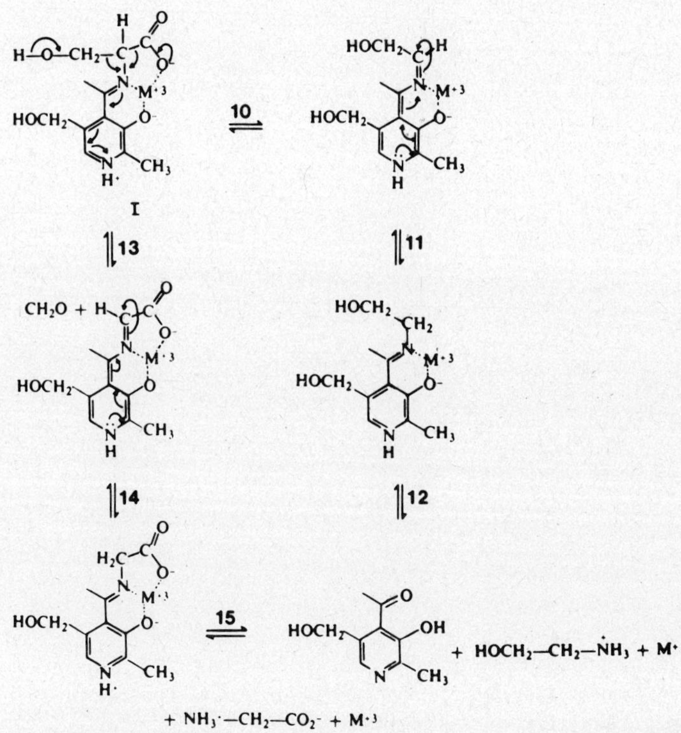

acyl residues in the protein furnish protons and facilitate removal of protons to and from the substrate, respectively. That is, the enzyme functions in general acid and base catalysis. Finally, the enzyme provides the substrate and product binding sites, thereby determining the substrate and product specificities of the reaction. Without these specificities the cellular catalytic activities would create a chaotic situation incapable of supplying the specific biosynthetic needs of the cell. In any reaction catalyzed by a PLP-dependent enzyme, the first step is therefore transimination with the formation of a Schiff's base between the coenzyme and the substrate, and the simultaneous displacement of the lysyl residue of the enzyme. Subsequently, enzymic amino acyl residues, in proper position relative to the substrate, then donate or remove protons or substrate moieties, provide charge neutralization, or otherwise stabilize intermediates. In so doing, they determine the course of the reaction.

The same principles are operative in each of the reactions shown in Figure 4.15. This figure depicts five reactions catalyzed nonenzymatically by pyridoxal in the presence of a metal ion, M^{+3}, at elevated temperatures, but the mechanisms are essentially the same for the PLP-dependent enzyme-catalyzed reactions, which additionally select stereochemically which sigma bond to the α-carbon will maximally overlap the withdrawing π system and be broken. First, a Schiff's base between substrate and cofactor is formed (reaction 1; structure I). Second, a bond to the α-carbon in serine is broken generating a carbanion, and the negative charge associated with the free electron pair is delocalized to the positively-charged ring nitrogen, the electron sink (reaction 2). This quinoid intermediate [structure II in Figures 4.15(a)] is stabilized by the neutralization of the positive and negative charges initially at the bottom and top of the molecule, respectively. Third, the free electron pair moves back up the molecule, restoring the aromatic character of the ring, and a new covalent bond with a proton is usually formed at some point in the substrate–coenzyme conjugate. Alternatively, the electron pair may be displaced to the electronegative hydroxyl group of serine which is rendered a good leaving group by protonation as in the dehydration reaction depicted in Figure 4.15(a). Fourth, the imine bond between substrate and coenzyme is broken by hydrolysis with water (for the nonenzymatic reactions) or by transimination (for the enzyme-catalyzed reactions) regenerating the free form of pyridoxal or the aldimine form of the coenzyme linked to the ϵ-amino group of a lysyl residue, respectively. Only in the case of the transamination reaction (aminotransfer reaction)

←

Figure 4.15 Reactions catalyzed by PLP-dependent enzymes which convert the amino acid, serine, to any one of several products, can actually be catalyzed by free pyridoxal in the presence of a metal ion (M^{+3}) at elevated temperatures without the participation of an enzyme. These reactions are illustrated as follows: (A) Racemization of D-serine to L-serine (reactions 1, 2, 3, and 4); transamination (or aminotransfer) of D-serine to give hydroxypyruvate and pyridoxamine (reactions 1, 2, 5, and 6) and deaminative dehydration of D-serine to pyruvate and ammonium ions (reactions 1, 2, 7, 8, and 9). Reaction 9 occurs spontaneously. All reactions involve the same resonance-stabilized intermediate (II). (B) Starting with the Schiff's base conjugate of D-serine and pyridoxal (upper left in figure B; intermediate II shown in figure A), decarboxylation proceeds via reactions 10, 11, and 12 while dealdolization precedes via reactions 13, 14, and 15. (Reproduced with permission from H. R. Mahler and E. H. Cordes, *Biological Chemistry,* Harper & Row, New York, 1966.)

is pyridoxamine or pyridoxamine phosphate generated. Finally, those newly generated intermediates which are unstable in aqueous solution will spontaneously rearrange to a more stable molecular configuration. To further clarify these reactions, each will now be discussed separately.

4.6.1 Racemization [Reactions 1, 2, 3, and 4 in Figure 4.15(a)]

When racemization is enzyme-catalyzed, labilization of the α-hydrogen of serine by general base catalysis generates a carbanion at the α-carbon. This carbanion is stabilized by a resonance structure in which the free electron pair is displaced to the positively charged nitrogen in the pyridinium ring, the electron sink (intermediate II in Figure 4.15). If the enzyme is not stereospecific with respect to the α-hydrogen, that is, if the amino acyl residue that functions as a general base to remove the α-hydrogen can flop from one position (in which it is adjacent to the α-hydrogen in L-serine) to an alternative position (in which it is adjacent to the α-hydrogen in D-serine), racemization is accomplished. All racemases, but few other enzymes, lack this sort of stereospecificity.

4.6.2 Decarboxylation [Reaction 1 in Figure 4.15(a) as well as reactions 10, 11, and 12 in Figure 4.15(b)]

Initially, exactly the same process occurs as in racemization except that the free electron pair giving rise to the α-carbanion is derived from the carbon–carbon bond linking the carboxyl group to the α-carbon. Loss of carbon dioxide and replacement of the carboxyl group by a proton gives the decarboxylated product after the covalent carbon–hydrogen bond is formed.

4.6.3 Transamination [Reactions 1, 2, 5, and 6 in Figure 4.15(a)]

Transamination (amino transfer) begins exactly as for racemization with the labilization of the α-hydrogen. Delocalization of the free electron pair is the same, generating the quinoid intermediate. However, when aromaticity is restored, that same electron pair forms a covalent bond with a proton adjacent to the 4′-carbon of the coenzyme. This event stabilizes the imine bond between the substrate α-carbon and the nitrogen atom of the Schiff's base so that hydrolysis gives an α-keto acid and pyridoxamine phosphate. The reverse of this entire process with another keto acid (for example α-ketoglutarate) restores the pyridoxal phosphate form of the coenzyme. The overall reaction is therefore: serine + α-ketoglutarate $\longrightarrow$ β-hydroxypyruvate + glutamate.

4.6.4 Dealdolization [Reaction 1 in Figure 4.15(a) as well as reactions 13, 14, and 15 in Figure 4.15(b)]

The dealdolization reaction is essentially the same as the other PLP-catalyzed reactions except that the bond broken to give the α-carbanion is the α,β-carbon–carbon single bond. Dissociation of the hydroxyl proton gives formaldehyde, and the α-carbanion is resonance stabilized as usual. In the enzyme-catalyzed reaction, dissociation of formaldehyde from the active site, and the appearance of a protonated amino acyl residue in its place, allows formation of the Schiff's base conjugate of glycine. Finally, glycine is displaced from the active site after transimination to form the Schiff's base conjugate between the active lysyl group of the enzyme and pyridoxal phosphate.

4.6.5 Dehydration [Reactions 1, 2, 7, 8, and 9 in Figure 4.15(a)]

The α-hydrogen is first removed to give an α-carbanion which is stabilized by resonance. However, when dehydration of serine occurs, molecular neutrality is restored in a different way: the hydroxyl group of serine is protonated to generate an oxonium ion, and the free electron pair which forms a π-bond between the α- and β-carbons provides the driving force for dehydration (loss of water). The molecule that results from this reaction sequence is unstable; hydrolysis of the Schiff's base with the coenzyme generates an unsaturated amine. This compound rearranges to an imine which spontaneously hydrolyzes in water to produce the final products, pyruvate and an ammonium ion.

It can be seen from these five reactions that virtually all of the PLP-catalyzed reactions use the same principles to effect very different net results. It is of further interest that in one of the PLP-catalyzed reactions depicted in Figure 4.15, dealdolization, the formaldehyde generated is normally transferred to the coenzyme to be discussed in the next section, tetrahydrofolate (FH_4). The details of this complex reaction sequence, which actually involves NADH and coenzyme B_{12} as well as PLP and FH_4, will be presented in greater detail in Chapter 9.

4.7 TETRAHYDROFOLATE (FH_4)

As noted in Section 4.1, tetrahydrofolate (FH_4) is derived from the vitamin, folate. A two-step reduction process using an NADH-dependent enzyme, dihydrofolate reductase, is involved. Folate deficiency (as with vitamin B_{12} deficiency) produces a macrocytic, megaloblastic anemia in mammals.

The generalized structure of FH_4 and its derivatives is shown in Figure 4.16. The active coenzyme consists of three moieties: a reduced, substituted pterin ring, *p*-aminobenzoic acid, and a chain of from one to seven L-glutamic acid residues linked by secondary amide bonds. The reactive portion of FH_4 consists of the two nucleophilic nitrogens, N^5 and N^{10}, both adjacent to aromatic rings. Because the electron pair of N^{10}, but not that of N^5, can be delocalized into its adjacent aromatic ring, N^5 is more nucleophilic and basic than N^{10}. FH_4 functions exclusively in one-carbon interconversion and transfer reactions.

As can be seen in Figure 4.17, several different derivatives of FH_4 result from the incorporation at N^5 and/or N^{10} of one-carbon fragments at the oxidation levels of formic acid, formaldehyde, and methanol. Thus, N^5-formyl, N^{10}-formyl, N^5-

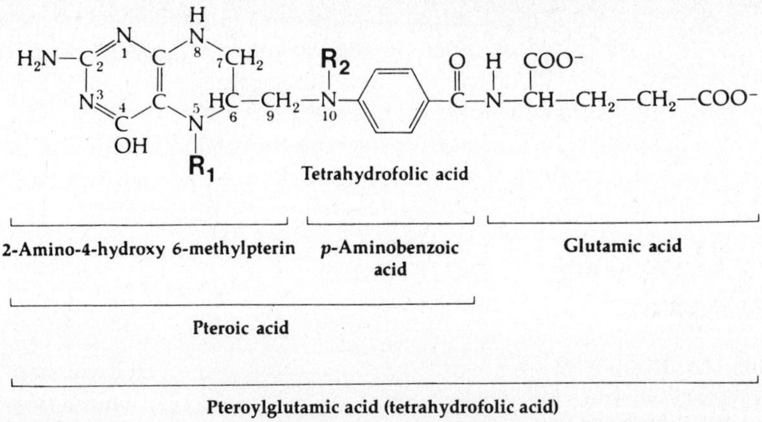

Figure 4.16 Generalized structure and nomenclature of tetrahydrofolate derivatives. The active, nucleophilic nitrogen atoms in the coenzyme are N^5 and N^{10}, both of which are activated by adjacent aromatic rings. The active coenzyme consists of three moieties: a reduced, substituted pterin ring, 2-amino-4-hydroxy-6-methylpterin, *p*-aminobenzoic acid, and a chain of from one to seven glutamyl residues. Only a single glutamyl residue is shown. R_1 and R_2 are either hydrogens (in FH_4 itself) or the one carbon fragments shown in Figure 4.17.

formimino, N^{10}-formimino, and N^5,N^{10}-methenyl FH_4 are all at the oxidation level of formic acid. A two electron-reduction of N^5,N^{10}-methenyl FH_4 with an NADPH-dependent enzyme gives N^5,N^{10}-methylene FH_4. This derivative is at the oxidation level of N^5-hydroxymethyl FH_4, N^{10}-hydroxymethyl FH_4, and formaldehyde. Reduction of N^5,N^{10}-methylene FH_4 by an NADH-dependent enzyme gives N^5-methyl FH_4, at the oxidation level of methanol. One-carbon compounds or one-carbon fragments can be transferred to or from various substrates at each of these three oxidation levels, usually in the presence of the appropriate enzyme.

To exemplify this fact, we shall consider the reactions whereby formic acid and formaldehyde are incorporated into FH_4. Because formic acid is relatively inert, it is first activated in an ATP-dependent phosphorylation reaction, and subsequent attack by the N^{10} atom of FH_4 on the carbon atom of formyl phosphate gives N^{10}-formyl FH_4. Subsequent spontaneous attack on the formyl group by the more nucleophilic N^5 atom and loss of water generates the methenyl derivative of FH_4 (see Figure 4.17; top right).

Formaldehyde is a highly reactive molecule which spontaneously reacts with the more nucleophilic N^5 atom of FH_4 to give the N^5-hydroxymethyl derivative (see Figure 4.17; middle, left). A second spontaneous reaction involving attack by N^{10} and displacement of water gives N^5,N^{10}-methylene FH_4. It appears that the different one-carbon derivatives of FH_4 at each oxidation level can interconvert spontaneously, but the enzymes which reduce or transfer the one-carbon substituents in FH_4 are highly specific for only one form.

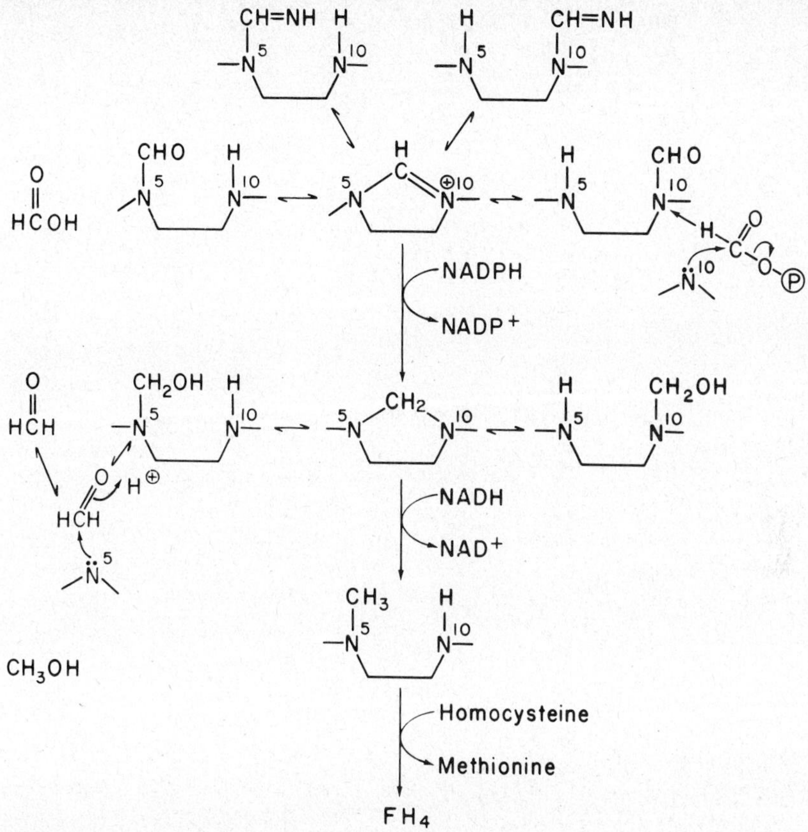

Figure 4.17 Interconversion of the various derivatives of tetrahydrofolic acid (FH_4). Vertical interconversions are catalyzed by $NADP^+$- and NAD^+-dependent enzymes as shown. Horizontal interconversions may occur spontaneously or be enzyme-catalyzed. The structures of formic acid (HCO_2H), formaldehyde (HCHO), and methanol (CH_3OH) are depicted on the left to indicate the oxidative state of the 1-carbon fragment(s) attached to FH_4. Reaction of an activated form of formic acid, the mixed anhydride derivative (top, right), and of formaldehyde (middle, left) with the free coenzyme (FH_4) are also shown.

4.8 COENZYME B_{12} (CoB_{12})

Coenzyme B_{12} was the last of the major coenzymes to be characterized and was the only coenzyme to be elucidated structurally by x-ray crystallographic techniques. Attempts to determine its structure by conventional chemical procedures had been thwarted by its complexity.

The principal form of the coenzyme, the deoxyadenosyl derivative, was not discovered until 1958, and elucidation of its structure followed three years later. The structure of 5′-deoxyadenosyl cobalamine is shown in Figure 4.18. It has a cobalt atom in a corrin ring system with 5′-deoxyadenosine linked covalently to the metal via a

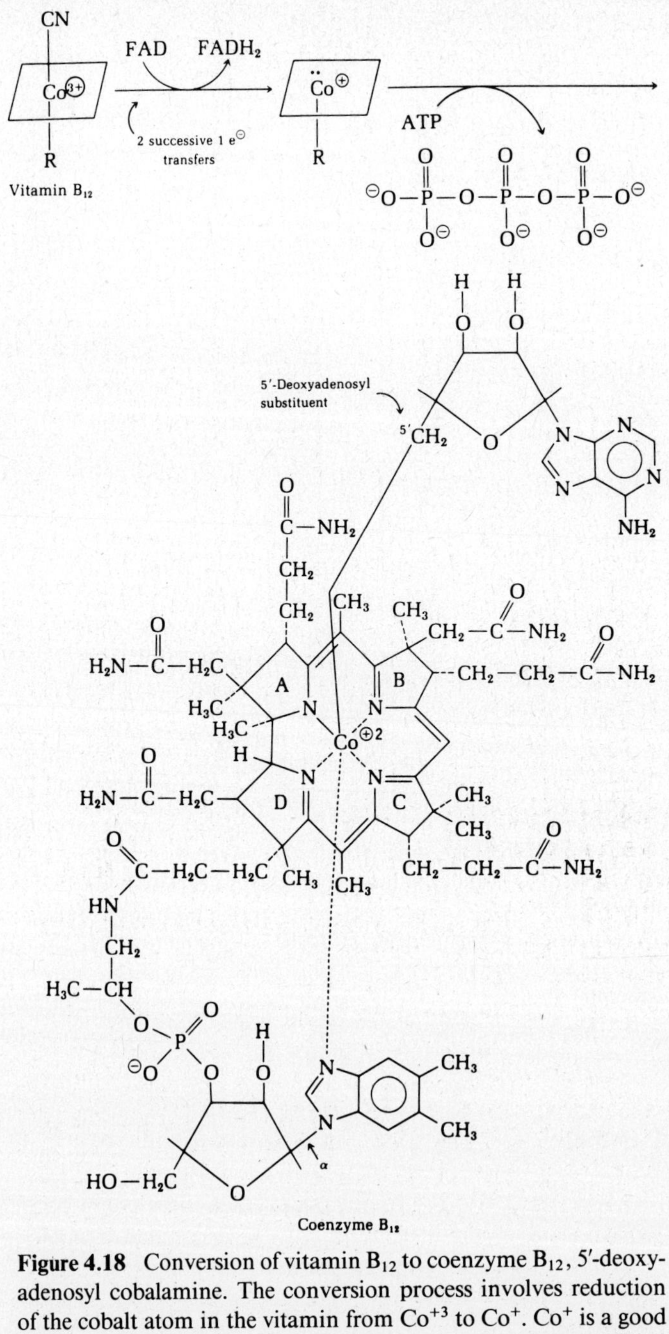

Figure 4.18 Conversion of vitamin B_{12} to coenzyme B_{12}, 5′-deoxyadenosyl cobalamine. The conversion process involves reduction of the cobalt atom in the vitamin from Co^{+3} to Co^{+}. Co^{+} is a good nucleophile which displaces the triphosphate moiety of ATP yielding 5′-deoxyadenosyl cobalamine (coenzyme B_{12}). The 5′-methylene group of the deoxyadenosyl substituent, which is covalently bound to the cobalt atom in the corrin ring, is the reactive moiety in most coenzyme B_{12}-dependent enzyme-catalyzed reactions.

carbon–cobalt bond. It was the first natural product to be isolated which had a stable cobalt–carbon bond. The valency of the cobalt atom can be considered to be Co^{+++}, in which case the C-5 atom of the deoxyadenosyl moiety must be considered to be a carbanion. Alternatively the bonding electron pair can be considered to be shared by the cobalt and carbon atoms, in which case cobalt assumes a valency of Co^{++}. Spectroscopic studies suggest a valency of Co^{++} with the bonding electron pair localized between the cobalt and carbon atoms, but more closely allied with carbon. For the sake of simplicity, we have designated the valency of the intact coenzyme as Co^{++} [see (4.2) and Figures 4.18 and 4.19]. The sixth coordination position of cobalt is filled by a ring nitrogen of a substituted benzimidazolyl ring in the coenzyme. The functional part of the molecule which participates in catalysis can be depicted as follows:

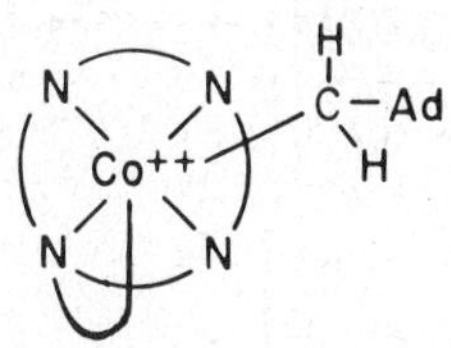

(4.2)

Vitamin B_{12} resembles the coenzyme except that the 5′-deoxyadenosyl group is replaced by a CN^-, OH^- or H_2O ligand. Conversion of the vitamin to the coenzyme occurs in a two-step process. First, an $FADH_2$-dependent enzyme reduces the cobalt atom from Co^{+++} to Co^+ in two successive one-electron transfers (Figure 4.18). Co^+ is a potent nucleophile, and the second step therefore involves attack at the 5′-carbon of ATP with displacement of the 5′-triphosphate group. The Co^{++}–carbon bond is long (2.0 nm) and labile, a fact that is of importance with respect to its biological activity.

De novo biosynthesis can be effected only by microorganisms. Neither plants nor animals have the capacity to make vitamin B_{12}. However, the amounts required for normal bodily functions are extremely small. Consequently, vitamin B_{12} deficiency does not readily result from an insufficient supply of the vitamin in the diet, except for vegetarians who do not supplement their diets with meat or other animal products. Rather, a pathological condition, called *pernicious anemia,* results from the inability to absorb the vitamin across the intestinal wall. Patients suffering from pernicious anemia lack a specific glycoprotein (intrinsic factor) in the gastric fluids which binds the vitamin. A ternary complex of intrinsic factor with vitamin B_{12} and Ca^{++} can be taken up by intestinal epithelial cells via an endocytic mechanism.

The types of reactions catalyzed by coenzyme B_{12}-dependent enzymes are shown in Table 4.3. These reactions fall into three major categories:

1. Internal oxido-reduction reactions involving exchange of atoms or molecular substituents on adjacent carbons;
2. An external oxido-reduction reaction which may function by the same mechanism; and
3. Methyl transfer reactions.

TABLE 4.3 REPRESENTATIVE REACTIONS CATALYZED BY COENZYME B_{12}-DEPENDENT ENZYMES

I. 1,2-shift reactions (internal oxido-reduction)

A. C—O bond broken: (diol dehydrase)

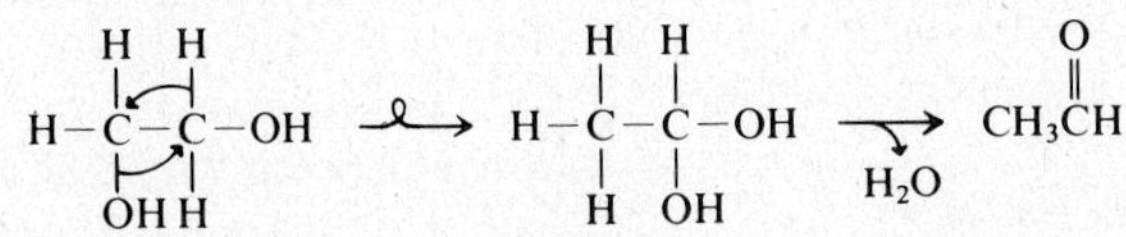

B. C—N bond broken: (ethanolamine ammonia lyase)

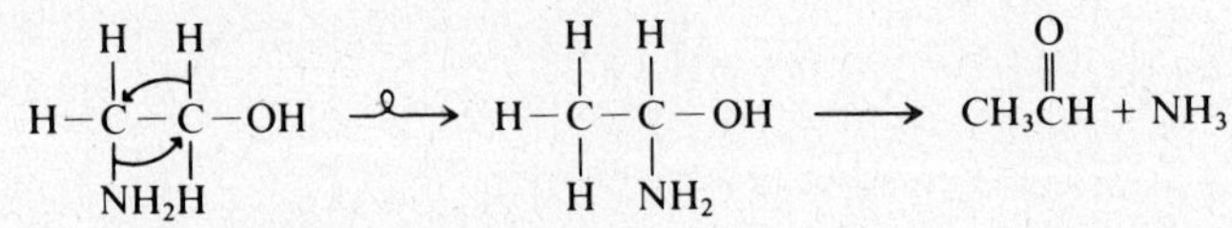

C. C—C bond broken: (methyl malonyl-CoA mutase)

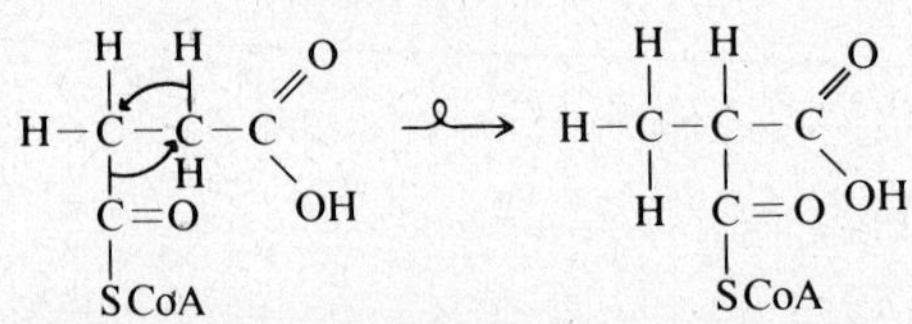

II. Shift reaction between two molecules (external oxido-reduction)

A. C—O bond broken: (ribonucleotide reductase)

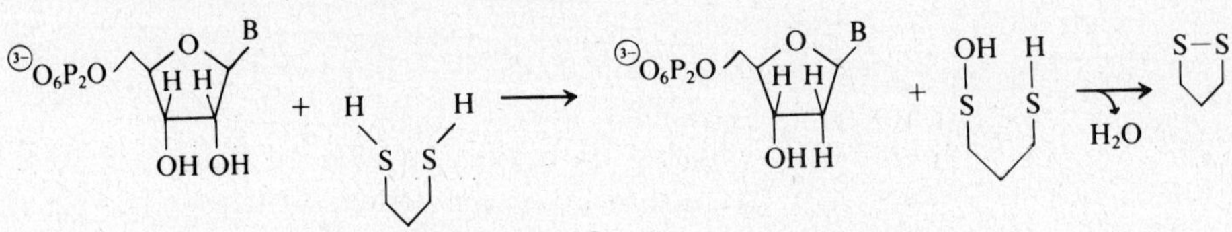

III. Methyl transfer reaction (methyl transferase)

A. C—S bond formed: (methionine synthase)

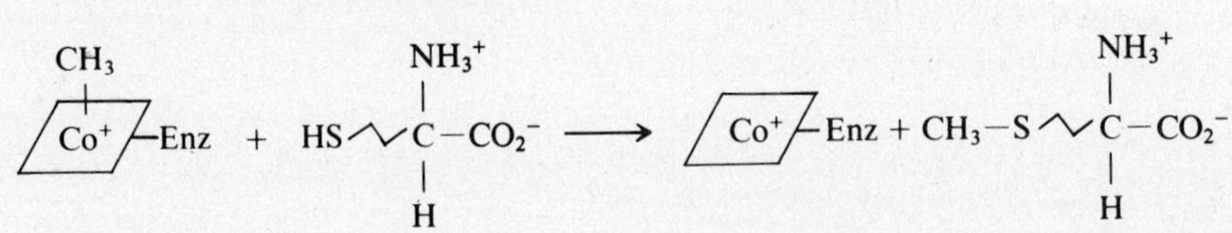

The first category occurs by a 1,2-shift of molecular groupings as follows:

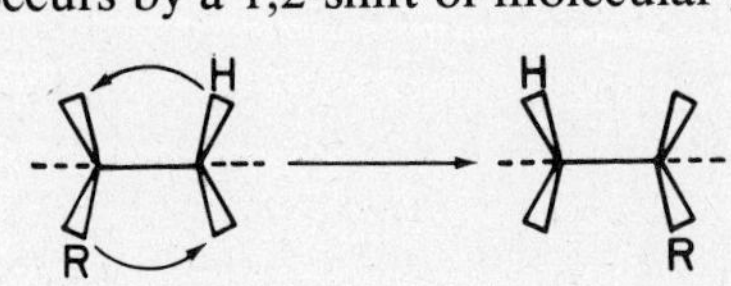

(4.3)

The hydrogen migrations in all coenzyme B_{12}-dependent rearrangements occur stereospecifically without isotopic exchange with water. For example, the migration of H in the diol dehydrase-catalyzed reaction occurs with inversion of configuration while the methyl malonyl-CoA mutase-catalyzed reaction occurs with retention of configuration.

A number of observations with diol dehydrase led to formulation of the mechanism of coenzyme B_{12}-catalyzed 1,2-shift reactions as illustrated in Figure 4.19. First, tritiated [1-^{3}H]1,2-propandiol gave rise to [1,2-^{3}H]propionaldehyde without loss of isotope to the solvent. Second, the tritium was transiently incorporated into both C-5′ hydrogen positions of the 5′-deoxyadenosyl moiety of the coenzyme. And third, free radical species (including Co^{++} in coenzyme B_{12} which has an unpaired electron) could be detected during reaction of substrate with enzyme.

On the basis of these observations, a reaction mechanism similar or identical to the one shown in Figure 4.19 is likely to account for the product formed. The first step shown involves formation of free radicals with separation of the two electrons of the bonding electron pair. Possibly a free electron is first associated with the 5′-carbon of deoxyadenosine before the tritium shown in Figure 4.19 is extracted from the one-carbon of the substrate. Transfer of the hydroxyl group on C-2 to C-1 then causes the free electron to appear on C-2. Finally, a second concerted transfer of a free electron from Co^{++} to the C-5′ position of deoxyadenosine provides the driving force for transfer of a hydrogen atom to the C-2 position of the substrate. The original coenzyme B_{12} is thereby regenerated, and the product need only dehydrate spontaneously to generate the aldehydic form. Other deoxyadenosyl coenzyme B_{12}-dependent enzymes, including ribonucleotide reductase, may function by a similar free radical mechanism. As shown in Table 4.3, the major difference between the reaction catalyzed by ribonucleotide reductase and those catalyzed by other deoxyadenosyl cobalamine-dependent enzymes may not reflect a fundamental mechanistic difference but merely the fact that group transfer occurs between two different molecules rather than within a single molecule.

Finally, a distinct but reactive form of coenzyme B_{12} is methylcobalamine in which a methyl group replaces the deoxyadenosyl moiety. Methionine synthase is a coenzyme B_{12}-dependent enzyme in which a methyl group from N^5-methyl FH_4 is transferred to Co^+ of the coenzyme and then to homocysteine (Table 4.3). The coenzyme must be maintained in the reduced state (Co^+) to be active. This reaction will be discussed further in Chapter 9. Methylcobalamine probably also functions in the reduction of methanol to methane and the synthesis of acetate from one-carbon compounds in bacteria.

4.9 COFACTORS WHICH ARE COVALENTLY BOUND TO PROTEINS

Lipoamide and biotin are enzyme cofactors which must first become covalently linked to lysyl residues in specific proteins in order to exhibit biological activity. The structures of these two protein-bound cofactors are shown in Figures 4.20(a) and (b), respectively. Phosphopantetheine is a third covalently linked protein cofactor which, however, also exists as a constituent of coenzyme A (Figure 4.21). These three cofactors will be presented briefly here and discussed in more detail in subsequent chapters.

The enzyme-bound cofactor shown in Figure 4.20(a) is lipoamide, derived from lipoate by condensation of the side-chain carboxyl group of the vitamin with the ϵ-amino group of a lysyl residue in the protein. The active moiety of this prosthetic group is attached to the protein backbone via an arm about 1.5 nm in length. This

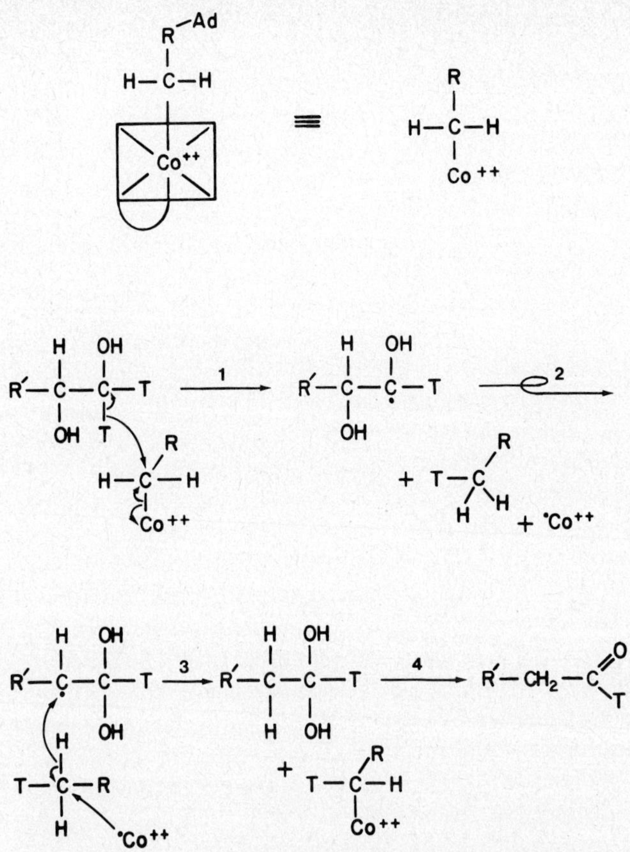

Figure 4.19 Proposed mechanism of the diol dehydrase reaction. A free radical mechanism is proposed. T in the figure represents a tritium (^3H) atom which in reaction 1 is transferred from the substrate to the 5′-methylene group in the coenzyme, generating two free radical species. The substrate then rearranges, resulting in transfer of the 2-hydroxyl group to the carbonyl carbon, C1 (reaction 2). Next, a hydrogen atom (H) is transferred to the substrate from the coenzyme while the cobalt free radical attacks the methyl group in the 5′-deoxyadenosyl moiety of the coenzyme (reaction 3). Because of the equivalence of the three hydrogen atoms in the methyl group of the 5′-deoxyadenosyl moiety, a tritium atom can be retained in the coenzyme as is shown. Finally, loss of water from the substrate (reaction 4) occurs spontaneously. Note that one third of the tritium atoms incorporated into coenzyme B_{12} from the 1-position of the substrate, propanediol, should be incorporated into the 2-position of propionaldehyde in a single stoichiometric transfer reaction involving a single substrate and a single enzyme molecule.

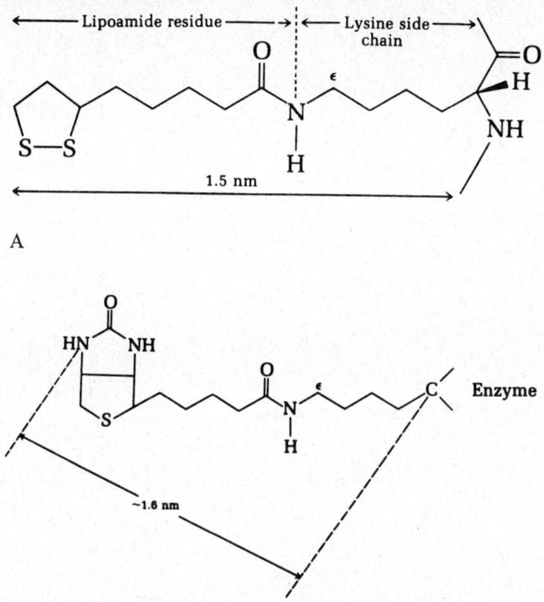

Figure 4.20 Structures of two enzyme cofactors which are covalently incorporated into proteins via protein lysyl residues. (A) Oxidized lipoate is covalently bound via a secondary amide linkage to an ϵ-amino group of a lysyl residue in the enzyme. (B) Biotin (vitamin H) is also linked via a secondary amide bond to an ϵ-amino group of a lysyl residue in a biotinyl carrier protein.

enzyme-bound cofactor functions to transfer electrons and activated acyl groups resulting from the decarboxylation and oxidation of α-keto acids. Three such keto acid dehydrogenase complexes are known: the pyruvate, α-ketoglutarate, and branched-chain α-keto acid dehydrogenase complexes found in bacteria and in the mitochondria of eukaryotes. The mechanism of action of the lipoamide moietites of these proteins is always essentially the same: the oxidized (disulfide) form of the lipoamide moiety is transiently reduced to dihydrolipoamide as it simultaneously accepts an activated acyl group and an electron pair. The acyl group is subsequently passed on to coenzyme A (see Figure 4.21) while the electron pair is used to reduce a flavoprotein, thus regenerating the oxidized form of the lipoamide derivative of the coenzyme. The reactions catalyzed by lipoamide-containing proteins will be discussed further in Chapter 6 when we consider the pyruvate and α-ketoglutarate dehydrogenase complexes.

As for lipoate, the side-chain carboxyl group of biotin (vitamin H) forms a secondary amide bond with the ϵ-amino group of a lysyl residue in the protein [Figure 4.2(b)]. The active moiety of this prosthetic group is therefore attached to the protein backbone via an arm about 1.5 nm in length. This enzyme-bound cofactor functions in six distinct ATP-dependent, enzyme-catalyzed carboxylation reactions. The first

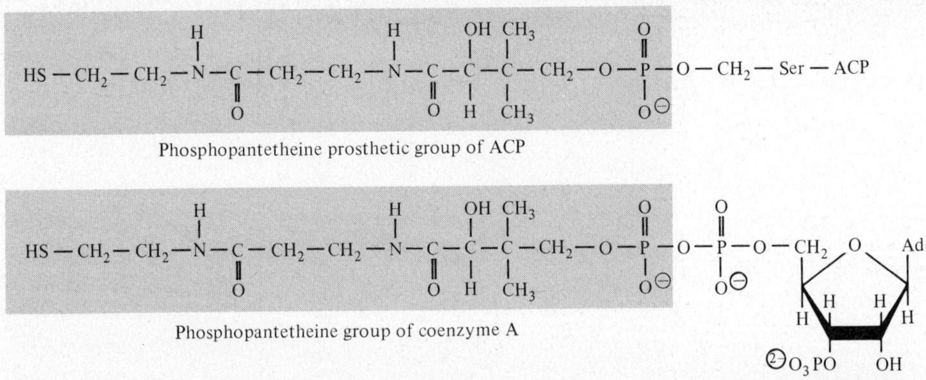

Figure 4.21 Structure of the phosphopantetheine group of the acyl carrier protein (ACP) (top) and coenzyme A (bottom). The prosthetic group of ACP is bound to a seryl residue in the protein via a phosphodiester linkage. The same moiety is bound to the 5′-position of adenosine-5′-phosphate (AMP) in coenzyme A via a pyrophosphoryl linkage.

two steps (activation of bicarbonate and carboxylation of the biotin-containing protein) are always the same:

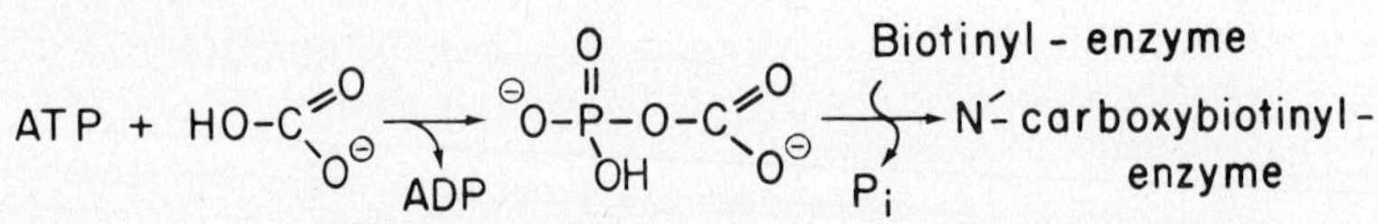

(4.4)

Subsequently, the carboxyl group is transferred from the activated biotinyl enzyme to the substrate for which the enzyme in question exhibits specificity. Reactions catalyzed by biotinyl enzymes such as that catalyzed by acetyl CoA carboxylase, will be discussed in Chapter 8 when we consider fatty acid biosynthesis.

The third protein-bound cofactor to be presented in this section is phosphopantetheine, derived from the vitamin, pantothenate. In some bacteria and many plants the cofactor is found as a constituent of a small protein, designated the acyl carrier protein (ACP) which serves to activate acyl groups by thioesterification (Figure 4.21; top). In other organisms this prosthetic group is found in larger proteins which fulfill the function of ACP as well as catalyze certain fatty acid biosynthetic reactions (see Chapter 8).

In both ACP and coenzyme A (which also functions to form thioesters with acyl groups and thereby to activate them for a variety of reactions) the sulfhydryl group of the cysteamine moiety of phosphopantetheine is the functional group (Figure 4.21). Like biocytin and lipoamide, the active moiety of the prosthetic group in ACP is attached to the protein via an arm, about 1.5 nm in length. All three of the protein cofactors described in this section therefore share a physical characteristic which allows the active cofactor moieties and the substrates to rotate about the protein-bound centers so that they can interact with other enzyme constituents of the enzyme complexes. The arm confers limited mobility to the activated substrate. The mode of action of phosphopantetheine in ACP and coenzyme A will be considered in greater detail in Chapter 8 when we discuss fatty acid oxidation and biosynthesis.

4.10 METAL IONS AS ENZYME COFACTORS

Metal ions activate enzymes and electron carriers by a wide variety of mechanisms and are present in very different microenvironments in the different proteins. About one-third of all enzymes contain at least one tightly bound metal ion, and in most of these cases the ion is required for optimal activity. Their functions include (a) to maintain an appropriate enzyme conformation for catalysis; (b) to participate in substrate binding at the active site; (c) to participate directly in the reaction as a catalyst; and (d) to participate in redox reactions, undergoing cyclic changes in oxidation state. The metal ion may be bound via side-chain carboxylate anions and histidyl imidazole functions in the protein, within a heme center or within an iron–sulfur center. Some metals (Fe^{++}, Cu^{++}, Zn^{++}, Mn^{++}, Co^{++}, Mo^{++}) are almost always tightly bound, forming *metalloenzymes,* while other metals (Mg^{++}, Ca^{++}, Mn^{++}) are usually loosely bound, forming *metal-activated enzymes.* With the former enzymes, the metal requirement may be difficult to demonstrate, but inclusion of a divalent metal ion chelator (EDTA or EGTA) with the latter enzymes invariably results in complete loss of activity. Some enzymes exhibit a specific requirement for Na^+, K^+ or an anion. These ions usually influence the protein conformation. However, they may function directly in the reaction mechanism as discussed in Section 6.2. Many metabolites such as ATP, exist as metal complexes (e.g., Mg · ATP), and these complexes are the true enzyme substrates. Finally, complexation of some enzymes with metals regulates the rates of enzyme synthesis and degradation.

Iron When iron is present in an electron carrier protein it is frequently complexed as part of the heme group of the protoporphyrin IX ring (Figure 4.22). Heme groups are the prosthetic groups of catalases and peroxidases that destroy hydrogen peroxide and alkyl peroxides, the latter employing reduced quinones and ascorbate. The reactions catalyzed by these two classes of enzymes are as follows:

$$2\ H_2O_2 \xrightleftharpoons{\text{catalase}} 2\ H_2O + O_2 \tag{4.5}$$

$$R{-}O{-}O{-}H + AH_2 \xrightleftharpoons{\text{peroxidase}} A + ROH + H_2O \tag{4.6}$$

Similar prosthetic groups are also found in the cytochromes which function in electron transport as well as in the oxygen carriers, myoglobin and hemoglobin.

Other electron carriers contain ferrous ions (Fe^{++}) complexed with inorganic sulfide in so-called iron-sulfur centers. Several iron–sulfur proteins are present within the electron transport chains of mitochondria and bacteria. Representative structures of these complexes are shown in Figure 4.23 and are discussed in more detail in Chapter 7.

Zinc Second in importance of the trace element activators of enzymes is zinc. Zinc is present at the active site of over a hundred well-characterized enzymes. This metal can only exist in the +2 oxidation state and therefore does not participate directly in redox reactions. Instead, it often functions to bind substrates to the active site. Zinc may form a coordination complex with the oxygen atom of a water molecule or

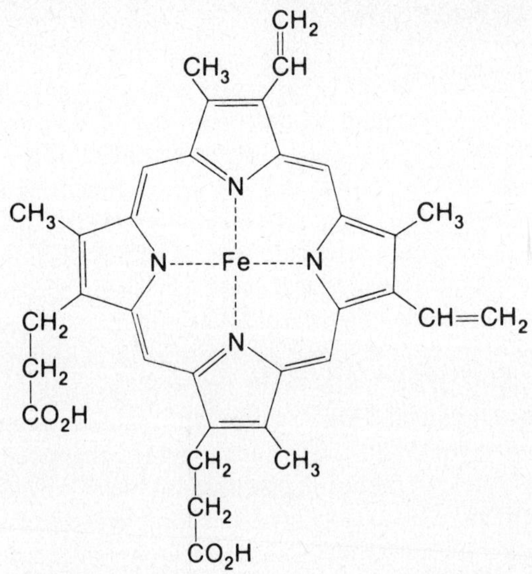

Figure 4.22 Structure of Fe-protoporphyrin IX. This prosthetic group, or variants of it, is found in enzymes such as the peroxidases that reduce peroxides, in oxygen-carrier proteins such as hemoglobin and myoglobin and in electron carrier proteins such as the cytochromes. (Reproduced with permission from P. A. Frey, "Structure and Function of Coenzymes," in *Biochemistry,* G. Zubay, ed., Addison-Wesley, Reading, MA, 1983.)

another electronegative atom in some molecular grouping thereby activating it for reaction. Among the zinc-containing enzymes are proteases, dehydrogenases, and hydroxylases. Carbonic anhydrase is an additional Zn^{++}-containing enzyme which functions to hydrate carbon dioxide to bicarbonate.

Copper The third most frequently occurring enzymic trace element is copper. Because it can exist either as the cuprous ion (Cu^{+}) or the cupric ion (Cu^{++}), and because these two states are readily interconvertible, this metal ion can participate directly in redox reactions. Copper is most often found in hydroxylases and oxidases which utilize molecular oxygen as the oxidizing substrate. Cytochrome oxidase, the terminal electron carrier complex in mitochondria and bacteria, is probably the best-known example of a copper-containing oxidase (Chapter 7).

Other Trace Elements In addition to these principal ions, several others can activate specific enzymes. These ions include Mn^{++}, Co^{++}, Ni^{++}, and Mo^{++}. Mg^{++}-activated enzymes are frequently active, although less so, when Mg^{++} is substituted by one of these other ions. Many Mg^{++}-dependent enzymes show relative activities with these ions in the following order: $Mg^{++} > Mn^{++} > Co^{++} > Ni^{++}$. Manganese and cobalt frequently bind to the magnesium binding site with much higher affinity than does

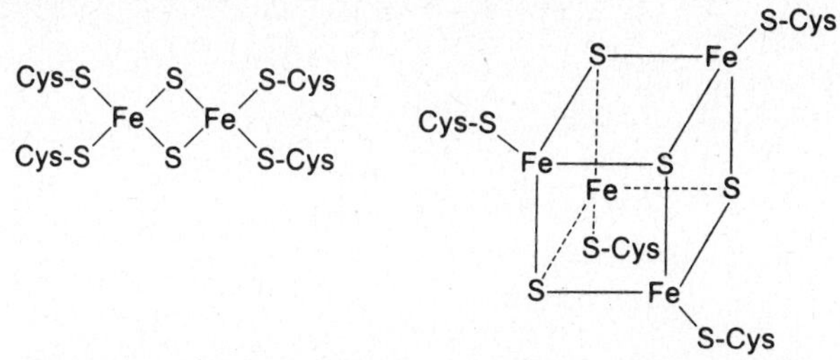

Figure 4.23 Structures of two common iron–sulfur clusters in the iron–sulfur electron carrier proteins of the mitochondrial or bacterial electron transport chains. The clusters consist of two (left) or four (right) iron atoms liganded to inorganic sulfide ions (*S*) as well as to cysteinyl–sulfhydryl groups of the protein (*cys-S*). (Reproduced with permission from P. A. Frey, "Structure and Function of Coenzymes," in *Biochemistry,* G. Zubay, ed., Addison-Wesley, Reading, MA, 1983.)

magnesium. Mo^{++} is found at the active sites of a few enzymes, an important one being nitrogenase, the enzyme which is responsible for all biological nitrogen fixation reactions.

Finally, calcium binds with high affinity to a number of eukaryotic calcium-binding proteins. These proteins frequently function in the regulation of various enzymatic reactions and cellular processes. The structure and function of one such calcium binding protein, calmodulin, was discussed in Chapter 2.

> *We cannot truly account for our acceptance of such theories without endorsing our acknowledgement of a beauty that exhilarates and a profundity that entrances us.*
>
> —*M. Polanyi*

BIBLIOGRAPHY

Abel, E. L., *Marihuana, Tobacco, Alcohol, and Reproduction,* CRC Press, Boca Raton (1983).

Babior, B. M., Ed., *Cobalamin, Biochemistry, and Pathophysiology,* Wiley, New York (1975).

Barker, B. M., and D. A. Bender, eds., *Vitamins in Medicine,* 4th edition, Heinemann, London (1980).

Blakley, R. L., *The Biochemistry of Folic Acid and Related Pteridines,* Elsevier/North Holland, Amsterdam (1969).

Boyer, P. D., ed., *The Enzymes,* Vol. 9, Group Transfer: Part B, Academic, New York (1973).

Branden, C. I., and H. Eklund, "Structure and Mechanism of Liver Alcohol Dehydrogenase, Lactate Dehydrogenase, and Glyceraldehyde-3-phosphate Dehydrogenase," in *Dehydrogenase Requiring Nicotinamide Coenzymes,* J. Jeffery, ed., *Experientia Supplementum* (1980).

Briggs, M. H., ed., *Recent Vitamin Research,* CRC Press, Boca Raton (1984).

Briggs, M. H., ed., *Vitamins in Human Biology and Medicine,* CRC Press, Boca Raton (1981).

Cowan, M. J., "Biotin Responsive Metabolic Disorders in Early Childhood," in *Recent Vitamins Research,* M. H. Briggs, ed., pp. 1–26, CRC Press, Boca Raton (1984).

Dolphin, D., B_{12}, Vols. I and II, Wiley, New York (1982).

Evangelopoulos, A. E., ed., *Chemical and Biological Aspects of Vitamin B_6 Catalysis: Proceedings of a Symposium held in Athens, Greece,* A. R. Liss, Inc., New York (1984).

Everse J., B. Anderson, and K. You, eds., *The Pyridine Nucleotide Coenzymes,* Academic, New York (1982).

Frey, P. A., "Structure and Function of Coenzymes," in *Biochemistry,* G. Zubay, ed., pp. 196–241, Addison-Wesley (1983).

Herbert, V., *Nutrition Cultism: Facts and Figures,* G. F. Stickley, Philadelphia (1980).

Hutchinson, D. W., *Nucleotides and Coenzymes,* Wiley, New York (1964).

Krampitz, L. O., *Thiamin Diphosphate and Its Catalytic Functions,* Marcel Dekker, New York (1970).

Krasnegor, N. A., ed., *Cigarette Smoking as a Dependence Process,* National Institute on Drug Abuse, Research Monograph Series #23, Rockville, MD (1979).

Kutsky, R. J., *Handbook of Vitamins, Minerals, and Hormones,* 2nd edition, Van Nostrand and Reinhold, New York (1981).

Massey, V., and C. H. Williams, eds., *Flavins and Flavoproteins: Proceedings of the Seventh International Symposium on Flavins and Flavoproteins,* Elsevier/North Holland, Amsterdam (1981).

McCormick, D. B., and L. D. Wright, eds., *Vitamins and Coenzymes Parts A–F,* in *Methods in Enzymology,* (Parts A–B) *Vol. 18* (1970); (Part C) *Vol. 18* (1971) (Part D) *Vol. 62* (1979); (Part E) *Vol. 66* (1980); (Part F) *Vol. 67* (1980), Academic, New York.

Robinson, F. A., *The Vitamin Cofactors of Enzyme Systems,* Pergamon, Oxford (1966).

Spiro, T. G., ed., *Zinc Enzymes,* Wiley, New York (1983).

Wagner, A. F., and K. Folkers, *Vitamins and Coenzymes,* Wiley, New York (1964).

Weiner, M., and J. Van Eys, *Nicotinic Acid: Nutrient–Cofactor–Drug,* Marcel Dekker, New York (1983).

Zagalak, B., and W. Friedrich, eds., *Vitamin B_{12}: Proceedings of the Third European Symposium on Vitamin B_{12} and Intrinsic Factor,* Gruyter, New York (1979).

Chapter 5

Anaerobic Carbohydrate Metabolism (Glycolysis)

> *Science is spectrum analysis; art is photosynthesis.*
>
> —KARL KRAUS

In the preceding chapters the molecular bases of enzyme catalysis and enzyme regulation were considered. Many of the examples chosen for scrutiny were enzymes involved in carbohydrate metabolism. The enzymes of glycolysis were probably among the first to evolve in primordial organisms, were among the first to be studied by early enzymologists, and are among the best characterized enzymes today. During the first 2 billion years of biological evolution, only prokaryotic organisms existed in an anaerobic environment. Molecular oxygen was not introduced into the atmosphere until after the advent of bacterial photosynthesis. The glycolytic pathway, more properly termed the *glycolytic cycle,* was undoubtedly the first extensive enzyme-catalyzed carbohydrate catabolic system to appear on earth. Its universal presence in virtually all living organisms shows that it was faithfully transmitted from organism to organism through evolution of the species.

In this chapter the glycolytic cycle and its constituent enzymes will be examined in detail. We shall also consider the pathways by which each of several simple sugars enter the glycolytic pathway and how these entry pathways are regulated. Since the initial steps of carbohydrate utilization usually involve transmembrane transport and phosphorylation of the exogenous sugar, these processes will be discussed first. It will be seen that there are several distinct mechanisms for transporting sugars into living cells, all of which are found in bacteria, but that the *principal* methods used by prokaryotes and eukaryotes differ. In bacteria, many of the simpler hexoses and hexitols are simultaneously transported and phosphorylated in a single step catalyzed by the phosphoenolpyruvate-dependent phosphotransferase system. In most animal cells the sugars are transported by a protein-mediated energy-independent process termed *facilitated diffusion.* Entry of the sugar into the cytoplasm is followed by phosphorylative capture by an ATP-dependent, hexokinase-catalyzed reaction. These differences between the sugar metabolic pathways of eukaryotes and bacteria may provide a basis for the development of new classes of antibacterial agents for future research endeavors and clinical uses.

5.1 STRUCTURES AND STEREOCHEMISTRY OF SIMPLE SUGARS

As illustrated in Figure 5.1, isomers are defined as different compounds with the same chemical formula. All of the sixteen aldohexoses (aldehydic sugars with six carbon atoms) are therefore isomers of each other (see Figure 5.2). The two fundamental types of isomers are termed structural isomers (which have different bond sequences) and stereoisomers (which have the same bond sequences but different atomic arrangements). An example of a pair of structural isomers is the keto acid, pyruvate

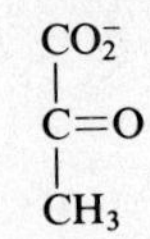

and its enol form, enolpyruvate

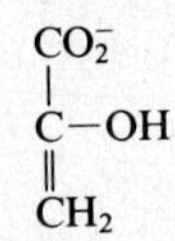

Because these two isomers are in rapid equilibrium in aqueous solution, they are termed *tautomers.*

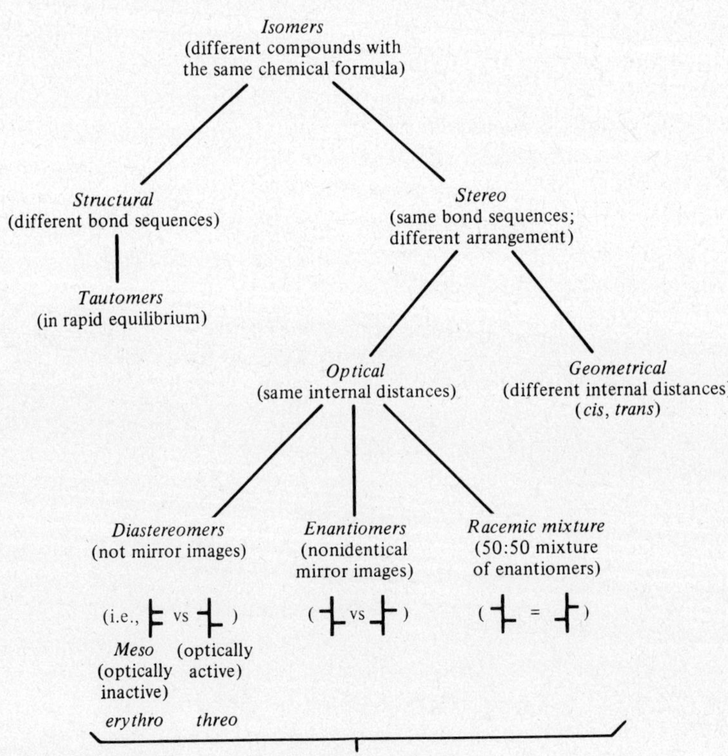

Figure 5.1 Definitions of different types of isomeric compounds.

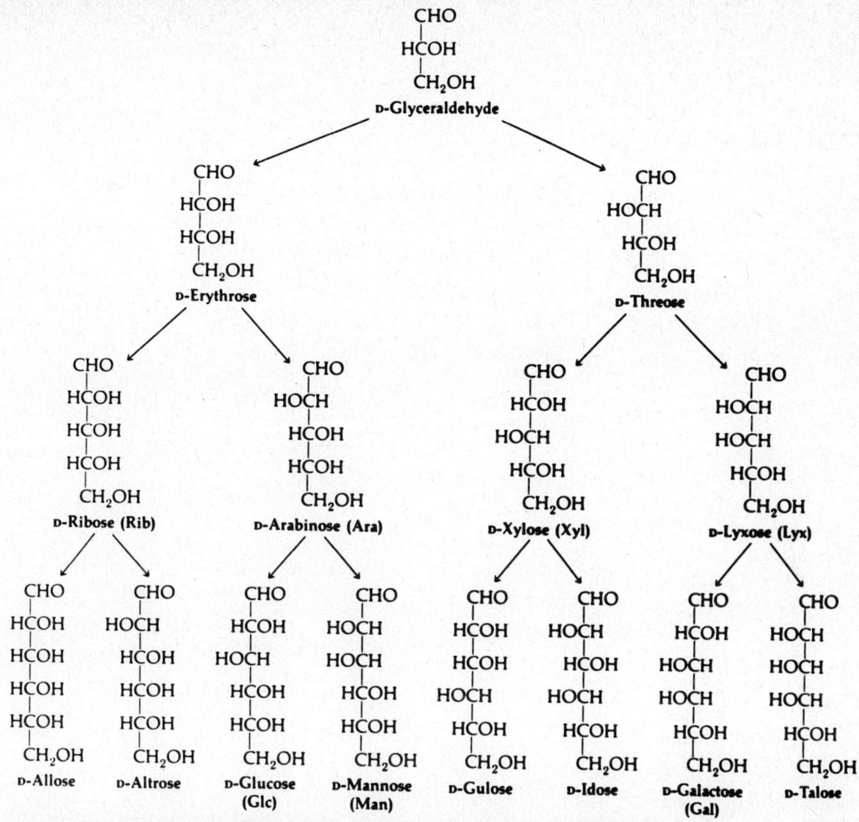

Figure 5.2 The family of D-aldoses having from three to six carbon atoms. The structures of the L-aldoses are the mirror images of the D-aldoses shown. The common three-letter abbreviations of the biologically important sugars are in parentheses. (Reproduced with permission from E. L. Smith et al., *Principles of Biochemistry,* Seventh Edition, McGraw-Hill, New York, 1983.)

Stereoisomers are either optical isomers or geometrical isomers. Geometrical isomers have different internal distances between atoms as is true of the two dicarboxylic acids, fumarate,

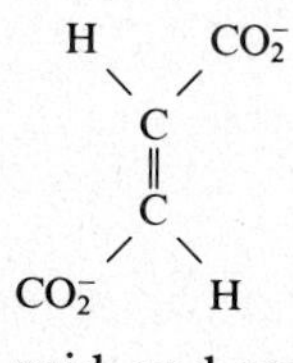

the trans isomer of this unsaturated acid, and maleate,

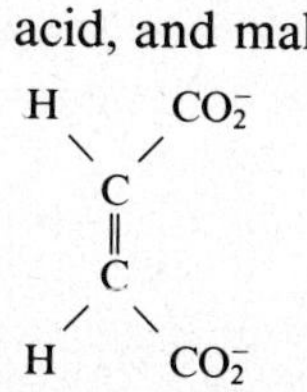

the cis isomer. Optical isomers have the same internal distances but possess at least one asymmetrical carbon atom. These include diastereoisomers, exemplified by the optically inactive sugar alcohol, erythritol,

$$\begin{array}{c} CH_2OH \\ | \\ H-C-OH \\ | \\ H-C-OH \\ | \\ CH_2OH \end{array}$$

and an optically active sugar alcohol with the same internal atomic distances, D-threitol,

$$\begin{array}{c} CH_2OH \\ | \\ HO-C-H \\ | \\ H-C-OH \\ | \\ CH_2OH \end{array}$$

They also include enantiomers, or enantiostereoisomers, such as D-threitol and L-threitol. These sugars are shown in Figure 5.1. When the hydroxyl group linked to the lowest *asymmetrical* carbon atom is to the right in the Fischer projection (as for all sugars shown in Figure 5.2) the sugar is said to be of the D-configuration. When this hydroxyl group is to the left, it is of the L-configuration. A 50:50 mixture of two enantiomers is termed a *racemic mixture.* A racemic mixture does not rotate plane-polarized light and results whenever a racemase is allowed to act on either of its two optically active enantiomeric substrates.

The structures of the D-aldoses of from three to six carbon atoms in length are shown in Fischer projection in Figure 5.2. It will be noted that while most biologically important amino acids are of the L-configuration, most naturally occurring sugars are of the D-configuration. Of these sugars, the single aldotriose, D-glyceraldehyde, the two aldotetroses, D-erythrose and D-threose, as well as the four pentoses, are all common in biological systems. Of the eight D-aldohexoses, only three, D-glucose, D-mannose, and D-galactose, are abundant in nature.

Figure 5.2 shows the sugars in straight-chain, open, Fischer projections. However they exist in aqueous solutions predominantly as five- and six-membered ring compounds. The different ring forms of a sugar are hemiacetals or hemiketals and therefore in rapid equilibrium with one another in aqueous solution. Five-membered ring sugars are termed *furanoses,* while six-membered ring sugars are termed *pyranoses.* Pyranoses, the more frequent ring structures of most of the hexoses, can be portrayed by any one of three conventions, termed *Fischer projections, Haworth projections,* and *conformational projections.* While the Fischer projections are probably most widely used, the Haworth and conformational projections more accurately depict the conformations of the ring sugars in aqueous solution.

Figure 5.3 illustrates the structures of the three principal aldohexoses found in nature: D-glucose, D-mannose, and D-galactose. In converting a straight-chain aldohexose to a six-membered ring hemiacetal, the electronegative hydroxyl group at carbon-5 attacks the carbonyl carbon at position 1, resulting in ring closure. The hydroxyl

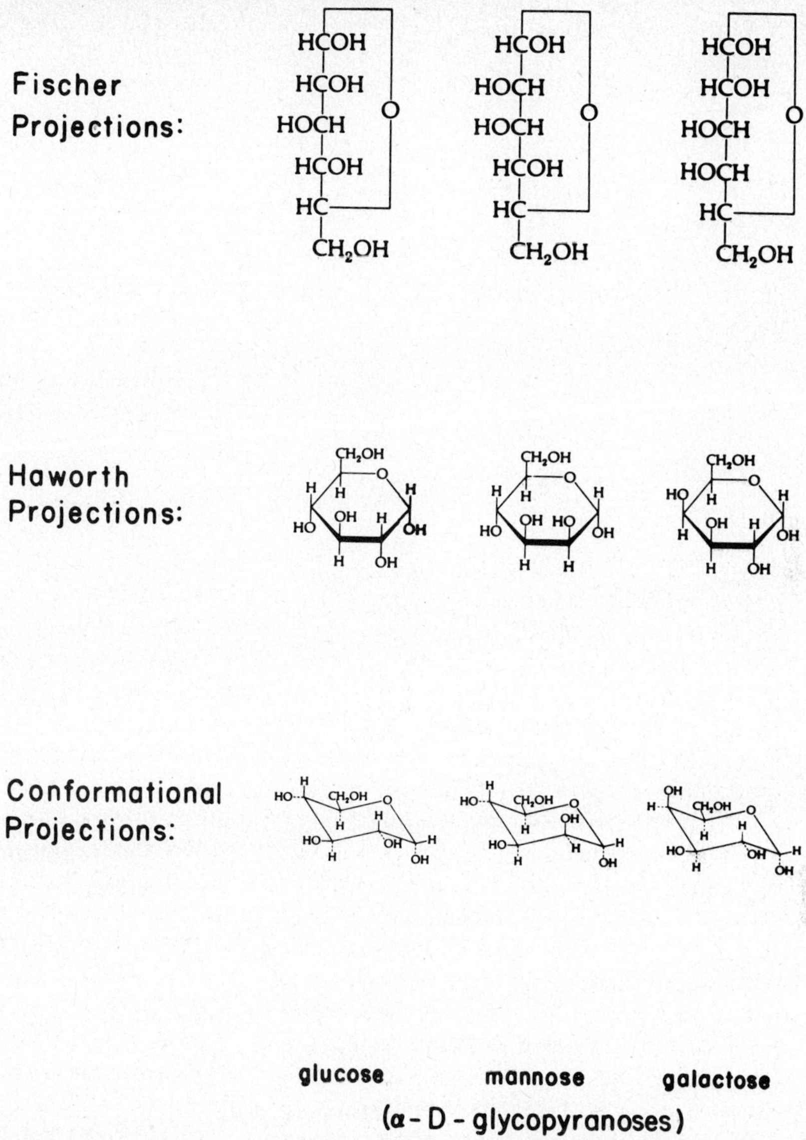

Figure 5.3 Depiction of the Fischer (top), Haworth (middle), and *N* (normal) chair-conformational (bottom) projections of the three common aldohexoses, D-glucose (left), D-mannose (middle), and D-galactose (right). Only the α-anomeric configurations of the hydroxyl groups at C-1 are indicated in the figure.

group at the 1-carbon can then assume either the α-anomeric configuration [projecting to the right in the Fischer projection shown in Figure 5.3, or to the left in the Fischer projection analogous to that shown in Figure 5.4(C)], or the β-anomeric configuration [projecting to the left in the Fischer projection shown in Figure 5.3, or up in the Fischer projection shown in Figure 5.4(C)].

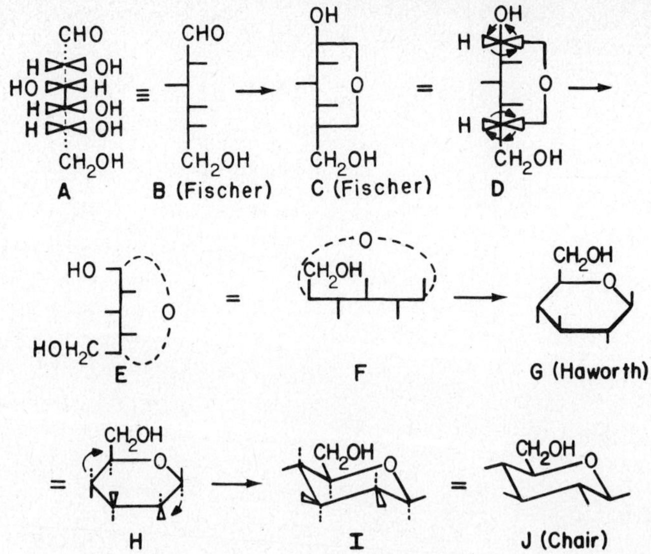

Figure 5.4 Interconversion of Fischer, Haworth, and conformational projections of β-D-glucopyranose (the six-membered ring structure of D-glucose with the anomeric hydroxyl group at position 1 in the β-configuration).

In order to understand the depiction of sugars by the three methods, the conventions of each must be understood. As shown in Figure 5.4, to draw a sugar in the open Fischer convention (B), the carbon skeleton of the sugar is drawn in a straight, vertical line. Recalling that each carbon atom exhibits tetrahedral symmetry with bond angles of 109°, this skeleton is really meant to curl back upon itself as shown in Figure 5.4(A). By this convention, all hydrogen atoms and hydroxyl groups project out toward us from the plane of the paper. Of the C—C bonds, only that between C_3 and C_4 is in the plane of the paper (solid line); the C_4—C_5 and C_2—C_3 bonds (dashed lines) project in back of the plane of the paper at 51° angles to the plane of the paper, and the C_1—C_2 and C_5—C_6 bonds (dotted lines) curl an additional 51° back, forming an angle of 102° with the plane of the paper. These bond angles place the C—5 hydroxyl group immediately behind C—1. Attack of the C—5 hydroxyl at C—1 and displacement of the π electron pair of C—1 and a proton to the carbonyl oxygen gives one of the two anomeric configurations (α or β). Only the β-anomer is shown in Figure 5.4(C), although the α-anomers are depicted in Figure 5.3.

In order to convert the Fischer projection (C) to the Haworth projection (G), free rotation about the C_2—C_1 bond (120° counterclockwise) and about the C_5—C_6 bond (120° clockwise) [as shown in (D)], puts the ring oxygen in back of the ring structure [Figure 5.4(E)]. Structure (E) (vertical Fischer) is then rotated 90° clockwise to give the horizontal Fischer projection (F), which is portrayed with bond angles between carbon atoms more closely approximating the correct angles as shown in the Haworth convention in (G). Note that the β-hydroxyl at C—1 is up in the Haworth projection while the α-hydroxyl group is down.

In order to interconvert the Haworth projection (G) and the conformational projection (which is a more or less true representation of the molecule in aqueous solution), the bonds between C and OH in (G) are drawn with solid lines while the C—H bonds are indicated by dotted lines. Then, rotating C_4 upward 71° about the $C_3—C_4$ and $C_4—C_5$ bonds while rotating C_1 downward 71° about the $C_1—C_2$ and C_1—ring O bonds as shown in structure (H) gives structure (I) in which all hydroxyl groups are shown as being in equatorial positions projecting out away from the ring while the hydrogen atoms are in axial positions. The bulky hydroxyl groups are each two to four times more stable in equatorial positions than in axial positions due to steric hindrance between axial substituents and axial hydrogens. An axial 6-hydroxymethyl group is very unstable, relative to the same group in the equatorial position. Consequently, the structure with this group in the equatorial position is called the normal (N) form of a sugar, while the alternative ring structure with the hydroxymethyl group axial is called the abnormal (or A) form. Figure 5.4(J) shows the normal chair configuration of β-D-glucopyranose. It is interesting to note that glucose, which is ordinary blood sugar and the sole constituent of glycogen and cellulose (the major storage and structural polysaccharides on earth), is the only aldopyranose to have all of its hydroxyl groups in equatorial positions. It is therefore the most stable of the hexoses, and its thermodynamic stability, which undoubtedly rendered it the most abundant sugar in the prebiotic sea, must have dictated its selection as the most important sugar in biological systems. The two other common aldohexoses, mannose and galactose, each possess a single axial hydroxyl group when the sugars are in the normal ring form of the β-D-glycopyranose structure. All other sugars except allose have two or three axial hydroxyl groups and are therefore of higher free energy or lower stability. Thermodynamic considerations therefore appear to account for the relative proportions of different sugars in biological systems.

5.2 THE GLYCOLYTIC CYCLE—AN OVERVIEW

The primary purposes of carbohydrate catabolism are to provide the cell with utilizable sources of energy and biosynthetic precursors. The first carbohydrate catabolic pathway to evolve was undoubtedly glycolysis [from the Greek, *glycos* (sweet) and *lysis* (splitting)]. The glycolytic cycle takes one mole of hexose, phosphorylates it twice to give fructose-1,6-diphosphate, splits the fructose-1,6-diphosphate into two moles of triosephosphate, and then oxidizes the triosephosphate to pyruvate, coupling the metabolic steps to ATP synthesis and NAD^+ reduction (Figure 5.5 and Table 5.1).

Let us consider the metabolism of glucose, the most abundant sugar in the biosphere. To a first approximation, the net equation for one turn in the glycolytic cycle is:

$$\text{D-glucose} + 2\ P_i + 2\ \text{ADP} + 2\ \text{NAD}^+ \rightarrow 2\ \text{pyruvate} + 2\ \text{ATP} + 2\ \text{NADH} \quad (5.1)$$

According to this equation, two molecules of ATP are generated and two NAD^+ molecules are reduced to NADH per molecule of glucose oxidized to pyruvate. While this equation partially reflects the needs of the cell under certain conditions, it is an oversimplification as discussed later in this section.

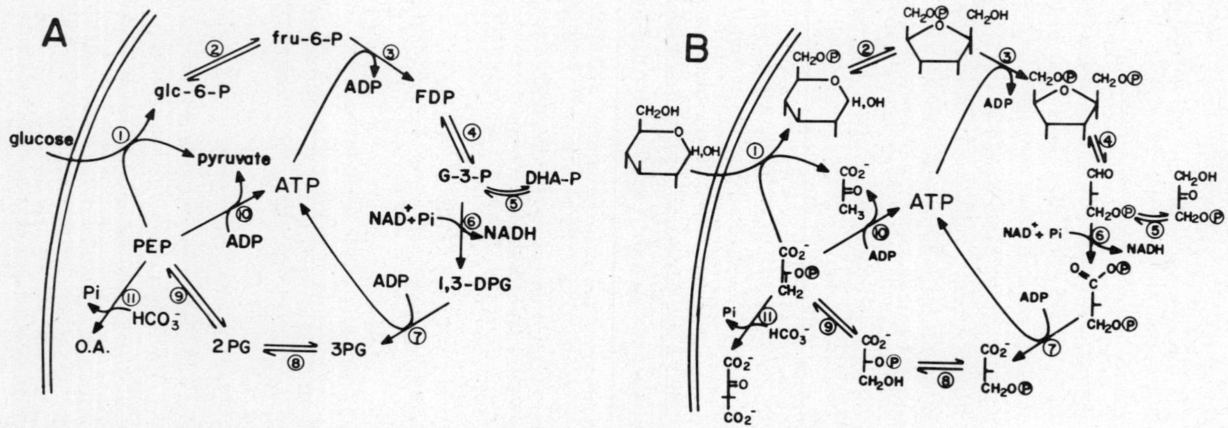

Figure 5.5 The glycolytic cycle as it occurs in bacteria such as *E. coli.* (A) The cycle is drawn using the standard abbreviations of the glycolytic intermediates. (B) The structures of the glycolytic intermediates are illustrated. The enzymes catalyzing the different reactions shown in the figure are: (1) the PEP:glucose phosphotransferase system (PTS); (2) phosphoglucoisomerase (PGI); (3) phosphofructokinase (PFK); (4) aldolase; (5) triose phosphate isomerase (TPI); (6) glyceraldehyde-3-P dehydrogenase (G3PDH); (7) phosphoglycerate kinase (PGK); (8) phosphoglycerate mutase (PGM); (9) enolase; (10) pyruvate kinase (PK); and (11) PEP carboxylase. Reactions 1–9 comprise the glycolytic cycle. Double-headed arrows indicate reversible reactions while single-headed arrows indicate essentially irreversible reactions. Reaction 7 has a large negative $\Delta G^{0\prime}$ and is therefore indicated as being irreversible. However, this reaction can be considered to be reversible by virtue of the endergonic nature of the reactions preceding and following step 7 (see Table 5.1).

TABLE 5.1 ENZYMES OF GLYCOLYSIS

Step	Systematic name	Trivial name	E.C. #	Abbreviation	Reactions	$\Delta G^{0\prime}$ (kcal/mole)	Cofactors	Essentially irreversible	Allosterically regulated	MW	Number of subunits	Source
1a	PEP:sugar phosphotransferase system (multicomponent)	Bacterial phosphotransferase system	2.7.3.9 and 2.7.1.69	PTS	Sugar + PEP → sugar-P + pyruvate	−10	Mg^{++}	Yes	Yes	$(60,000 + 8,000)_2$ and $(68,000)_2$	Multiple	Bacteria
1b	ATP:hexose 6-phosphotransferase	Hexokinase	2.7.1.1	HK	Hexose + ATP → hexose-P + ADP	−4	Mg^{++}	Yes	Yes	100,000 100,000	1 2	Mammals, yeast
2	Glucose-6-phosphate isomerase	Phosphoglucoisomerase	5.3.1.9	PGI	Glc-6-P → fru-6-P	+0.4	None	No	No	132,000 120,000	2 2	Mammals, yeast
3	ATP:D-fructose-6-phosphate-1-phosphotransferase	Phosphofructokinase	2.7.1.11	PFK	Fru-6-P + ATP → FDP + ADP	−4	Mg^{++}	Yes	Yes	320,000 900,000	4 4	Mammals, yeast
4	Fructose-1,6-diphosphate aldolase	Aldolase	4.1.2.13		FDP → DHAP + gly-3-P	+5	None	No	No	160,000 80,000	4 2	Mammals, yeast
5	Triosephosphate isomerase	Triosephosphate isomerase	5.3.1.1	TPI	DHAP → gly-3-P	+2	None	No	No	50,000	2	Mammals, and yeast
6	D-Glyceraldehyde-3-phosphate:NAD^+ oxidoreductase (phosphorylating)	Glyceraldehyde-3-phosphate dehydrogenase	1.2.1.12	G3PDH	Gly-3-P + NAD^+ + Pi → 1,3-DPG + NADH	+1.5	NAD^+, Zn^{++}	No	No	143,000	4	Mammals, and yeast
7	ATP:3-phospho-D-glycerate 1-phosphotransferase	Phosphoglycerate kinase	2.7.2.3	PGK	1,3-DPG + ADP → 3PG + ATP	−5	Mg^{++}	No	No	45,000	1	Mammals, and yeast
8	2,3-Diphospho-D-glycerate:2-phospho-D-glycerate phosphotransferase	Phosphoglyceromutase	2.7.5.3	PGM	3PG → 2PG	+1	2,3-DPG	No	No	55,000 110,000	2 4	Mammals, yeast
9	2-Phospho-D-glycerate hydro-lyase	Enolase	4.2.1.11		2PG → PEP + H_2O	+0.4	M^{++}	No	No	82,000 88,000	2 2	Mammals, yeast
10	ATP:pyruvate 2-*O*-phosphotransferase	Pyruvate kinase	2.7.1.40	PK	PEP + ADP → pyruvate + ATP	−7.5	K^+, Mg^{++}	Yes	Yes	240,000	4	Mammals

The glycolytic cycle can be somewhat arbitrarily divided into two parts. The first is the preparatory or energy-utilizing phase in which glucose is converted to two molecules of glyceraldehyde-3-P at the expense of two ATP molecules in animal cells or of one molecule of PEP and one molecule of ATP in bacterial cells (reactions 1–5 in Figure 5.5). The second is the energy-yielding phase (reactions 6–10 in Figure 5.5). The energy released by converting glyceraldehyde-3-P to phosphoenolpyruvate is partially conserved by the chemically coupled synthesis of ATP in steps 6 and 7 and the generation of reduced NAD^+ in step 6. Since two triosephosphates are generated from the cleavage of fructose-1,6-diP in step 4, there are two NAD^+ molecules reduced (step 6), two ATP molecules synthesized (step 7), and two PEP molecules generated (step 9) per molecule of glucose metabolized. In the preparatory activating phase of glycolysis, PEP is responsible for uptake and phosphorylation of the sugar in bacteria yielding cytoplasmic glucose-6-P (step 1). ATP is utilized in the third step to convert fructose-6-P to fructose-1,6-diP (step 3). The complete reaction as it occurs in bacteria can therefore be written:

$$\text{glucose} + \text{PEP} + \text{ATP} + 2\ \text{NAD}^+ + 2\ \text{P}_i + 2\ \text{ADP} \rightarrow 2\ \text{PEP} + \text{pyruvate} + \text{ADP} + 2\ \text{NADH} + 2\ \text{ATP} \quad (5.2)$$

The net reaction is:

$$\text{glucose} + 2\ \text{NAD}^+ + 2\ \text{P}_i + \text{ADP} \rightarrow \text{PEP} + \text{pyruvate} + 2\ \text{NADH} + \text{ATP} \quad (5.3)$$

In animal cells, where ATP is used for both preparatory phosphorylation reactions, the overall reaction can be written:

$$\text{glucose} + 2\ \text{NAD}^+ + 2\ \text{P}_i \rightarrow 2\ \text{PEP} + 2\ \text{NADH} \quad (5.4)$$

In the latter case, the sugar is transported into the cell by a protein-mediated, energy-independent process, and the sugar is phosphorylated in an ATP-dependent kinase-catalyzed reaction. The two ATP molecules synthesized in step 7 cycle back to activate glucose in steps 1B (hexokinase) and 3 (phosphofructokinase).

It is important to remember that the glycolytic cycle depicted in Figure 5.5 occurs in both bacteria and animal cells, and that the net reactions recorded in equations (5.3) and (5.4) are gross oversimplifications. The net PEP generated can be utilized for any of several purposes. For example, it can be utilized for ATP synthesis in the pyruvate kinase-catalyzed reaction (step 10 in Figure 5.5); it can be utilized to make the Krebs cycle intermediate, oxaloacetate in the PEP carboxylase-catalyzed reaction (reaction 11 in Figure 5.5); or it can be utilized for the biosynthesis of tryptophan, phenylalanine, and tyrosine. The importance of these shunt pathways is illustrated by the fact that without some source of a Krebs cycle intermediate, this cycle can not function as the sole source of carbon and energy, even under aerobic conditions. When *E. coli* is grown on glucose as the sole source of carbon, the conversion of PEP to oxaloacetate is an obligatory step. Also, the utilization of PEP for the biosynthesis of tryptophan, phenylalanine, and tyrosine is required unless these amino acids are supplied.

Equations (5.3) and (5.4) as well as Figure 5.5 are oversimplifications of glycolysis for yet another reason: some of the glucose utilized via glycolysis is never converted to PEP. Instead, various intermediates are drained off for biosynthetic purposes. For example, L-serine is biosynthesized from 3-phospho-D-glycerate, while α-glycerol phosphate, an intermediate of phospholipid biosynthesis, is made by reduction of dihydroxyacetone phosphate.

There are three reasons why glycolysis should be thought of as a cycle rather than a linear pathway. First, one of the two PEP molecules that results from glucose catabolism (step 9 in Figure 5.5) is actually used to initiate glucose metabolism (step 1 in Figure 5.5) in bacteria. The bacterial system probably most closely resembles the primordial system. Second, the ATP synthesized in step 7 is utilized for phosphorylation of fructose-6-P, and third, the P_i and ADP utilized for ATP synthesis (steps 6 and 7) must be regenerated in order for the glycolytic cycle to continue to operate. ATP hydrolysis or utilization, which can occur by several pathways, allows the regeneration of P_i and ADP. Considerable evidence suggests that under certain circumstances the rate-limiting step for glycolysis is the availability of ADP and inorganic phosphate.

Another important fact to be noted is that PEP is a much more energetic molecule than is ATP. It releases about twice as much energy upon hydrolysis to pyruvate and inorganic phosphate than does ATP when hydrolyzed to ADP and P_i. The free energies of hydrolysis for these and many other compounds of biological interest are summarized in Table 5.2. These values and their physiological significance will be discussed later in this and subsequent chapters.

The enzymes of the glycolytic cycle, the reactions catalyzed by each of these enzymes, and the thermodynamic properties of the reactions are summarized in Table

TABLE 5.2 STANDARD FREE ENERGIES OF HYDROLYSIS AT pH 7 OF VARIOUS ENERGY-RICH BONDS OF BIOLOGICAL INTEREST[a]

Compound	Type of bond	$-\Delta G^{0\prime}$ (hydrolysis) (kcal/mole)
Glycerol-3-phosphate Glucose-6-phosphate Glucose-1-phosphate Seryl-, threonyl-, or tyrosyl-phosphate in a protein	Phosphoryl ester	2–5
Pyrophosphate (P_2) ATP GTP	Phosphoanhydride	7–8
Acyl-Coenzyme A Acyl-ACP	Thioester	7–8
Phosphocreatine Phosphoarginine	Phosphoramidate	10–11
Acetyl phosphate 3-phosphoglyceroyl-1-phosphate Carbamoyl-phosphate Aspartyl- or glutamylphosphate in a protein	Mixed anhydride	11–12
Histidyl–phosphate in a protein	Phosphoramidate	14–15
Phosphoenolpyruvate (PEP)	Phosphoryl-*enol*-ester	14–15

[a] With the exception of the thioester bonds, hydrolysis of the compounds listed above gives inorganic phosphate as one of the products.

5.1. The cycle is essentially the same in bacteria (*E. coli*) and mammals in all respects except for the initiation of glucose metabolism.

In bacteria, glucose uptake and phosphorylation are coupled in a single process. The free energy of sugar phosphorylation with PEP as the phosphoryl donor is about −10 kcal/mole. In animal cells, the sugar is reversibly transported across the membrane but is irreversibly phosphorylated using ATP as the phosphoryl donor. Similarly, step 3 is essentially irreversible ($\Delta G^0 = -4.5$ kcal/mole). The next three steps show positive ΔG^0 values, but the equilibrium is shifted toward the right by the large negative value of the phosphoglycerate kinase reaction. Finally, the pyruvate kinase- and PEP carboxylase-catalyzed reactions are physiologically irreversible. It is worth noting that every essentially irreversible reaction in glycolysis is subject to allosteric control, while none of the enzymes catalyzing reversible reactions are regulated in this fashion. The only exception is the phosphoglycerate kinase-catalyzed reaction which, as discussed in the legend to Figure 5.5, functions to counteract the positive free energy of the previous three reactions in the cycle. The nature of the allosteric control mechanisms will be discussed in greater detail when the individual enzymes are considered.

5.3 HISTORICAL PERSPECTIVES OF THE STUDY OF GLYCOLYSIS

The glycolytic cycle was one of the first metabolic pathways to be understood biochemically. The student of biochemistry is frequently confronted with a given set of facts which are accepted as established dogma. However, a great deal of confusion usually shrouds investigations probing new fields of study, and this was certainly true of the early studies of glycolysis. In this section, some of the highlights of the historical developments will be presented in approximate chronological order.

1. In 1905, the study of yeast fermentation was begun by Harden and Young. In their early studies these workers discovered sugar phosphates, showed a need for inorganic phosphate and a "coenzyme," and proposed a scheme for the direct oxidation of glucose to ethanol without obligatory phosphorylation. In 1929, Harden received the Nobel prize for his work in this area. In his Nobel lecture, he defended his theory of fermentation in which sugar phosphorylation was merely a side reaction or "coupled" reaction which allowed glucose to enter the pathway.
2. In 1913, Newberg proposed that methyl glyoxal, a highly toxic compound, was an intermediate in glucose metabolism. It was later shown that methyl glyoxal arose from glyceraldehyde 3-phosphate in a nonenzymatic side reaction.
3. In 1920, the composition of Harden and Young's "coenzyme" was determined. It was shown to be an impure mixture of inorganic phosphate, magnesium, and probably ATP. Pure ATP was not isolated until 1929.
4. In 1924, hexose phosphates were first isolated from muscle leading to the suggestion that sugar metabolism in yeast and animals might exhibit similarities. Three years later, hexose diphosphate was isolated. Lohmann showed that it gave rise to an acid-stable and an acid-labile compound in the presence of fluoride. The former was probably phosphoglycerate, but Lohmann assumed it was merely a more stable form of hexose diphosphate and did not bother to isolate it. In that same year, Embden suggested that hexose phosphates are true intermediates of glucose metabolism which

he called *lactacidogens,* but his idea was not accepted. Meyerhof, for example, stated in 1930 that hexose phosphates were "stabilization products of more reactive species having the characteristics of free radicals."

5. In 1933, Nilsson incubated hexose diphosphate with "yeast juice" in the presence of fluoride and obtained phosphoglycerate as a major product. Nevertheless, he assumed that a side reaction gave rise to this product.

6. In a preliminary report in 1933, Embden and two coworkers proposed a novel metabolic sequence which corresponded in some respects to the glycolytic pathway as we know it today. Carl Cori wrote of Embden in 1983: "Embden alone, not unlike the child in the story of the Emperor's new clothes, believed what he saw and drew the right conclusions from the available clues." Embden died in 1933, the year in which his article was published.

In evaluating the salient features of the proposal of Embden, there are four major points;

1. Fructose-1,6-diphosphate is split into one molecule each of dihydroxyacetone phosphate and D-glyceraldehyde-3-phosphate.
2. A dismutation of the two triosephosphates to α-glycerophosphate and 3-phosphoglyceric acid takes place.
3. Phosphoglyceric acid is split to pyruvate and inorganic phosphate.
4. An oxido-reduction between pyruvate and α-glycerophosphate yields lactate and glyceraldehyde 3-phosphate which enters reaction 2 and so on.

Scrutinizing these four proposals, point 1 has been shown to be absolutely correct. Fructose-1,6-diphosphate is, in fact, split into dihydroxyacetone-P and D-glyceraldehyde-3-P. This proposal was the major conceptual advance put forth by Embden in 1933. However, points 2–4 are incorrect when applied to glycolysis. Point 2: Dismutation of triosephosphates can occur, but not as part of the glycolytic pathway. Instead, D-glyceraldehyde-3-P is oxidized to give 1,3-diphosphoglycerate (Figure 5.5, step 6). Point 3: Phosphoglycerate is not split to pyruvate and inorganic phosphate but is converted to phosphoenolpyruvate which *can* (but need not) be utilized for ATP synthesis with pyruvate as a by-product. Point 4: No oxido-reduction process between pyruvate and α-glycerophosphate occurs. Embden was apparently not as insightful as Cori gave him credit for.

Between 1935 and 1940, the intermediates and enzymes of glycolysis were identified, mostly in Meyerhof's laboratory. Because of the major contribution of Embden and Meyerhof in elucidating the glycolytic scheme, it is sometimes called the Embden–Meyerhof pathway. It can be seen from this discussion how much confusion can be associated with the scientific process. It is sometimes only after years of intensive research that it can be stated that we understand the molecular details of a biochemical process to a reasonable level of sophistication.

5.4 SUGAR TRANSPORT AND PHOSPHORYLATION IN BACTERIA

Bacteria fall into two fundamentally different structural types, the Gram-negative bacteria and the Gram-positive bacteria. The envelopes of these two bacterial classifications are shown in Figure 5.6. Both groups of organisms possess cytoplasmic membranes surrounded by a peptidoglycan-containing cell wall to which is attached carbohydrate containing polymers. These polymers are teichoic acids in Gram-positive bacteria and lipopolysaccharides in Gram-negative bacteria (Figure 5.6). The membrane of the Gram-positive bacterial envelope shows invaginations as illustrated in Figure 5.6, right, and the mesosomes so formed house a number of extracytoplasmic enzymes involved in the hydrolysis of membrane impermeable nutrients. The Gram-negative bacterium lacks mesosomes but contains a second, outer, lipopolysaccharide-containing membrane which, like the inner cytoplasmic membrane, serves as a barrier for the diffusion of nutrients and other compounds.

In order to allow passage of these nutrients into the space between the two membranes of Gram-negative bacteria, which is called the *periplasmic space,* or *periplasm,* proteins are imbedded in the outer membrane that function as hydrophilic pores of various diameters through which water soluble solutes can diffuse. The periplasm contains about 5% of the total cellular protein. These proteins include a special class of digestive enzymes that cleave membrane-impermeable nutrients into cellular building blocks which can traverse the cytoplasmic membrane by virtue of the presence in this structure of specific transport systems or permeases. Hundreds of these permeases are present in the cytoplasmic membrane, and they exhibit specificities for the amino acids, salts, sugars, vitamins, mono-, di-, and tricarboxylic acids, nucleosides, purine and pyrimidine bases, and other compounds of nutritional value to the cell.

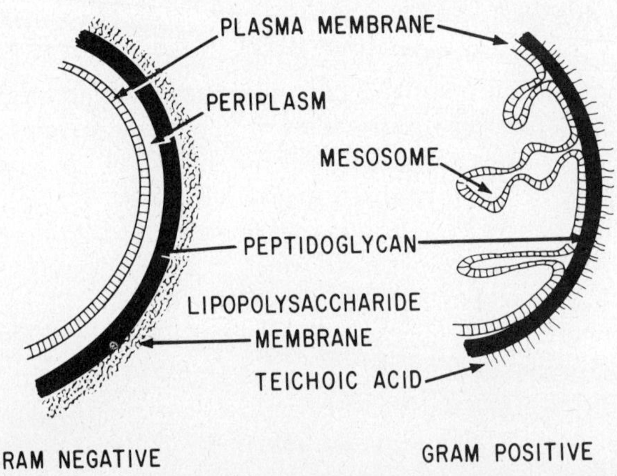

Figure 5.6 Schematic depiction of the structures of the Gram-negative (left) and Gram-positive (right) bacterial envelopes. Both envelopes consist of a cytoplasmic membrane surrounded by a rigid peptidoglycan layer. The Gram-negative bacterial envelope also possesses an outer membrane containing species-specific lipopolysaccharide. The space between the inner and outer membranes is called the periplasm. Gram-positive bacteria lack an outer membrane but have species-specific teichoic acids covalently bound to their peptidoglycan layer. (Reproduced with permission from M. H. Saier, Jr. and C. D. Stiles, *Molecular Dynamics in Biological Membranes,* Springer Verlag, New York, 1975.)

The carbohydrate transport systems in the inner cytoplasmic membrane of *E. coli,* a Gram-negative bacterium, fall into five major classes as illustrated in Figure 5.7. Glycerol crosses the membrane barrier via a proteinaceous pore of inner diameter equal to about 0.4 nm. Only uncharged, straight-chain compounds can pass through this aqueous channel. Because the process is not linked to metabolic energy, a solute transported by this type of system cannot be accumulated against a gradient. Any transport system that involves protein facilitation by an energy-independent process is termed *facilitated diffusion.* Lactose, a β-galactoside, containing one molecule of glucose and one of galactose, enters the *E. coli* cell by a carrier-type mechanism in a translocation process in which each molecule of lactose is obligatorily transported with one proton. Because of the tight coupling of lactose and proton transport, the flux of protons down their electrochemical gradient can drive the active accumulation of lactose in the cytoplasm against a 1000-fold concentration gradient. In a similar fashion, the Na^+ electrochemical gradient can be utilized to drive the active accumulation of melibiose, an α-galactoside, in the cell cytoplasm because uptake of each molecule of this sugar is coupled to the uptake of a Na^+ ion. This type of *chemiosmotic coupling* will be discussed in greater detail in Chapter 7.

The fourth transport system shown in Figure 5.7 is responsible for the transport of maltose across the cytoplasmic membrane. Maltose is an α-1,4-linked disaccharide of glucose derived from the partial hydrolysis of glycogen and starch. Four proteins function in concert to catalyze irreversible transport of maltose via this system. It is probable that two of these proteins [F and G in Figure 5.7(D)] span the membrane and serve as a stereospecific transmembrane channel, possibly with one solute binding site associated with each transmembrane protein. The other two proteins [E and K in Figure 5.7(D)] are localized to the periplasmic and cytoplasmic sides of the membrane, respectively. While the E protein is involved in solute recognition and induces the changes that promote solute transport, the K protein appears to function in energy coupling and regulation of permease activity. The energy source and energy-coupling mechanism for this transport system are completely unknown.

The fifth and last transport system depicted in Figure 5.7 is called the mannitol permease. This permease is part of the complex phosphoenolpyruvate (PEP):sugar phosphotransferase system (PTS). Like the maltose transport system, the PTS is a multicomponent system. Three proteins of the PTS are shown in Figure 5.7(E). Enzyme I and HPr are the general energy-coupling proteins of the PTS, while the Enzymes II are the sugar-specific permeases. There are about a dozen Enzymes II in the *E. coli* cell, each specific for a different sugar. Thus, Enzymes II specific for glucose, mannose, fructose, glucitol (reduced glucose), and mannitol (reduced mannose) are all known as are several other Enzymes II. In some cases, but not others, an Enzyme II functions in conjunction with a sugar-specific energy-coupling protein of the PTS called an Enzyme III. For example, the glucose or glucitol permease each functions with an Enzyme III, but the mannitol permease does not.

Of all of the permease types shown in Figure 5.7 and of the various PTS permeases, the mannitol permease, a phosphotransferase permease, is probably the best understood structurally and mechanistically. This protein has been solubilized from the membrane, purified to homogeneity, and its transport function has been reconstituted in spherical artificial membranes called *liposomes.* The gene (DNA) encoding this protein has been cloned and sequenced so that the entire amino acid sequence of

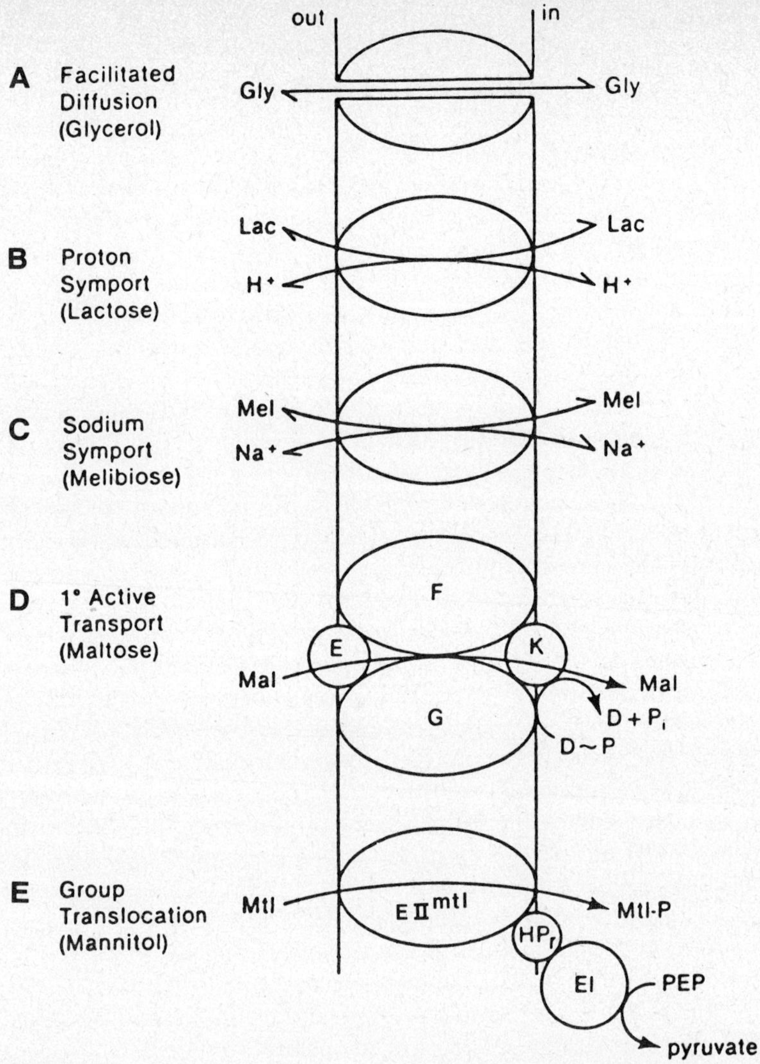

Figure 5.7 Permease-mediated transmembrane carbohydrate transport processes that occur in *E. coli.* Glycerol (Gly) crosses the membrane by passive diffusion through a nonstereospecific protein pore. Lactose (Lac) and melibiose (Mel) enter the cell by cation symport involving protons and sodium ions, respectively. Each of these three transport processes is probably catalyzed by a single protein species encoded by a specific gene on the bacterial chromosome. Maltose (Mal) transport may involve the hydrolysis of a high-energy phosphoryl donor (D ~ P) which drives the active accumulation of the sugar. Four distinct proteins, encoded by four different genes within the *mal* regulon, are required for transport. Finally, the transport of mannitol (Mtl) involves three proteins of the phosphotransferase system, the general energy coupling proteins of the system, Enzyme I (EI) and HPr, as well as the integral Enzyme II specific for mannitol (EII^{Mtl}). Each of these proteins is sequentially phosphorylated at the expense of phosphoenolpyruvate (PEP) before translocation of mannitol and its coupled phosphorylation can occur. (Reproduced with permission from M. H. Saier, Jr. and G. R. Jacobson, *The Molecular Basis of Sex and Differentiation,* Springer-Verlag, New York, 1984.)

the protein is known. This protein consists of a chain of 637 amino acyl residues with a total molecular weight of 67,893.

Hydropathy analyses have been performed on this protein employing computer techniques which have shown that the N-terminal half of the protein is largely embedded within the phospholipid matrix of the membrane. (See Section 2.4 in Chapter 2.) α-Helical segments within the N-terminal half of the polypeptide chain probably span the membrane at least seven times. Between each of these hydrophobic transmembrane α-helices are hydrophilic β-turns which allow the polypeptide backbone to turn around in the aqueous environment and to again traverse the membrane in the opposite direction. These seven transmembrane α-helical segments as well as several shorter hydrophobic segments which may span the membrane as many as four times as β-structure, may constitute the channel or pathway through which the sugar passes as it traverses the membrane.

Computer analyses of the amino acyl sequence of the C-terminal half of the Enzyme II^{mtl} and comparison of the analyses with those of a large number of soluble proteins has led to the suggestion that most of this domain consists of short α-helical segments which fold back upon themselves into a globular structure. One region of the polypeptide chain may form a small β-pleated sheet. While the N-terminal half of the molecule is clearly associated with transport function, the C-terminal half couples the transmembrane translocation step to metabolic energy. Many of the details of this energy-coupling process are known and will be discussed in subsequent paragraphs.

The structure of the mannitol Enzyme II is schematically illustrated in Figure 5.8 (top) as is that proposed for a related system responsible for the transport of glucitol (Figure 5.8, bottom). The glucitol permease appears to possess a structure similar to that of the mannitol permease with at least two principal differences. First, the sugar-binding site must differ substantially so that the orientation of the hydroxyl group at the 2 position of the sugar is distinguished. Presumably, one or a few differences in amino acyl residues at the sugar binding site could account for this difference. Second, while the mannitol permease is a single protein (the Enzyme II^{mtl}), the glucitol permease consists of two distinct proteins (the Enzyme II^{gut}–Enzyme III^{gut} pair). Analyses of the molecular weights of these proteins show that the sum of the molecular weights of the glucitol Enzymes II and III equals that of the mannitol Enzyme II. This observation can be accounted for if it is assumed that a chain termination signal was introduced into the evolving glucitol permease gene but not into the evolving mannitol permease gene. A common evolutionary origin of these two proteins is suggested from these and other observations.

Figure 5.8 also reveals an important functional aspect of the PTS. Each of the energy-coupling proteins of the PTS is actually a phosphoryl carrier protein. Phosphoenolpyruvate first phosphorylates Enzyme I on the N-3 position of the imidazole ring of a histidyl residue; the phosphoryl moiety of phospho-Enzyme I is then transferred to the N-1 position of a histidyl residue in the small heat-stable protein, HPr, and phosphoHPr functions to phosphorylate the N-3 position of a histidyl residue in a sugar-specific protein, either in the C-terminal half of the Enzyme II^{mtl} (Figure 5.8, top) or in the Enzyme III^{gut} (Figure 5.8, bottom). The fourth phosphoryl transfer reaction probably involves transfer to the phosphate group from N-3 of one histidyl residue in Enzyme II^{mtl} to the N-1 position of a different histidyl residue within the

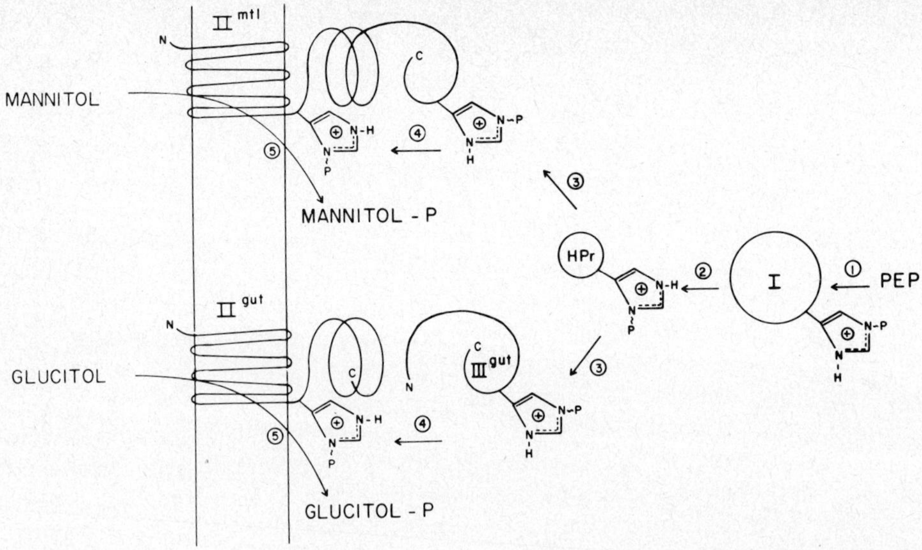

Figure 5.8 Sequential protein phosphorylation reactions of the phosphoryl transfer chains for mannitol (Mtl) and glucitol (Gut) in *E. coli.* The figure shows five phosphoryl transfer reactions which result in the phosphorylation of four distinct protein sites as well as the sugar substrate of the system. Phosphoenolpyruvate (PEP) phosphorylates Enzyme I on the N-3 position of a histidyl residue; Enzyme I then phosphorylates the heat-stable phosphocarrier protein of the PTS, HPr, on the N-1 position of a histidyl residue; the first phosphorylation site on the Enzyme II^{Mtl} and the phosphorylation site on Enzyme III^{Gut} are N-3 histidyl residues, while the second phosphorylation site on the Enzyme II^{Mtl} and the phosphorylation site on Enzyme II^{Gut} are thought to be N-1 histidyl residues. The last phosphoryl transfer reaction involves transfer of the phosphoryl moiety from the N-1 position of a histidyl residue in the Enzyme II to the incoming sugar. The Enzyme II^{Gut}–III^{Gut} pair is shown to be structurally and functionally equivalent to the Enzyme II^{Mtl}. It is proposed that all Enzymes II and Enzyme II–III pairs of the PTS exhibit similar structural features, involve the same sequence of phosphoryl transfer reactions, and catalyze sugar transport by essentially the same mechanisms as illustrated in the figure. These proposals result from their common evolutionary ancestry. (Reproduced with permission from M. H. Saier, Jr., *Mechanisms and Regulation of Carbohydrate Transport in Bacteria,* Academic, New York, 1985.)

N-terminal half of the protein, or in the case of the glucitol system, from N-3 of a histidyl residue in Enzyme III^{gut} to the N-1 position of a histidyl residue in Enzyme II^{gut}. Finally, the last step involves transfer of the phosphoryl group on N-1 histidine of the Enzyme II to the sugar as the latter passes through the membrane.

Structural and functional analyses of many of the proteins of the PTS have led to the realization that all of the sugar-specific proteins, and maybe the general energy-coupling proteins of the system as well, are evolutionarily related. This proposal is shown schematically in Figure 5.9. The complex phosphotransferase system found in *E. coli* may have evolved from a much simpler system, possibly a phosphoenolpyruvate-dependent sugar kinase which, by virtue of its hydrophobic amino acid composition, became membrane-associated in a fashion that allowed the active site to span the

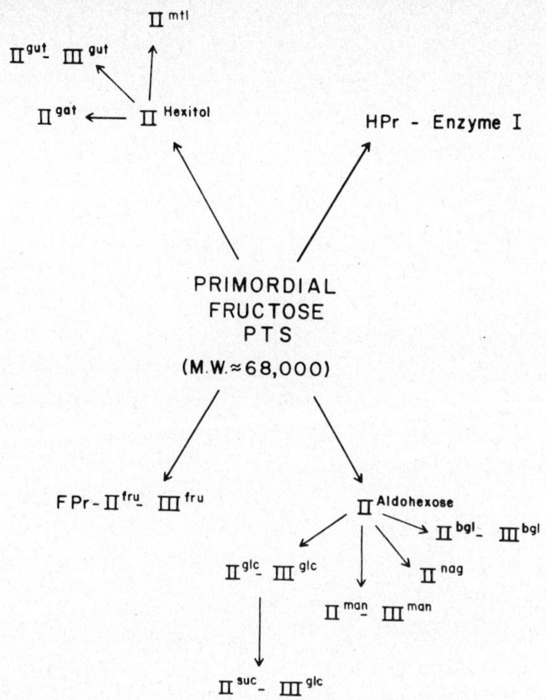

Figure 5.9 Proposed pathway for the evolution of the enzymatic constituents of the phosphotransferase system in *E. coli* and *S. typhimurium*. This scheme is based primarily on the apparent relatedness of the Enzymes II and Enzyme II–III pairs of the *E. coli* PTS. The scheme indicates directionality in the evolutionary process with a fructose PTS (middle) as the primordial system, giving rise to the present-day fructose (*fru*)-specific system (bottom left); to the energy-coupling proteins of the PTS, Enzyme I and HPr (top right); to the hexose-specific systems, including those specific for β-glucosides (*bgl*), *N*-acetylglucosamine (*nag*), mannose (*man*), glucose (*glc*), and sucrose (*suc*) (bottom right); and to the hexitol-specific systems, including those specific for mannitol (*mtl*), glucitol (*gut*), and galactitol (*gat*) (top left). FPr is a fructose-inducible HPr-like protein of the PTS. (Reproduced with permission from M. H. Saier, Jr., *Mechanisms and Regulation of Carbohydrate Transport in Bacteria,* Academic, New York, 1985.)

membrane. Thus, it became possible for the sugar substrate to bind to a portion of the enzyme surface localized to the external leaflet of the phospholipid bilayer, even though the sugar phosphate product was released into the cytoplasm of the cell. In this way, vectorial phosphorylation was accomplished. The anaerobic environment of early biotic earth and the evolution of glycolysis as the first carbohydrate catabolic pathway were responsible for the fact that phosphoenolpyruvate (the end-product of glycolysis) instead of ATP served as the primary phosphoryl donor for sugar uptake. By virtue of the use of this phosphoryl donor for sugar uptake, the PTS plus the enzymes of glycolysis comprise a glycolytic cycle as shown in Figure 5.5.

Early evolutionary events leading to a more complex phosphotransferase system may have involved intragenic duplications, gene duplications (possibly resulting from whole operon duplications) or even entire genome duplications. Gene segmentation events, giving rise to a multigenic system encoding a number of distinct energy-coupling and transport proteins, may have followed.

The proposed pathway for the evolution of the enzymes of the PTS reproduced in Figure 5.9 suggests that the primordial PTS exhibited specificity toward fructose and that it was the duplication of the fructose phosphotransferase gene(s) which led to all of the present-day genes encoding phosphotransferase proteins. These include the *pts* operon, encoding Enzyme I and HPr; the fructose regulon, encoding Enzyme II^{fru} and III^{fru}; the three hexitol phosphotransferases encoded within the three hexitol operons (*mtl, gut,* and *gat*), and the five aldohexose phosphotransferases (Figure 5.9). The central role of fructose in glycolysis, the presence of fructose-specific phosphotransferases in numerous Gram-negative bacteria including primitive photosynthetic, nitrogen-fixing, and heterotrophic bacteria, and the presence of a fructose-inducible HPr-like molecule which is lacking in the other sugar-specific operons encoding PTS proteins—all argue in favor of this postulate.

Mechanistic studies have led to the proposal that the simplest possible mechanism of sugar transport via the phosphotransferase system may be as outlined in Figure 5.10. According to the proposal depicted, there are two routes of sugar phosphorylation: (1) either sugar can bind to the external sugar binding site of the unphosphorylated Enzyme II followed by phosphorylation of the N-1 histidyl residue in the Enzyme II, or (2) phosphorylation may precede sugar binding. Only with sugar bound to the

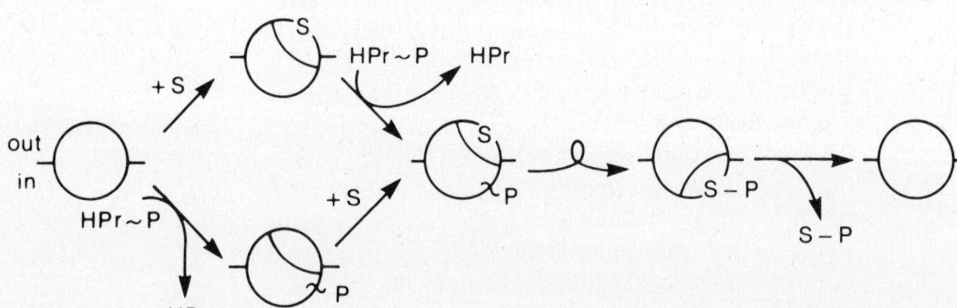

Figure 5.10 Simple mechanism proposed for the transport of a sugar, catalyzed by an Enzyme II of the bacterial phosphotransferase system (PTS). This proposal suggests the involvement of a single protomeric enzyme that can exist either in the free or the phosphorylated state. A more complicated model involves a dimeric enzyme which functions by a half-of-sites mechanism (see text for details). Abbreviations: HPr, heat-stable phosphocarrier protein of the PTS; *S,* sugar substrate of the PTS; *P,* phosphate group. The circle represents an Enzyme II of the PTS which spans the cytoplasmic membrane and can alternately possess a sugar binding site on the external side of the membrane and a sugar–phosphate binding site on the cytoplasmic side of the membrane.

external binding site of the phosphorylated Enzyme II can translocation of sugar across the membrane occur. As shown, the transport event may accompany a conformational change in the enzyme which exposes the sugar and the sugar binding site to the cytoplasmic face of the membrane. This conformational change may, in fact, involve a simple molecular movement of one membrane-imbedded domain of the protein relative to another such domain in a fashion similar to that observed for many soluble proteins. This conformational change presumably occurs concomitantly with and may be driven by the transfer of the phosphoryl moiety from the histidyl residue in the protein to the sugar. The final step is dissociation of the sugar phosphate from the enzyme complex into the cytoplasm so that the enzyme can resume its original conformation and repeat the cycle.

The mechanism proposed in Figure 5.10 may actually be an oversimplification of the true situation. This suggestion results from the interpretation of kinetic studies which led to the conclusion that monomeric Enzyme II may be inactive or at least possess low activity relative to the dimeric enzyme. If the dimer is the active species, then a half-of-sites-type mechanism may be operative. That is, the dimer may be an asymmetric dimer in which the two protein monomers must be catalyzing different reactions at any one time. For example, considering the simplified mechanism shown in Figure 5.10, it may be that one subunit must always have its sugar binding site exposed on the external (periplasmic) side of the membrane, while the other has its substrate-binding site exposed on the internal (cytoplasmic) side of the membrane. This could be a static situation in which case transport would involve transfer of sugar from the binding site on subunit 1 to that on subunit 2. Alternatively, it could be a dynamic situation, in which case each subunit would catalyze the entire cycle shown in Figure 5.10, but the other subunit in the dimeric enzyme would catalyze the opposite reaction. In other words, when the external substrate-binding site of subunit 1 undergoes the conformational change that brings it to the internal surface, subunit 2 must undergo the reverse conformational change which translocates the binding site from its internally exposed location to the external locale. It should be clear that a thorough understanding of these conformational events as they occur in various transport proteins comprise the molecular details of the transport processes.

The evolutionary arguments depicted in Figure 5.9 provide unity to a large number of observations made with the proteins of the PTS and allow one to extrapolate results from one sugar-specific permease to another. To elucidate the mechanism of one PTS permease will probably reveal the mechanisms of them all, because all of these enzymes probably function by essentially the same mechanism. This sort of extrapolation reveals the value of the evolutionary argument and the basis for the enthusiasm and excitement that scientists feel toward the elucidation of evolutionary pathways. Moreover, one should not set one's sights too low. There are numerous suggestions that certain proteins of dissimilar function may also have evolved from a common ancestry. The evolutionary pathways outlined in Figure 5.11 illustrate this important point.

In the preceding discussion, the proteins of the PTS were shown to be bifunctional. They serve both as PEP-dependent sugar kinases (enzymes, E) and sugar permeases (P). The situation is really much more complex, however. Each Enzyme II of the PTS also functions as a chemoreceptor (C) for its sugar substrate because the binding of a

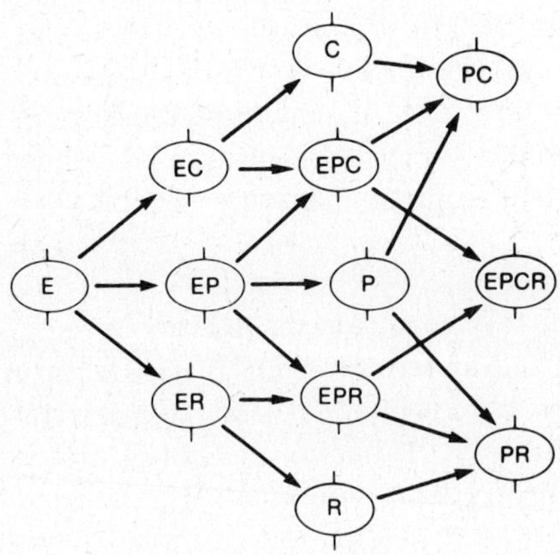

Figure 5.11 Possible pathways for the evolutionary appearance of permeases (P), chemoreceptors (C), regulatory proteins (R), and multifunctional proteins possessing more than one of these functions. All proteins are assumed to be derived originally from metabolic enzymes (E) present in evolving primordial cells. It is proposed that an evolving protein may gain a new function before its original function is lost. Such an event gives rise to multifunctional proteins. Examples of most of the multifunctional proteins depicted are known in present-day organisms. The proteins shown may have evolved as soluble proteins, membrane-associated proteins, or integral constituents of the membrane. Mechanisms allowing evolution of genes coding for proteins of divergent functions may have included (1) nucleotide substitution, (2) gene duplication followed by divergence, and (3) gene fusion and splicing events. (Reproduced with permission from M. H. Saier, Jr., and G. R. Jacobson, *The Molecular Basis of Sex and Differentiation,* Springer-Verlag, New York, 1984.)

sugar substrate to the Enzyme II causes a signal to be transmitted to the bacterial flagellum (the organelle of motility). This signal "informs" the bacterium that a nutrient is present, and that it should swim up the concentration gradient of the sugar. Additionally, the Enzymes II function in a regulatory capacity (R) both to control the activities of other types of carbohydrate permeases in the cell and to be regulated by various stimuli. A single protein therefore functions as an enzyme (E), a permease (P), a chemoreceptor (C), and a regulatory protein (R). Other proteins are known that possess one, two, or three of these functions. Some of these proteins [such as the E protein in Figure 5.7(D)] are permease proteins and chemoreceptors that retain no catalytic or regulatory functions. Others [such as the K protein in Figure 5.7(D)] may possess enzymatic, permease, and regulatory functions but no chemoreception function. These observations lead to the possibility that many proteins serving diverse functions in the cell may show similar structures and even carry out their divergent functions by related mechanisms. This same evolutionary theme will reoccur in future discussions in this chapter and in subsequent chapters in this book.

5.5 REGULATION OF SUGAR TRANSPORT IN BACTERIA

As transmembrane permeation represents the first step in the catabolism of exogenous sugars, one would expect the process to be subject to stringent regulatory control. Five distinct mechanisms are currently recognized for the regulation of sugar uptake in *E. coli.* These mechanisms are illustrated schematically in Figure 5.12(A)–(E).

Since the end-products of sugar metabolism are utilizable sources of intracellular carbon and energy, the ideal situation would be one in which the permeases could sense the energy states and metabolite levels of the cell. These agents would exert negative control over permease function by mechanisms that would be analogous to feedback inhibition of enzyme action. They would prevent the uptake of carbohydrates in excess of the needs of the cell. Bacterial permeases are, in fact, responsive to two

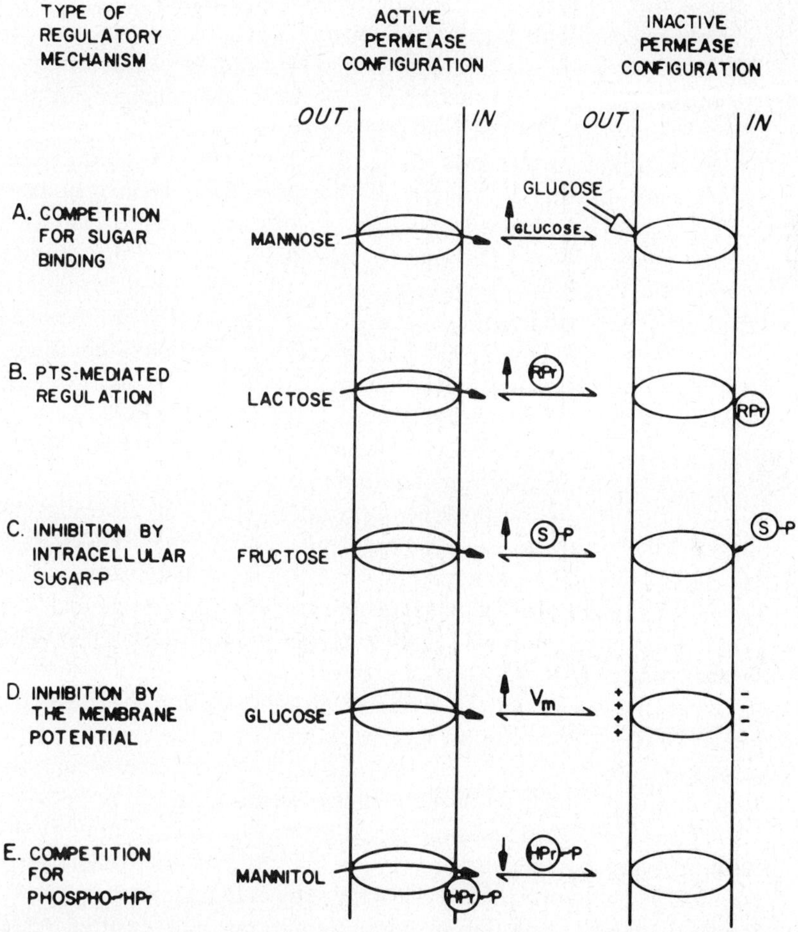

Figure 5.12 Proposed carbohydrate transport regulatory mechanisms in bacteria. Representative examples occur in *E. coli* (see text for explanation). Abbreviations: HPr, histidine-containing protein of the PTS; PTS, phosphoenolpyruvate:sugar phosphotransferase system; RPr, regulatory protein [glucose Enzyme III (Enzyme III^{glc}) of the PTS]; Sugar-P, sugar phosphate; V_m, membrane potential (possibly the proton electrochemical gradient). (Reproduced with permission from S. S. Dills, A. Apperson, M. R. Schmidt, and M. H. Saier, Jr., "Carbohydrate Transport in Bacteria," *Microbiological Reviews,* **44:** 385–418 (1980).

forms of cellular energy, the proton electrochemical gradient, or the electrical component of this gradient, the membrane potential [Figure 5.12(D); see Chapter 7], and a variety of intracellular metabolites such as sugar phosphates and fructose-1,6-diphosphate [Figure 5.12(C)]. Moreover, each extracellular carbohydrate can inhibit the uptake of other carbohydrates by at least three additional mechanisms illustrated in Figure 5.12(A), (B), and (E).

If two sugars bind to the active site and are transported by the same permease protein, then increasing the concentration of one of these two sugars will inhibit the uptake of the second by a simple competitive process. A case in point is the mannose permease, the mannose Enzyme II of the PTS, which binds and transports both mannose and glucose. The presence of glucose in the extracellular medium in which *E. coli* is growing will inhibit mannose uptake [Figure 5.12(A)].

It might be expected that bacterial cells would benefit from mechanisms that allow them to set up a hierarchy of preferred carbon sources. To a first approximation, a preferred carbon source would be one that is readily available and feeds into a major catabolic pathway after a minimal number of metabolic conversions which are catalyzed by inducible enzymes. According to this assumption, glucose is preferred to glycerol or lactose in *E. coli* because the former sugar is concomitantly transported and phosphorylated in a single process, catalyzed by the PEP-dependent phosphotransferase system, and further metabolism is catalyzed by constitutively synthesized enzymes. Lactose, maltose, melibiose, and glycerol, on the other hand, enter the cell by mechanisms that do not couple phosphorylation to transport (see Figure 5.7), and several enzyme-catalyzed metabolic steps are required before these carbohydrates feed into glycolysis. Thus, glucose should regulate the rates of uptake of these carbohydrates by a nonreciprocal mechanism. As we shall see, this is, in fact, the case.

Genetic analyses of this type of transport regulation have suggested the scheme shown in Figure 5.13. A regulating sugar substrate of the PTS appears to interact with a specific membrane protein, the Enzyme II responsible for the transport and phosphorylation of that sugar. Thus, mannitol can interact with the mannitol-specific Enzyme II, glucose interacts with its Enzyme II, and fructose interacts with the Enzyme II specific for fructose. Any one of these interactions is presumed to lead to a change in a central regulatory protein, RPr, and, in some fashion, RPr regulates the activities of the permeases that transport lactose, maltose, melibiose, and glycerol. These interactions occur in a fashion such that the activities of these permeases are inhibited whenever a sugar substrate of the PTS is present in the culture medium.

This scheme was originally based on the analyses of mutant strains that were resistant to transport regulation. In one such mutant that lacked the Enzyme II for mannitol, all transport systems normally subject to regulation by the PTS were found to be insensitive to inhibition by mannitol but were still sensitive to regulation by the other sugar substrates of the PTS. In an analogous mutant that lacked the Enzyme II specific for fructose, all transport systems were resistant to inhibition by fructose, but mannitol and other sugar substrates of the PTS still exerted their normal regulatory effects. These characteristics implicated the Enzymes II as sugar-specific components of the regulatory system.

In a second class of mutants, all transport systems were insensitive to regulation by all sugar substrates of the PTS. These mutants lacked, or were defective for, the

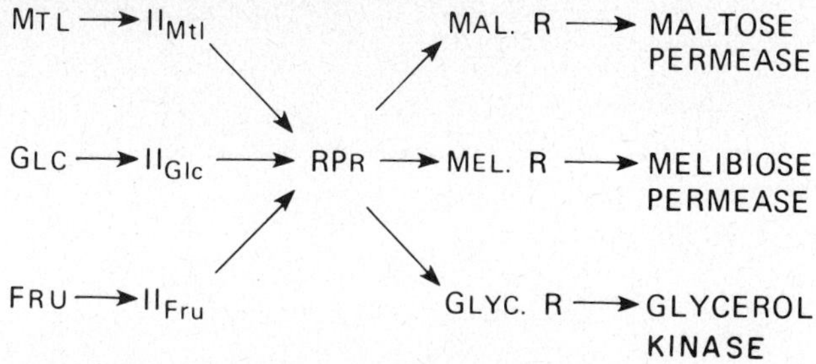

Figure 5.13 Proposed scheme for PTS-mediated transport regulation in bacteria. The scheme suggests that a sugar substrate of the PTS [mannitol (Mtl), glucose (Glc), fructose (Fru)] interacts with the Enzyme II complex in the membrane specific for that particular sugar. The interaction of the sugar with the Enzyme II causes a change in a central regulatory protein, RPr, known to be the Enzyme III^{glc} of the PTS. Finally, RPr interacts with allosteric regulatory domains of the target permeases or catabolite enzymes to control the activities of these transport systems. (Reproduced with permission from M. H. Saier, Jr., and C. D. Stiles, *Molecular Dynamics in Biological Membranes,* Springer-Verlag, New York, 1975.)

central regulatory protein, RPr, which was identified as the glucose Enzyme III, a small, heat-stable, cytoplasmic protein (MW = 20,000). Finally, in a third class of mutants, a single uptake system became resistant to inhibition by all sugar substrates of the PTS, but the other transport systems retained normal sensitivity to inhibition. For example, the lactose permease system specifically was rendered resistant to transport regulation by one such mutation, whereas another mutation abolished regulation of maltose permease activity. Genetic results proved that this last class of mutants resulted from genetic defects in the allosteric regulatory sites associated with the individual permease proteins.

Further genetic and physiological studies showed that mutant strains with reduced cellular levels of Enzyme I or HPr were *hypersensitive* to regulation; exceptionally low concentrations of a sugar substrate of the PTS were sufficient to inhibit transport activity. This observation would be anticipated if the phosphorylation of a cellular constituent catalyzed by Enzyme I and HPr in the presence of PEP *relieved* inhibition. The observations provided evidence for the mechanism shown in Figure 5.14, and subsequent biochemical analyses established the mechanistic features shown in the figure. RPr exists in either of two forms; one is phosphorylated, the other is not. Phosphorylation of RPr can occur as a result of phosphate transfer from phosphoHPr. Only nonphosphorylated RPr interacts with the permeases to inhibit their activities. The regulatory protein, RPr, is normally phosphorylated in energy-sufficient cells that contain PEP but which are growing in a medium that does not contain a sugar substrate of the PTS. Consequently, the transport systems are in their active conformations. However, addition of a PTS-substrate promotes dephosphorylation of RPr, converting it to the free form that can interact with the allosteric regulatory site of the sensitive permeases, thereby inhibiting their activities. In other words, the catalytic activities

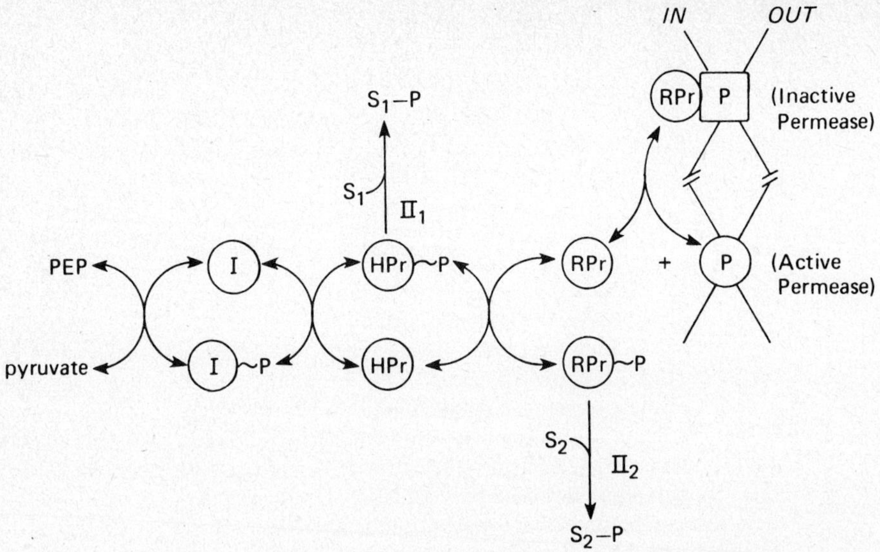

Figure 5.14 Mechanism for the PTS-mediated regulation of permease function in bacteria. The figure illustrates the phosphorylation of the central regulatory protein (RPr), as a result of sequential transfer of phosphate from phosphoenolpyruvate (PEP) to enzyme I (I), to a heat-stable phosphate carrier protein (HPr), and, finally, to RPr. RPr interacts with an allosteric regulatory site on the permease to inhibit its activity. The phosphorylated form of RPr does not bind to or inhibit the permease. Addition of a sugar substrate of the PTS (S_1 or S_2) drains phosphate away from phospho-RPr, converting it to free RPr which interacts with the target permease to inhibit its activity. (Reproduced with permission from M. H. Saier, Jr., and C. D. Stiles, *Molecular Dynamics in Biological Membranes,* Springer-Verlag, New York, 1975).

of the PTS proteins are responsible for the regulation of non-PTS carbohydrate uptake activity.

While the permeases responsible for the uptake of lactose, melibiose, and maltose are the direct targets of RPr action, the glycerol permease is not. Instead, the first enzyme of glycerol metabolism, glycerol kinase, is the target of RPr inhibition. Because glycerol kinase effectively "traps" the cytoplasmic glycerol by phosphorylating it (see Section 3.9), RPr controls glycerol uptake.

Because its conversion to fructose-1,6-diphosphate is catalyzed by constitutively synthesized enzymes, glucose is also preferred to other sugar substrates of the phosphotransferase system such as mannitol and glucitol. A distinct mechanism for setting up a hierarchy of preferred PTS substrates involves competition for the common phosphoryl carrier protein of the PTS, phosphoHPr [Figure 5.12(E)]. The preferred carbon sources are those that are transported by the predominant sugar-specific permeases and possess high affinity for phosphoHPr. Because the basal level of the glucose-specific system is relatively high, and because this system apparently has high affinity for phosphoHPr, glucose is utilized preferentially to other sugar substrates of the PTS.

Experiments conducted with Gram-positive bacteria have shown that protein kinase-catalyzed, ATP-dependent phosphorylation of a seryl residue in HPr can selectively inhibit utilization of one PTS sugar relative to another and that PTS permeases themselves are allosterically regulated. Because the protein kinase is specifically activated by fructose-1,6-diphosphate, inhibition of PTS-function is actually sensitive to the levels of metabolites present in the cytoplasm of the cell. The inhibitory effects of phosphorylation of the regulatory seryl residue in HPr on sugar uptake via the PTS is a novel type of feedback inhibition mediated by a metabolite-sensitive protein kinase. The complete feedback loop is shown in Figure 5.15.

When ATP is generated anaerobically via glycolysis or when electrons are allowed to flow down the electron transport chain of the bacterium, a transmembrane proton electrochemical gradient, the electrical component of which is termed the *membrane potential* is generated. It has been long recognized that many permease activities in bacteria are controlled by this *chemiosmotic* source of energy. For example, most of the Enzymes II of the PTS are inhibited when the magnitude of the proton electrochemical gradient is large. Although the mechanism of this regulatory interaction is not known, one simple explanation is that the electrical dipole moments of the Enzymes II interact with the membrane potential in a way which influences the conformation of the protein. This possibility is illustrated in Figure 5.16. The form of the protein with the vectorial component of its dipole moment more parallel but opposite in sign to the transmembrane electric field must be the less active conformation.

Another possible mechanism recently proposed involves the membrane potential-driven oxidation of a pair of sulfhydryl groups in the enzyme. According to this hypothesis, while the reduced form would be expected to possess maximal activity, the

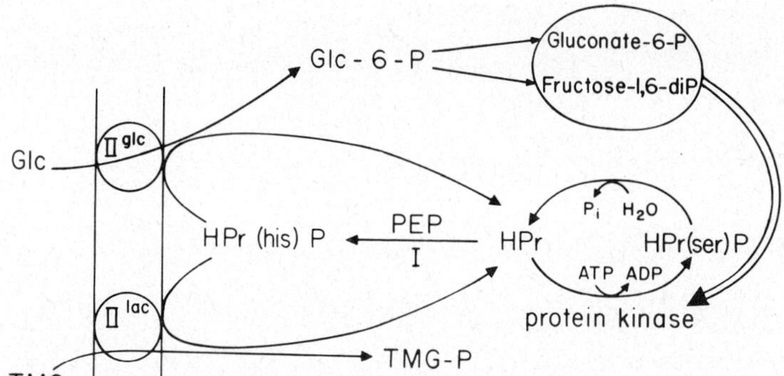

Figure 5.15 Feed-back loop controlling sugar uptake via the phosphotransferase system in Gram-positive bacteria. External sugar [glucose (Glc)] enters the cell and is phosphorylated to glucose-6-P at the expense of phosphoryl-histidyl-HPr, [HPr(his)P]. Glucose-6-P is converted to fructose-1,6-diphosphate and gluconate-6-P which activate a protein kinase. The kinase phosphorylates a seryl residue in HPr, thereby preventing phosphorylation of the histidyl residue in HPr by PEP and Enzyme I (I). Consequently, the uptake of various sugar substrates of the phosphotransferase system such as glucose and TMG (thiomethyl-β-galactoside, a nonmetabolizable analogue of lactose) is inhibited by the protein kinase. An HPr(ser)P phosphatase hydrolyzes the HPr(ser)P bond to regenerate free HPr.

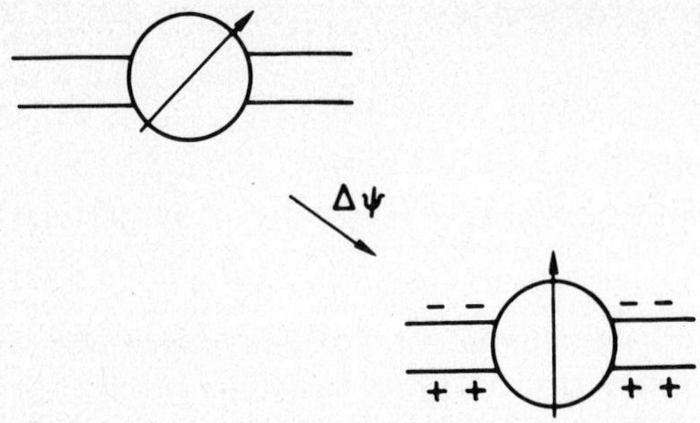

Figure 5.16 Theoretical effect of an imposed membrane potential on the dipole moment of a transmembrane protein. If the electrical dipole of the protein is nonperpendicular to the plane of the membrane, imposition of an electrical potential ($\Delta\psi$) across the membrane will tend to convert the protein to a conformation with its dipole more perpendicular to the plane of the membrane. If these two conformations differ in biological transport activity, the permease or channel protein will be regulated by the membrane potential. The figure is meant to imply a conformational change in the protein, not rotation of the protein in the phospholipid bilayer. (Reproduced with permission from *The Molecular Basis of Sex and Differentiation,* by M. H. Saier, Jr. and G. R. Jacobson, Springer-Verlag, New York, 1984).

oxidized form would be inactive or less active. Further experimentation will be required to determine if sulfhydryl oxidation accounts for the chemiosmotic control of permease function.

5.6 HEXOSE TRANSPORT AND PHOSPHORYLATION IN EUKARYOTES

Eukaryotes (unicellular eukaryotic protists, fungi, plants, and animals) do not possess a phosphotransferase system. Instead, glucose and other hexoses are transported across the membrane without modification by transport carriers. Kinetic analyses have revealed that there are three types of sugar carriers in eukaryotes. First, *facilitators* stereospecifically bind the sugar substrates and equilibrate the sugar across the membrane without accumulating it against the concentration gradient. This process is not coupled to metabolic energy. Well-characterized species of yeast, most animal cell types, and some plant cells transport glucose by this mechanism. A second mechanism involves *sugar:Na^+ cotransport* analogous to that catalyzed by the melibiose permease in *E. coli* [Figure 5.7(C)]. Some intestinal and kidney epithelial cells accumulate sugars cytoplasmically because tight coupling of Na^+ transport to sugar transport allows the flow of Na^+ down its concentration gradient to be coupled to the active accumulation of sugar, up its concentration gradient. Finally some algal and fungal cells accumulate sugars by *sugar:H⁺ symport* (cotransport) as is illustrated for the *E. coli* lactose permease in Figure 5.7(B).

As noted above, hexose transport into most animal cells is mediated by a protein-facilitated, energy-independent, stereospecific, saturable process. The permease responsible for this activity is a transmembrane glycoprotein of about 55,000 molecular weight with about 20% of its mass as carbohydrate chains attached to that part of the polypeptide which is localized to the external face of the membrane. The protein appears to associate to form a dimer or a tetramer in the phospholipid bilayer of native membranes.

A limited number of sugar permease proteins are present in the plasma membranes of animal cells, the number ranging from about 2,000 to about 100,000 transport proteins per μm^2 of membrane surface area, depending on the tissue type. In some tissues (mammalian liver, bone, erythrocytes) the transport rate is rapid relative to the sugar phosphorylating activity of the cellular hexokinases. In these tissues the intracellular glucose level is high, kinase activity is rate limiting for metabolism, and transport is not regulated. In other tissues (mammalian muscle and fat tissues, nucleated erythrocytes) transport is slow relative to kinase activity, the intracellular glucose levels are low, and transport is subject to metabolic and hormonal regulation. For example, in mammalian muscle and fat, insulin greatly stimulates transport activity, while in muscle and avian erythrocytes, metabolite depletion stimulates transport. Insulin stimulation of transport is rapid and results in an increased V_{max} due to the translocation of *cryptic* intracellularly localized permeases to the cell surface upon exposure of the cell to insulin. The mechanism by which insulin effects this regulatory change is unknown, but a protein kinase-mediated phosphorylation event has been proposed to be involved. This proposal is strengthened by the demonstration that a tyrosyl protein kinase activity is associated with the insulin receptor.

Some studies point to ATP as the metabolite controlling metabolite-sensitive glucose transport in muscle and nerve cells as well as in avian erythrocytes. In contrast to the effects of insulin, regulatory responses to ATP appear to alter the Km of the permease for the substrate sugar, sometimes by several fold. Because nonmetabolizable ATP analogues could not effect these changes, a phosphorylation mechanism has been proposed. It is clear, however, that more extensive biochemical studies, preferably with purified, reconstituted transporter, will be required to establish the regulatory mechanisms involved.

Another kinetically well-characterized glucose facilitator is found in the yeast, *Saccharomyces cerevisiae* (common brewer's, or baker's, yeast). In yeast, as in mammalian tissues, the activity of the facilitator is subject to regulatory control, but by a unique mechanism which apparently couples the activity of the facilitator to that of the sugar kinase. Sugar entry can occur by both a low-affinity process and a high-affinity process. Genetic evidence has been presented suggesting that both processes are mediated by the same transport protein. When a sugar kinase is associated with the cytoplasmic face of the facilitator, uptake exhibits high-affinity kinetics; when no kinase is associated with the facilitator, low-affinity kinetics are observed. It is not known whether binding of the kinase to the facilitator *allosterically* controls the conformation and activity of the transporter, or if the facilitator and kinase function in conjunction, by a *concerted* mechanism to bring sugar into the cell. Several studies have shown that low-affinity sugar transport is accompanied by release of free, externally derived sugar into the cytoplasm, while high-affinity transport results in the release of the sugar phosphate into the cytoplasmic pool. A tightly coupled process of transport and ATP-dependent phosphorylation, mediated by a complex of the facilitator and kinase seems likely. Thus, the process of sugar transport in yeast may resemble that mediated by the phosphotransferase system in bacteria from a physiological standpoint, even though the enzymatic machinery and mechanism are entirely different.

5.7 INITIATION OF SUGAR METABOLISM IN PROKARYOTES AND EUKARYOTES

Due to the presence of the phosphotransferase system (PTS) in most bacteria that can ferment sugars anaerobically via the glycolytic cycle and the absence of any such system in eukaryotic organisms, the pathways for the initial metabolism of these sugars in the two major cell types are markedly different. Some of these pathways are summarized in Table 5.3. All bacteria that utilize fructose via the PTS phosphorylate this sugar on the 1-hydroxyl group. By contrast, eukaryotes and bacteria lacking a phosphotransferase system transport the free sugar across the membrane and phosphorylate it on the 6-hydroxyl employing ATP and a hexokinase or fructokinase. In bacteria

TABLE 5.3 DIFFERENCES BETWEEN SUGAR METABOLIC PATHWAYS IN BACTERIA AND MAMMALIAN CELLS[a]

Substrate sugar	Bacteria	Mammalian cells
Fructose	Fructose ↓ PTS Fructose-1-P ↓ Fructose-1-P kinase Fructose-1,6-di-P	Fructose ↓ Hexokinase Fructose-6-P ↓ P-Fructokinase Fructose-1,6-di-P
N-Acetylglucosamine	*N*-Acetylglucosamine ↓ PTS *N*-Acetylglucosamine-6-P ↓ NAG-6-P deacetylase Acetate + glucosamine-6-P	*N*-Acetylglucosamine ↓ NAG deacetylase Acetate + glucosamine ↓ Hexokinase Glucosamine-6-P
Hexitols (glucitol, mannitol, galactitol)	Hexitol ↓ PTS Hexitol-P ↓ Hexitol-P dehydrogenase Hexose-P	Hexitol ↓ Hexitol dehydrogenase Hexose ↓ Hexokinase Hexose-6-P
Sucrose	Sucrose ↓ PTS Sucrose-P	Sucrose ↓ Sucrase Fructose + glucose

[a] Bacteria which do not catabolize sugars via the phosphotransferase system employ metabolic pathways resembling those found in mammalian cells.

possessing a fructose-specific PTS, the enzyme, fructose-1-P kinase phosphorylates the 1-monophosphate ester to fructose-1,6-diphosphate (FDP). Phosphofructokinase (fructose-6-P kinase), a distinct enzyme, converts the 6-monophosphate ester of fructose to FDP whenever fructose-6-P arises.

In bacteria, *N*-acetylglucosamine is first phosphorylated via the PTS and then deacetylated to glucosamine-6-P. This derivative is then deaminated to fructose-6-P, which can be phosphorylated to FDP. In mammals *N*-acetylglucosamine is first deacetylated and then phosphorylated. Because all hexokinases catalyze phosphorylation of this hexosamine, usually at rates appreciably slower than the rates of glucose phosphorylation, a distinct kinase is not required.

In bacteria hexitols are phosphorylated via the PTS to hexitol phosphates and then oxidized. Glucitol-6-P and mannitol-1-P, for example, are both oxidized in NAD^+-dependent, dehydrogenase-catalyzed reactions to fructose-6-P. By contrast, galactitol-6-P is oxidized to a similar hexose phosphate, D-tagatose-6-P which differs from fructose-6-P only with respect to the orientation of the 4-hydroxyl group. Phosphofructokinase is responsible for phosphorylating tagatose-6-P to tagatose-1,6-diP. A novel aldolase, called hexose diphosphate aldolase, different from the usual FDP aldolase, then cleaves tagatose-1,6-diP to dihydroxyacetone-P and glyceraldehyde-3-P. Galactitol is therefore metabolized via a pathway which initially functions in parallel with the usual glycolytic enzymes. In eukaryotes and bacteria lacking a PTS, hexitols are first oxidized to hexoses and then phosphorylated by the appropriate ATP-dependent kinase.

The last sugar listed in Table 5.3 is sucrose. The phosphotransferase system phosphorylates sucrose on the 6-hydroxyl of the glucose moiety as the disaccharide is transported across the membrane. Subsequently, the sucrose phosphate is hydrolyzed to glucose-6-P and fructose. Eukaryotic cells utilize this common sugar by a pathway that first involves hydrolysis of the disaccharide to glucose and fructose. Hexokinases then phosphorylate these sugars.

The comparisons noted in Table 5.3 suggest that the phosphotransferase system may be useful for the development of novel antibiotics which are innocuous to animals. Any sugar analogue that can be transported and phosphorylated by the PTS but not by animals may be toxic to pathogenic bacteria without harming the host organism. Because of the wide range of substrates utilized by the PTS, this approach may be of great value in attempts to control bacterial infections.

5.8 HEXOKINASE

The second process, or first chemical reaction, in the glycolytic cycle in all eukaryotic cells and in some bacteria, is the phosphorylation of glucose to glucose-6-phosphate in a reaction that involves transfer of the γ-phosphoryl moiety of ATP to the sugar (Section 5.1). Because the equilibrium of this reaction lies far to the right ($\Delta G^{0\prime} = -4.0$ kcal/mole), the reaction is essentially irreversible. The phosphorylation of hexoses serves two purposes: first, it allows metabolites of glucose to be trapped within the cytoplasm—phosphorylated glucose cannot cross the cell membrane because no transport system in the plasma membranes of eukaryotic cells recognizes this compound, and, second, this phosphorylation event as well as the one catalyzed by phosphofructokinase (Figure 5.5, step 3), activates the 6-carbon sugar molecule for its eventual cleavage into two triose phosphates, glyceraldehyde-3-phosphate and dihydroxyacetone phosphate.

Enzymes that phosphorylate glucose, fructose, and mannose with comparable specific activities are called hexokinases (HK). Those that are most active with glucose are designated glucokinases and those that are most active with fructose are called fructokinases. Thus, the nomenclature for these enzymes corresponds to their preferences for sugar substrates. Mammalian tissues house four kinases which act on hexoses. Three of these are present in most mammalian tissues with differing levels of activity. HKI predominates in brain and red blood cells; HKII possesses its highest specific activity in muscle, and HKIII is most active in the liver, lung, and spleen. Glucokinase is present only in the liver. Yeast hexokinases appear in two native forms. A third yeast enzyme is specific for glucose.

Bacteria also contain a variety of hexokinases. For example, *E. coli* contains two such enzymes. One is a glucokinase which phosphorylates only glucose and to a lesser extent glucosamine. The other is a mannofructokinase which phosphorylates the four hexoses with the following order of efficiency: Mannose > fructose > glucose > glucosamine. This enzyme cannot be considered to be an ordinary hexokinase because glucose is phosphorylated only 10% as well as mannose. In contrast to the situation in eukaryotic cells, the kinases present in *E. coli* possess activities that are insufficient to allow maximal growth rates on exogenous hexoses. The phosphotransferase system functions in the utilization of exogenous hexoses, and the sole function of the hexose kinases is phosphorylation of endogenously generated hexoses; that is, hexoses generated from the cytoplasmic hydrolysis of disaccharides such as maltose, lactose, and sucrose, oligosaccharides such as the maltooligosaccharides, and polysaccharides such as glycogen.

The structure–function relationships of all known hexo- and glucokinases are similar. The binding sites of these proteins consist of a deep cleft between two asymmetrically situated lobes. Asymmetric association of these domains allows for nonsymmetrical interaction with both the sugar and ATP. Asymmetry may also be important for purposes of control. Upon binding of a sugar substrate, the upper lobe rotates about 12° relative to the lower lobe, trapping the substrate in its binding site. This conformational change serves to insure substrate specificity because only the correct substrate, a hexose, will allow proper closing of the cleft.

Rotation of the lobes of hexokinases is also necessary for catalysis. As the lobes come together, they promote binding of ATP to the upper lobe so that it is brought within range for nucleophilic attack by the C—6 hydroxyl group of the sugar substrate. When the lobes close, only the 6-hydroxyl group, to which the γ-phosphoryl group of ATP will be transferred, remains exposed to the aqueous environment.

The phosphoryl transfer reactions catalyzed by all hexokinases occur by essentially the same mechanism. The ATP phosphoryl donor is situated above the captive substrate so that an in-line addition–elimination reaction will occur. This means that the nucleophile (the electronegative 6-hydroxyl group of the sugar) attacks the phosphorous atom directly opposite the bond to the leaving group (ADP). A pentavalent intermediate is formed (Figure 5.17) which has a trigonal bipyrimidal configuration. The nucleophile

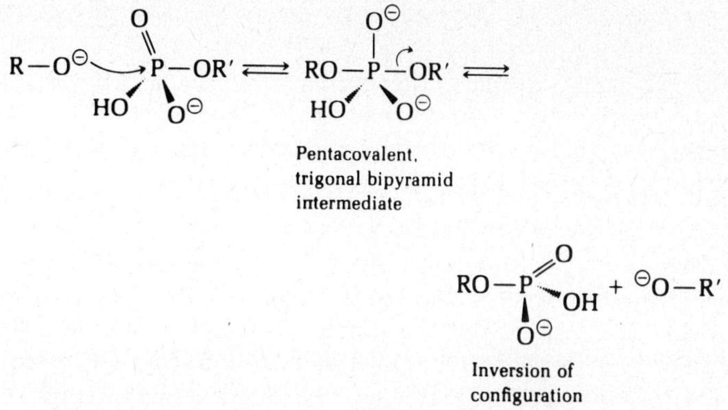

Figure 5.17 In-line mechanism for addition–elimination in a nucleophilic substitution reaction at tetravalent phosphorous. The reactions catalyzed by hexokinase, phosphofructokinase, and glycerate kinase are representative of this mechanism. This sequential reaction mechanism always proceeds via a pentacovalent trigonal bipyramid intermediate with inversion of configuration as shown. The anionic form of the attacking hydroxyl group is shown.

and the leaving group occupy apical positions. Loss of ADP results in inversion of configuration of the phosphoryl group (Figure 5.17).

The two yeast hexokinases exist both as active monomers and active dimers, but the dimers exhibit higher catalytic potential than the monomers. The kinetic mechanism of all hexokinase reactions is essentially an ordered, bi–bi sequential mechanism with the formation of the appropriate ternary complex of enzyme, sugar, and MgATP leading to product formation. The affinity and rate of nucleoside triphosphate binding are enhanced by the presence of enzyme-bound sugar. Further, sugar binding renders the γ-phosphoryl group of ATP more labile. For example, the binding of xylose, which structurally resembles the first five carbons of glucose, stimulates ATP hydrolysis. It is presumed that glucose induces a conformational change in the enzyme which promotes ATP binding and reactivity. An "induced fit"-type mechanism is implied.

There are two distinct types of ATP binding sites associated with yeast hexokinase, one which functions in allosteric regulation (the I site) and the other which functions catalytically (the A site). While there is one catalytic binding site per subunit, a single I site lies between the subunits of the dimer. It binds allosteric activators and is believed to function by promoting stabilization of the more active dimeric form.

A comparison of yeast and mammalian hexokinases reveals a number of interesting differences. For instance, while the yeast enzymes are active both as monomers and as dimers with a monomer molecular weight of 50,000, mammalian hexokinases are single polypeptide enzymes with molecular weights of 100,000. It has been hypothesized that the mammalian enzymes arose from ancestors resembling the yeast enzymes as a result of gene duplication and fusion.

The regulation of brain hexokinase (HKI), the most carefully characterized of the mammalian hexokinases, differs from that of the yeast enzymes. First, it appears that brain hexokinase is allosterically inhibited by ADP which binds to a regulatory site distinct from the catalytic site. Second, an inhibitory effect of glucose-6-P is lessened by inorganic phosphate. While noncompetitive inhibition by the nucleotide pool provides coarse control of glycolysis in mammalian brain cells, the delicate interaction between glucose-6-P and inorganic phosphate may provide a means to more finely control glycolysis in response to the energy needs of the cell.

5.9 PHOSPHOGLUCOISOMERASE (PGI)

Phosphoglucoisomerase (PGI) catalyzes the second glycolytic reaction, transforming glucose-6-P, an aldose phosphate, into fructose-6-P, a ketose phosphate. This reaction frees the C—1 hydroxyl group of the sugar for phosphorylation in the next step in the cycle. The enzyme is specific for glucose-6-P and fructose-6-P, and cannot isomerize other sugars. Although PGI utilizes straight-chain sugars, the ring sugars are probably the preferred substrates.

The first step in the PGI reaction is the opening of the pyranose ring of glucose-6-P (Figure 5.18). In this step, the 1-hydroxyl group loses a proton to the medium to produce the straight-chain aldose. In order to facilitate this ring opening, a cationic lysyl residue donates a proton to the ring oxygen generating a hydroxyl group on C—5 [Figure 5.18, step (a)].

Once the aldehydic form of the substrate has been generated, isomerization can proceed. The next step, common to all aldose–ketose isomerization reactions, involves the formation of a *cis*-enediol anionic intermediate [Figure 5.18, step (b)]. The nucleophile is an imidazole nitrogen of a histidyl residue. A proton is extracted from C—2 of the substrate adjacent to the newly generated carbonyl (C—1), leaving a free electron pair to form a double bond between C—2 and C—1. The π electron pair of the carbonyl group at C—1 is displaced to oxygen in the process. The negatively charged oxygen then extracts a proton from the medium. This 1-hydroxyl group will be phosphorylated in the next step of glycolysis.

The isomerization reaction is continued in a general acid-catalyzed reaction involving a protonated, active site histidyl residue of the enzyme [Figure 5.18, step (c)]. An electron pair on the C—2 oxygen forms the new carbonyl bond, and the π electron pair of the C—C double bond is displaced to C—1. The resulting carbanion then extracts a proton from the active-site histidyl residue in the enzyme. This completes the tautomerization reaction. The success of this isomerization reaction rests on the ability of the enediol intermediate to tautomerize freely between aldo- and keto-configurations.

In the final step of this reaction [Figure 5.18, step (d)], the straight-chain fructose-6-P molecule cyclizes by nucleophilic attack of the C—5 hydroxyl group on the carbonyl generated in the preceding step. A proton is transferred to the lysyl residue which originally participated in the ring opening. The enzyme preferentially catalyzes closure of the ring to form the α-anomer of fructose-6-P. Thus, the furanose product is generated, and the participating amino acyl residues are properly restored to their original forms. Because the change in free energy of this reaction is small, the reaction is freely reversible. The enzyme does not appear to play a regulatory role in glycolysis although

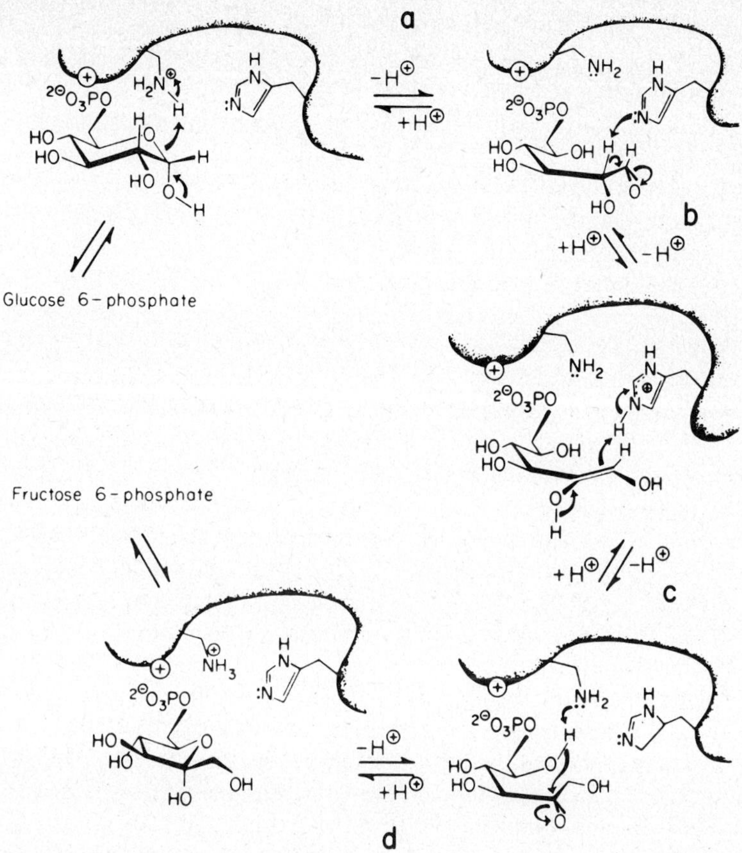

Figure 5.18 Stepwise mechanism for the reaction catalyzed by phosphoglucoisomerase. (Reproduced with permission from E. A. Noltmann, "Aldose-ketose isomerases," in *The Enzymes,* Vol VI, Third Edition, p. 300, P. D. Boyer, ed., Academic, New York, 1972.)

several intermediates of the pentose phosphate pathway (see Chapter 6) inhibit its activity.

All known phosphoglucose isomerases are dimeric proteins consisting of two identical subunits. There are no isozymic forms of PGI in mammals, so the enzyme derived from different tissues is the same. There are three yeast PGI isozymes, but they exhibit no striking differences in their physicochemical or catalytic properties.

5.10 PHOSPHOFRUCTOKINASE (PFK)

Phosphofructokinase (PFK) phosphorylates β-D-fructose-6-phosphate with MgATP to yield β-D-fructose-1,6-diP and ADP. This reaction represents the first step that is general to all of the sugars metabolized via glycolysis. It is a physiologically irreversible step which is subject to strict regulatory control in virtually all living organisms. Uptake of the sugar from the extracellular medium, initial phosphorylation, and the PFK-catalyzed reaction probably represent the most important allosteric control points within the glycolytic cycle.

PFK exhibits a sequential reaction mechanism suggesting that both substrates bind simultaneously to the surface of the enzyme before reaction can occur. The in-line phosphoryl transfer reaction catalyzed by this enzyme is mechanistically analogous to that catalyzed by hexokinase and glucokinase (Section 5.8). PFK exhibits broad specificities for the sugar phosphate–phosphoryl acceptor, the nucleoside triphosphate–phosphoryl donor, and the activating divalent cation. β-D-Fructofuranose-6-P and ATP are the preferred substrates, while Mg^{++} gives maximal activation. A few bacteria and eukaryotic microorganisms utilize pyrophosphate instead of ATP as the phosphoryl donor. These enzymes may be remnants of primordial PFKs which utilized this inorganic, high-energy phosphoryl donor to phosphorylate their substrate.

The regulatory constraints imposed on phosphofructokinases are species specific. For example, ATP is an allosteric inhibitor of the enzymes in virtually all animal and plant tissues as well as in yeast and *E. coli,* but PFKs from many microorganisms are not regulated by this indicator of cellular energy state. AMP, ADP, and inorganic phosphate (P_i) are allosteric activators of ATP-inhibitable PFKs, counteracting the inhibitory effect of ATP. Citrate, an intermediate of the Krebs cycle, may be an allosteric inhibitor of the enzymes in animal and plant tissues but those of many microorganisms are insensitive to this compound. In general, microbial PFKs are controlled by fewer effectors than are those of higher organisms.

When PFKs from most animal and plant sources as well as those from yeast and *E. coli* are studied kinetically, a plot of reaction rate versus fructose-6-P concentration gives a sigmoidal curve. This observation suggests cooperative interactions between subunits. Native PFK from mammalian tissues is a tetramer of 320,000 molecular weight which dissociates to inactive dimers (MW = 160,000) and monomers (MW = 80,000). All substrates and positive allosteric effectors have been shown to promote association to the tetramer, but the physiologically relevant regulatory properties of mammalian PFKs are probably inherent to the tetramer. Dissociation–association phenomena are too slow to account for the conformational changes induced by effectors.

Virtually all living organisms that have been examined contain more than a single isozyme of PFK. Human tissues contain at least four PFK isozymes, while *E. coli* contains two. Of the mammalian PFKs, that from liver is more sensitive to inhibition by ATP than is the muscle enzyme, and the PFK from brain is least sensitive of all. Only citrate and isocitrate of the Krebs cycle intermediates inhibit the muscle enzyme, but brain PFK is inhibited by *cis*-aconitate, malate, succinate, and α-ketoglutarate as well. These Krebs cycle intermediates act synergistically with ATP. Moreover, a variety of phosphorylated compounds affect the activity of the enzyme either positively or negatively. While fructose-6-P and fructose-1,6-diP activate the enzyme, phosphocreatine, 3-phosphoglycerate, 2-phosphoglycerate, 2,3-diphosphoglycerate, and phosphoenolpyruvate all inhibit in the presence of ATP by a synergistic mechanism. The synergism apparently results from the cooperative binding of these agents. The binding of ATP enhances the affinity of the enzyme for the Krebs cycle and glycolytic intermediates, and vice versa.

Direct binding studies have established that each subunit of the tetrameric muscle PFK binds fructose-6-P and ATP at the substrate-catalytic site. There are at least three distinct regulatory binding sites. One is the ATP-regulatory site, the second is specific for Krebs cycle intermediates, and the third binds inorganic phosphate and possibly the glycolytic intermediates. Phosphorylated adenosine activators (AMP and ADP) probably bind to the ATP regulatory site but induce a different conformational change. The synergism noted between ATP and citrate, AMP and FDP, and ADP and P_i have been shown to be due to actual increases in the binding affinity of the enzyme for the first effector when the second member of the pair is added to the enzyme–effector complex.

In order to account for these regulatory effects, specific models have been proposed. Because the principles are essentially the same for PFKs from a variety of biological sources, a single model will be presented. This model is based on the enzyme from yeast which does not undergo association–dissociation reactions, is sensitive to fewer regulatory agents than the mammalian enzyme, and has been characterized in considerable kinetic detail.

Although the yeast PFK resembles the mammalian enzyme mechanistically and is simpler in terms of its kinetic behavior, its structure is actually more complex. It has a net molecular weight of about 900,000 and contains two immunologically non-crossreacting types of subunits designated α (MW = 118,000) and β (MW = 112,000). It is apparently an octamer containing four α and four β subunits. Four identical subunits form a tetrameric core, and the other four subunits are peripherally located (i.e., $\alpha_2\beta_4\alpha_2$ or $\beta_2\alpha_4\beta_2$). Like the mammalian enzyme, there are both catalytic and regulatory binding sites for ATP, AMP, and ADP. The latter two adenine nucleotides counteract the inhibitory effect of ATP. Fructose-6-P relieves the inhibition by ATP. Unlike the mammalian enzyme, however, yeast PFK is insensitive or only slightly sensitive to regulation by FDP and citrate. Another difference between the yeast and mammalian enzymes is the fact that the cooperative (sigmoidal) nature of the velocity *versus* fructose-6-P concentration curve for yeast PFK is not altered by adenine nucleotides (ATP, AMP, or ADP).

In general, PFKs from various sources are believed to exist in either of two principal conformations, R or T, at any one time. Each of these two principal conformations has at least two and possibly more subconformations, designated, R_1, R_2, . . . , R_n and T_1, T_2, . . . , T_n. While multiple subconformations are likely, and a non-concerted mechanism of subunit interconversion best fits the data for at least some of the mammalian enzymes, a simpler model with just two subconformations and concerted interconversions adequately describes the kinetic data for the yeast enzyme (Figure 5.19).

In the proposed mechanism, the substrate, fructose-6-P, binds to R_1 and T_1, but not to R_2 or T_2. The former two conformations of the enzyme exhibit different affinities for fructose-6-P but identical maximal activities. ATP as substrate appears to bind to all four forms of the enzyme with equal affinity. As a negative effector, ATP binds only to R_2 and T_2. The addition of ATP therefore inhibits PFK by shifting the equilibrium in favor of R_2 and T_2, which do not bind fructose-6-P and therefore are catalytically inactive. By contrast, AMP and ADP activate PFK because they bind to the active R_1 and T_1 forms with higher affinity than to the inactive R_2 and T_2 forms.

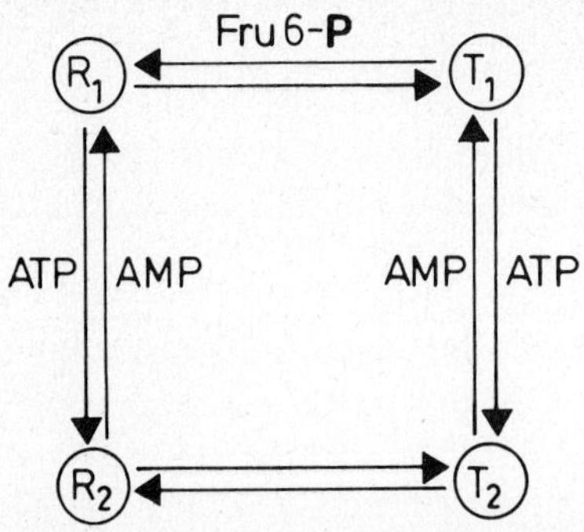

Figure 5.19 Schematic depiction of a four-state model explaining the allosteric transitions of yeast phosphofructokinase. R and T are the two principal conformations of the enzyme. Each of these principal conformations can exist in either of two subconformations (1 and 2). (Reproduced with permission from E. Hofmann and G. Kopperschlager, "Phosphofructokinase in Yeast," in *Methods in Enzymology,* Vol. 90, Carbohydrate Metabolism, Part E, W. A. Wood, ed., Academic, New York, 1982.)

Consequently, they oppose and can reverse the inhibitory effect of ATP. The effect of ADP in counteracting ATP inhibition is much less pronounced than that of AMP, first because it binds to the enzyme less tightly, and second because the difference in its affinity for R_1 and T_1 versus R_2 and T_2 is only slight. Thus, the allosteric equilibrium between R and T is influenced primarily by fructose-6-P whereas the adenine nucleotides influence only the equilibria between the subconformations.

In *E. coli* two distinct genes encode the two phosphofructokinases found in the cytoplasm of this organism. These two genes, designated *pfkA* (encoding PFK1) and *pfkB* (encoding PFK2) map at opposite sides of the circular bacterial chromosome, at 87 min. and 38 min., respectively. To account for these and other "coincidental" map positions it has been hypothesized that the primordial bacterial chromosome was once one-quarter of its present size, and it duplicated twice, giving rise to the four quadrants of the present-day chromosome which could independently diverge and evolve. If this hypothesis is correct, the two *pfk* genes may have arisen from a single primordial gene following the second chromosomal duplication. The similar subunit sizes and substrate K_M values of the two enzymes provide support for this hypothesis. However, the enzymes also exhibit differences. PFK1 is a nondissociable tetramer, while PFK2 is a dimer that can associate to a less-active tetramer in the presence of nucleoside di- and triphosphates. Dissociation to the PFK2 dimer occurs in the presence of fructose-6-P. The two enzymes show little immunological cross-reactivity and do not hybridize to form heterooligomers.

The mechanism of *E. coli* PFK1 regulation is analogous to that of the mammalian and yeast enzymes although less complex. The enzyme appears to undergo a concerted transition between a T_4 and an R_4 state. R_4 has greater affinity for fructose-6-P than does T_4, accounting for the sigmoidal activity response to fructose-6-P concentration in the presence of ATP. Both T_4 and R_4 are presumed to bind ATP with equal affinity. PFK2 does not exhibit sigmoidal kinetics with respect to fructose-6-P concentration, presumably because the T_4 to R_4 transition does not occur.

The two enzymes differ not only in their regulatory properties but also with respect to the regulation of their syntheses. PFK1 is synthesized in larger amounts under anaerobic conditions in the presence of a sugar such as glucose. PFK2 is synthesized constitutively, so that the rate of its synthesis is not influenced by the composition of the growth medium. Consequently, PFK1 is thought of as the anaerobic enzyme (involved in glycolysis under anaerobic conditions) while PFK2 may function aerobically in glycolysis and gluconeogenesis (see Chapter 6).

5.11 INVOLVEMENT OF FRUCTOSE-2,6-DIPHOSPHATE IN THE REGULATION OF GLYCOLYTIC CARBOHYDRATE METABOLISM

In 1980, a unique sugar diphosphate, β-D-fructofuranose-2,6-diphosphate (F-2,6-DP) was discovered and shown to play an important regulatory role in glycolysis and gluconeogenesis in all mammalian tissues, in plants, and in various microorganisms. F-2,6-DP was discovered during studies on the effect of the hormone glucagon on PFK activity in crude extracts from liver. The compound activates PFK, and the addition of glucagon to liver cells (hepatocytes) dramatically reduces the F-2,6-DP cytoplasmic concentration. F-2,6-DP is also a potent inhibitor of the gluconeogenic enzyme fructose-1,6-diphosphatase (FDPase) (see Section 6.7). F-2,6-DP acts synergistically with AMP in both of these actions. These two compounds overcome the inhibitory effects of ATP and citrate on the mammalian PFK. It is probable that F-2,6-DP is the most important effector of PFK and FDPase in the intact cell: it exerts reciprocal effects on PFK and FDPase, the two key regulatory enzymes controlling the direction of carbon flow. Consequently, it is a crucial regulatory molecule controlling glycolysis and gluconeogenesis.

The mode of action of F-2,6-DP on the enzyme from mammalian liver has been extensively studied. The cytoplasmic concentration of the compound is in the micromolar range and is responsive to dietary and hormonal control. Its concentration decreases in diabetes and starvation; glucagon and β-adrenergic agents such as adrenaline lower its concentration by a cyclic AMP-mediated mechanism, and insulin exerts an opposing effect.

A single enzyme with two distinct catalytic sites appears to catalyze F-2,6-DP synthesis and hydrolysis. These two reactions proceed as follows:

$$\text{F6P} + \text{ATP} \rightarrow \text{F-2,6-DP} + \text{ADP} \tag{5.5}$$

$$\text{F-2,6-DP} + H_2O \rightarrow \text{F6P} + P_i \tag{5.6}$$

Reaction (5.5) is catalyzed by 6-phosphofructo-2-kinase (ATP:D-fructofuranose-6-phosphate 2-phosphotransferase). The reverse reaction is catalyzed by fructose-2,6-diphosphatase (F-2,6-DPase). As noted above, a single bifunctional protein catalyzes these two reactions. This enzyme is a dimer of two 50,000-dalton subunits. It is regulated by a covalent phosphorylation reaction in which a cyclic AMP-dependent protein kinase transfers the γ-phosphoryl moiety of ATP to a seryl residue in each of the two subunits in the dimer. This phosphorylation event inhibits the kinase activity while activating the F-2,6-DPase activity of the enzyme.

The enzyme moiety responsible for F-2,6-DP synthesis apparently functions in a two-step process which involves a phosphoenzyme intermediate as does that responsible for F-2,6-DPase activity. This suggestion was first put forth when it was demonstrated that the enzyme catalyzes ADP/ATP and F6P/F-2,6-DP exchange reactions as follows:

$$[^{14}\text{C}]\text{ADP} + \text{ATP} \rightleftharpoons [^{14}\text{C}]\text{ATP} + \text{ADP} \tag{5.7}$$

$$[^{32}\text{P}]\text{F6P} + \text{F-2,6-DP} \rightleftharpoons 6\text{-}[^{32}\text{P}]\text{F-2,6-DP} + \text{F6P} \tag{5.8}$$

The phosphoenzyme intermediate responsible for reaction (5.8) was subsequently shown to be a 3-phosphohistidyl protein. Considerable evidence argued for two active sites, each catalyzing one of the two reactions of F-2,6-DP synthesis and hydrolysis. Such a bifunctional enzyme could have arisen during evolutionary history from a simple kinase site by partial gene duplication which left a larger fused gene product with two active sites per polypeptide chain. It should be recalled that the evidence for two distinct active sites is not yet conclusive.

The occurrence of a single enzyme that catalyzes both the forward and reverse reactions in a regulatory cascade has been established in several instances. Adenylylation and deadenylylation of *E. coli* glutamine synthase (Chapter 9), the uridylylation and deuridylylation of the P regulatory protein of the glutamine synthase cascade (Chapter 9), and the enzyme responsible for the phosphorylation and dephosphorylation of *E. coli* isocitrate dehydrogenase (Chapter 6), are all examples of this type of bifunctional protein. It is interesting to note that all four of these enzymes play a direct and exclusive role in metabolic regulation.

5.12 ALDOLASE

Fructose-1,6-diphosphate aldolase catalyzes the cleavage of FDP into dihydroxyacetone phosphate (DHAP) and glyceraldehyde-3-phosphate (Glyc-3-P) in a reversible, base-catalyzed aldol cleavage reaction. There are two general types of aldolases, and they are assumed to have arisen and evolved independently. Class I aldolases are Schiff's base-forming enzymes which function with the aid of strategically placed lysyl residues. These proteins are irreversibly inhibited by hydride-donating agents such as sodium borohydride ($NaBH_4$) but are unaffected by metal chelators (e.g., EDTA). They require no cofactor for catalytic activity. Class I aldolases from rabbit tissues yield three isozymes, A, B, and C. Type A is associated with muscle and is the best characterized of all aldolases. Type B is found in the liver, while type C is located in the brain. Class I vertebrate aldolases from different sources have very similar molecular weights (between 150,000 and 160,000) and are tetramers.

Class II aldolases, common to prokaryotes, are metalloaldolases. These proteins require a divalent metal cation as a cofactor and are reversibly inhibited by metal-chelating agents such as EDTA. Usually this metal ion is a tightly-bound Zn^{2+} ion, but in some cases more loosely-bound Fe^{2+} or Co^{2+} ions are used. Metalloaldolases are not affected by $NaBH_4$, but they are strongly inhibited by reagents which react with sulfhydryl groups. Class II aldolases exist as dimers with molecular weights of 70,000–80,000.

In class I aldolases, a Schiff's base imine, formed between the ϵ-amino group of a lysyl residue in the enzyme and the carbonyl group of FDP, functions as an electron sink. As pictured in Figure 5.20, FDP enters the active site and is held in place by electrostatic interactions between the two negatively charged phosphoryl groups of the substrate and positive or partially positive residues in the enzyme. Loss of water generates a Schiff's base, characteristic of class I aldolases. The rate-limiting reaction in the cleavage of FDP is the removal of a proton from the 4-hydroxyl group. An anionic sulfhydryl residue that loses a proton to an amino group (probably lysine) is responsible for this deprotonation. This same amino group also functions electrostatically to bind the 6-phosphoryl group of FDP. Carbons 4–6 of the original FDP molecule dissociate

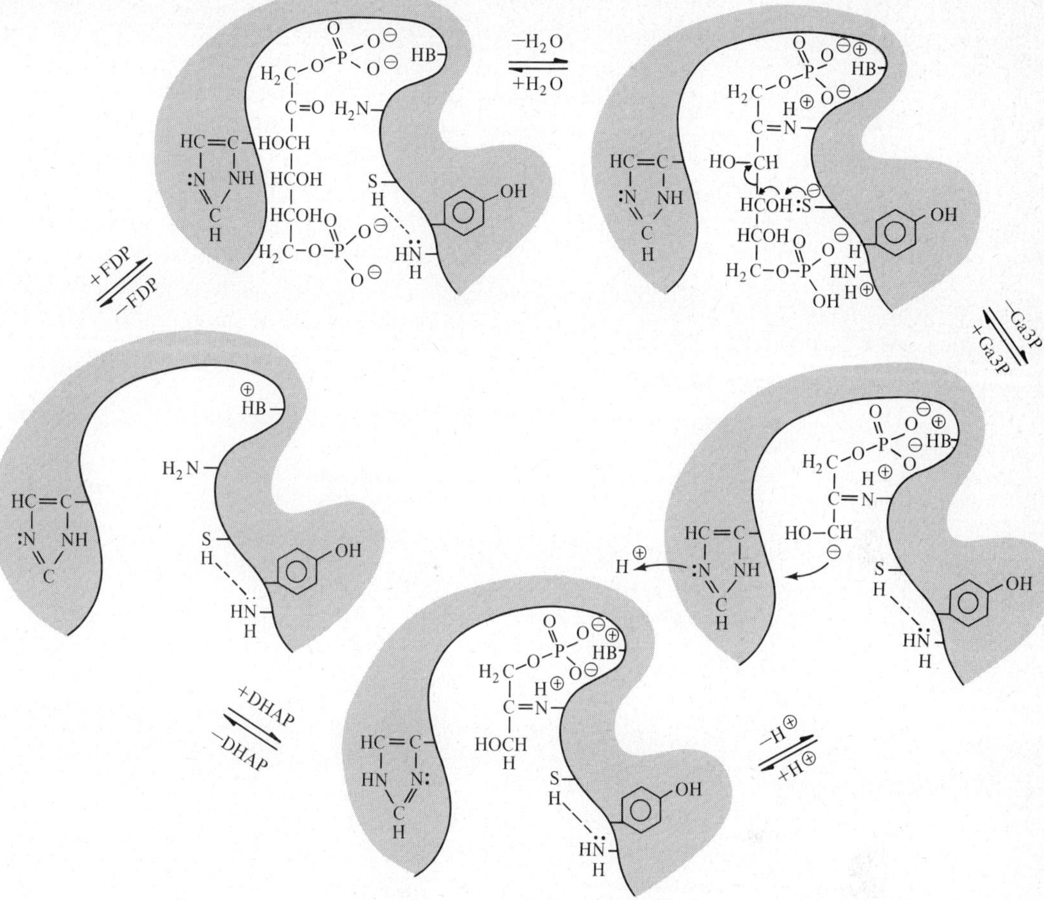

Figure 5.20 Mechanism of action of Schiff's base-forming aldolases (class I aldolases). Fructose-1,6-diphosphate (FDP) binds to the active site of the enzyme (left, top), and condensation with the ϵ-amino group of an enzymic lysyl residue creates a Schiff's base between enzyme and substrate. Aldol cleavage is followed by dissociation of glyceraldehyde-3-phosphate (Ga3P) from the active site. Subsequently, the Schiff's base hydrolyzes, and dihydroxyacetone phosphate (DHAP) dissociates, leaving the free enzyme.

from the binding cleft as glyceraldehyde-3-phosphate. The carbanionic precursor of DHAP, which is stabilized by resonance, picks up a proton, possibly from an active-site histidyl residue, and hydrolysis yields DHAP and the free enzyme.

Figure 5.21 illustrates the mechanism of action of metalloaldolases. As shown, the metal ion serves as the electron sink which enhances the electron-withdrawing ability of the carbonyl group so that the α-hydrogen becomes more acidic. The metal cofactor also serves to stabilize the negative charge on the DHAP carbanion by forming a resonance-stabilized intermediate which exists in equilibrium with the carbanionic form. While the metal cofactor acts as a charge stabilizer and electron sink, a general base (B) catalyzes the formation of the carbanionic form of DHAP by accepting a

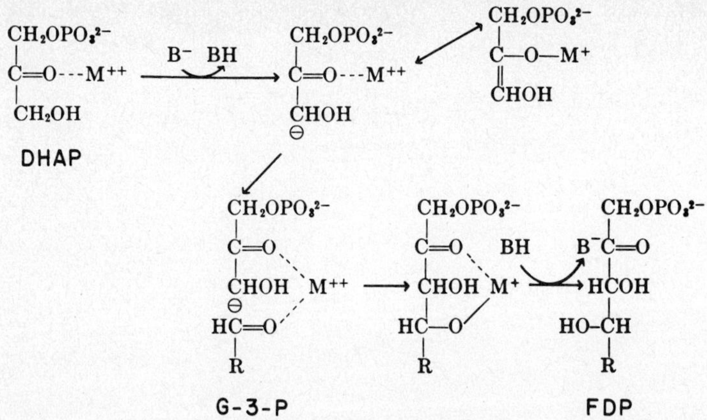

Figure 5.21 Mechanism of action of metalloaldolases (class II aldolases). The metal ion functions as an electrophilic catalyst. B^- (top, left) serves as a general base catalyst while BH serves as a general acid catalyst (bottom, right). The reaction is drawn in the reverse direction of that shown in Figure 5.20. The abbreviations are as follows: DHAP: dihydroxyacetone phosphate; G-3-P: glyceraldehyde-3-P; FDP: fructose-1,6-diphosphate. (Reproduced with permission from D. E. Morse and B. L. Horecker, "The Mechanisms of Action of Aldolase," in *Advances in Enzymology,* F. F. Nord, ed., **31:** 130, 1968.)

proton from the 3-carbon and then donating a proton to the anionic form of the 4-hydroxyl group of FDP generated after condensation of the two triose phosphates. It is likely that two different bases catalyze the deprotonation and protonation events.

The reaction catalyzed by aldolase is endergonic (see Table 5.1), but it is drawn toward the formation of DHAP and glyc-3-P by the exergonic formation of FDP and the continual oxidation and depletion of the glyceraldehyde-3-phosphate pool.

5.13 TRIOSEPHOSPHATE ISOMERASE

Triosephosphate isomerase (TPI) accomplishes the interconversion of dihydroxyacetone phosphate and D-glyceraldehyde-3-phosphate. This enzyme is active as a dimer (MW = 50,000), catalyzes a reversible reaction, is not allosterically regulated, and exists in most higher organisms as multiple isozymes. It is a symmetrical, barrel-shaped enzyme, with an inner cylinder consisting of eight strands of parallel β-pleated sheets surrounded by an outer cylinder of antiparallel, predominantly helical strands which are coaxial to the inner core.

The enzyme catalyzes the interconversion of its triose phosphate substrates in a reaction mechanistically similar to that catalyzed by phosphoglucoisomerase (PGI) (see Section 5.9). As with PGI, the transformation of DHAP into D-glyceraldehyde-3-phosphate centers on the formation of an enediol intermediate (Figure 5.22). It is known that an active-site glutamyl residue, acting as a base, is responsible for the stereospecific transfer of a proton from C—2 of glyceraldehyde 3-phosphate to C—1

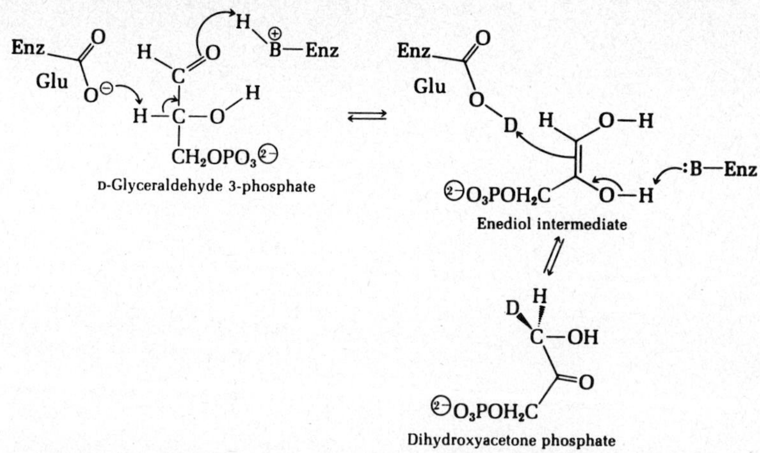

Figure 5.22 Mechanism of action of triosephosphate isomerase. The interconversion of glyceraldehyde-3-phosphate and dihydroxyacetone phosphate involves an enediol intermediate as shown. A glutamyl residue in the enzyme and an additional residue (B:) serve as general base catalysts. The figure illustrates the stereospecific transfer of a deuteron (D) to the enediol intermediate yielding dihydroxyacetone phosphate.

of the enediol intermediate to generate dihydroxyacetone phosphate. Although in aqueous solution dihydroxyacetone phosphate and glyceraldehyde-3-phosphate are 45% hydrated and 97% hydrated, respectively, the enzyme utilizes only unhydrated substrates. The rate-determining step in the TPI reaction is the binding of substrate to the enzyme, and the reaction is therefore diffusion limiting.

5.14 GLYCERALDEHYDE-3-PHOSPHATE DEHYDROGENASE

Glyceraldehyde-3-phosphate dehydrogenase (G3PDH) is responsible for the oxidation and phosphorylation of D-glyceraldehyde-3-phosphate to 1,3-diphospho-D-glycerate (1,3-DPG). The oxidation of the aldehydic substrate is highly exergonic—enough so to drive the reduction of NAD^+ to NADH and to create a high-energy phosphoanhydride bond. Although the overall reaction is slightly endergonic, it is drawn in the desired direction by the energy released in the next reaction.

The enzyme requires NAD^+ as a coenzyme and differs from all other enzymes in the glycolytic cycle by utilizing inorganic phosphate (P_i) as a substrate. In the first step of the G3PDH reaction, the sulfhydryl group of an active site cysteyl residue acts as a nucleophile, attacking the C—1 aldehydic carbon and generating a thiohemiacetal intermediate [Figure 5.23(A)].

In the next step, a hydride ion, transferred directly from C—1 of the thiohemiacetal, reduces the enzyme-bound NAD^+ and creates a high-energy thioester [Figure 5.23(B)]. In this reaction, an active-site histidyl residue participates as a general base. The NADH remains bound to the enzyme and is reoxidized by a free NAD^+ molecule.

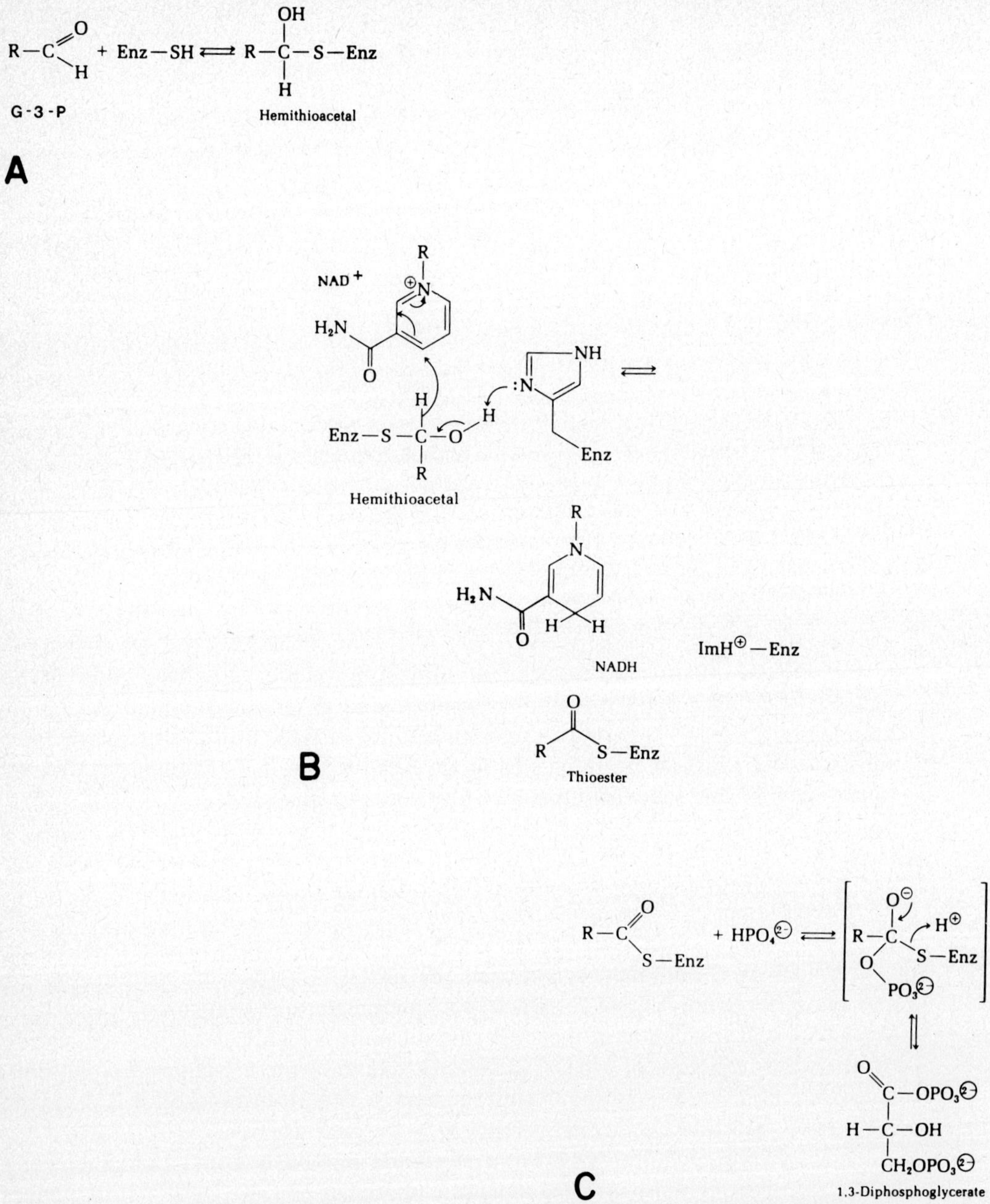

Figure 5.23 Three-step mechanism for the reaction catalyzed by glyceraldehyde-3-phosphate dehydrogenase (G3PDH). Step A: formation of the enzyme–substrate hemithioacetal. Step B: Oxidation of the hemithioacetal to the enzyme–substrate thioester employing NAD^+ as oxidant. Step C: Displacement of the enzymic thiol by inorganic phosphate. G-3-P: glyceraldehyde-3-phosphate.

In the final step of this reaction, the enzyme-bound thioester intermediate is displaced from the active site by the nucleophilic attack of an inorganic phosphate molecule. This phosphorolytic reaction conserves the energy of the thioester bond in a new high-energy compound, the mixed anhydride product, 1,3-DPG [Figure 5.23(C)].

Glyceraldehyde-3-phosphate dehydrogenase is a tetrameric protein composed of four identical subunits, each of which is capable of binding one coenzyme and one substrate molecule. Each subunit consists of two domains, one which binds the coenzyme and the other, the substrate. The NAD^+-binding domain is a large, hydrophobic pocket that allows the coenzyme to be bound in a number of different conformations. The other domain is responsible for substrate binding and specificity. The active site lies in a cleft between the two domains. The transfer of a hydride ion to NAD^+ requires a nonaqueous environment. It is likely that conformational changes that close off the active site and exclude water help meet this requirement.

G3PDH is inactivated by alkylating agents such as iodoacetate, and most isozymes are inhibited by the product, 1,3-DPG. At one time it was believed that the muscle dehydrogenase exhibited negative cooperativity in response to substrate binding. However, this was shown to be an artifact arising during enzyme purification. The yeast dehydrogenase, on the other hand, exhibits positive cooperativity with respect to the binding of substrate.

5.15 PHOSPHOGLYCERATE KINASE

The first ATP-yielding reaction in glycolysis involves the transfer of the 1-phosphoryl group from 1,3-DPG to ADP, generating 3-phosphoglycerate (3-PG) and ATP. The enzyme that catalyzes this transfer is phosphoglycerate kinase (PGK), named for the reverse reaction. Since two molecules of triosephosphate are produced per molecule of glucose entering the glycolytic sequence, two molecules of ATP are generated at this step, and the net energy expended in activating the sugar equals that produced. The PGK-catalyzed reaction is reversible, although highly exergonic (see Table 5.1). In fact, this reaction is sufficiently exergonic to overcome the preceding energetically unfavorable two reactions catalyzed by TPI and G3PDH. The transfer of phosphate from 1,3-DPG to ADP proceeds by a straightforward reaction mechanism involving nucleophilic attack by the terminal phosphoryl group of ADP on the phosphoryl moiety in the C—1 position of 1,3-DPG.

Phosphoglycerate kinase is the only monomeric enzyme in the glycolytic cycle. It has a bilobal structure with one domain responsible for MgADP binding and the other domain responsible for 1,3-DPG binding. Because the two substrates of PGK are bound to the two different lobes of the enzyme, a substantial conformational change must accompany binding, bringing them into proper orientation for the phosphoryl transfer reaction. The enzyme is inhibited by nucleoside monophosphates such as AMP and GMP. In some organisms PGK is closely associated with glyceraldehyde-3-phosphate dehydrogenase, and the product of the latter enzyme may be passed directly to the active site of PGK. Some evidence suggests that at least in some animal cells these and other glycolytic enzymes are present in a complex in association with the plasma membrane. Such an occurrence might facilitate catalysis by minimizing the need for diffusion between enzyme active sites.

5.16 PHOSPHOGLYCERATE MUTASE

Phosphoglycerate mutase (PGM) catalyzes the interconversion of 3-PG and 2-phosphoglycerate (2-PG). Transfer of the phosphoryl moiety from the C—3 position to C—2 prepares the substrate for conversion into the high-energy compound, phosphoenolpyruvate, a reaction catalyzed by enolase. Phosphoenolpyruvate can then be utilized in the final ATP-producing reaction which is catalyzed by pyruvate kinase, or it can enter a number of alternative metabolic pathways. Although the PGM-catalyzed interconversion is slightly endergonic (see Table 5.1) the large amount of free energy released in the pyruvate kinase or PEP carboxylase reaction readily draws this reaction in the desired direction.

Two types of phosphoglycerate mutases are found in nature. The enzymes from yeast and mammalian tissues require 2,3-diphosphoglycerate (2,3-DPG) as a cofactor and catalyze intermolecular phosphoryl transfer (Figure 5.24). The type of PGM found in many plants, on the other hand, does not require 2,3-DPG and catalyzes an intramolecular transfer reaction.

The imidazole side chains of two histidyl residues lie alongside the substrate, 3-PG, at the active site of the yeast enzyme. One of these two histidyl residues functions in nucleophilic catalysis and becomes transiently phosphorylated. The phosphohistidinyl protein first donates its phosphoryl group to a 3-PG molecule generating enzyme-bound 2,3-DPG (Figure 5.24). The 3-phosphoryl moiety of 2,3-DPG is then transferred to the enzyme, and 2-PG is released. The second histidyl residue at the active site of the enzyme probably functions in general acid-base catalysis.

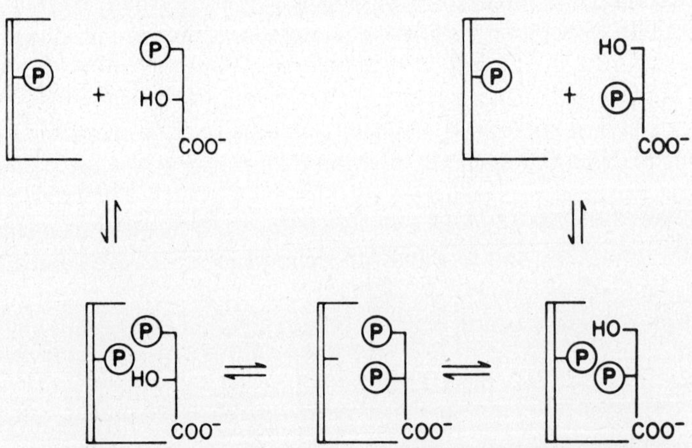

Figure 5.24 Pathway for phosphoryl transfer in the reaction catalyzed by 2,3-diphosphoglycerate-requiring phosphoglycerate mutases. The phosphorylated enzyme (left, top) transfers its phosphoryl group to 3PG, giving rise to dephospho-PGM and 2,3-DPG (bottom, middle). The 3 phosphoryl group of 2,3-DPG is then transferred to the enzyme yielding the phosphorylated enzyme and 2-PG. Free 2-PG dissociates from the active site (top, right). (Reproduced with permission from W. A. Blattler and J. R. Knowles, *Biochemistry,* **19,** 738–743, 1980.)

Although dissociation of 2,3-DPG from the enzyme surface can occur, such an occurrence cannot account for the *de novo* synthesis of this essential cofactor because the dephosphoenzyme is essentially inactive unless rephosphorylated at the expense of 2,3-DPG. Instead, the principal pathway leading to 2,3-DPG involves the conversion of 1,3-DPG to 2,3-DPG in a reaction catalyzed by diphosphoglycerate mutase (DPGM). It is this *shunt* reaction that provides the 2,3-DPG cofactor for the PGM-catalyzed reaction.

In mammalian tissues PGM exists as a dimer (MW = 55,000) of two identical subunits. Each subunit carries an active site. The yeast enzyme is a tetramer (MW = 110,000) which apparently possesses nonidentical subunits.

5.17 ENOLASE

Enolase is responsible for the dehydration of 2-PG to yield phosphoenolpyruvate (PEP), a high-energy compound that feeds into several metabolic pathways. This reaction is reversible ($\Delta G^{0\prime} = +0.4$ kcal/mole) and is drawn in the desired direction by the availability or depletion of PEP.

In the enolase-catalyzed reaction, 2-PG undergoes the net α,β-elimination of a water molecule, which has the effect of transforming the substrate into the enol tautomer of phosphorylated pyruvate. First, the α-proton is removed from 2-PG with the aid of a general base at the active site, generating a carbanion on C—2. The free electron pair of the carbanion then forms a π-double bond between C—2 and C—3, ejecting the β-hydroxyl group, possibly to an enzymic manganese or magnesium atom (Figure 5.25). Because of the phosphoryl group bonded to C—2, PEP cannot tautomerize into the more stable keto form of pyruvate, and it is trapped in the thermodynamically unstable enol form. Thus, a simple dehydration reaction transforms 2-PG, a phosphorylated compound with a relatively low free energy of hydrolysis, into PEP, a compound with one of the highest free energies of hydrolysis of all biologically important metabolites (see Table 5.2).

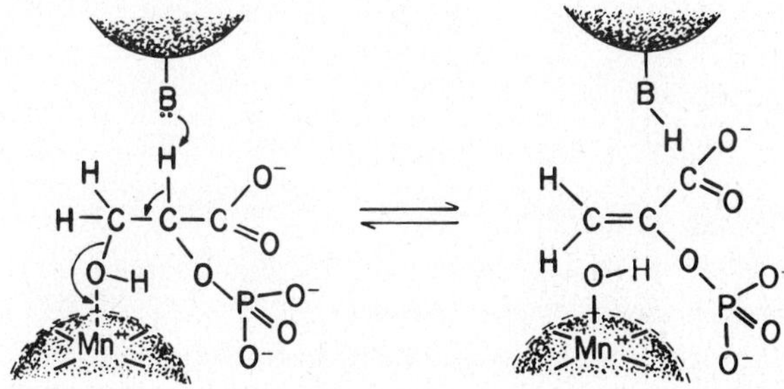

Figure 5.25 The mechanism of action of enolase. Enzyme-bound 2-phosphoglycerate (2PG) is shown on the left. Nucleophilic attack by an enzymic general base (B) initiates the conversion of 2PG to phosphoenolpyruvate (PEP) shown on the right. Shaded regions denote participatory regions of the active site of the enzyme.

Enolase is a dimeric enzyme composed of identical, spherical subunits. Each subunit binds two divalent metal cations (Mn^{2+} and Mg^{2+} or two Mg^{2+}), one of which is required to stabilize the active dimeric form of the enzyme and the other which functions catalytically in an enzyme-substrate-M^{2+} complex. The substrate, 2-PG, is believed to be held in precise alignment at the active site, facilitating removal of the slightly acidic α-hydrogen. Interaction of the substrate β-hydroxyl group with active site residues presumably aids in abstraction of the α-proton by holding the substrate in correct orientation relative to an amino acyl residue which acts as a general base.

From the preceding discussion, it can be appreciated that the glycolytic cycle, which evaded elucidation by the scientific community for several decades, is now the best understood biological carbohydrate catabolic pathway. Its central role in anaerobic metabolic processes during the first 2 billion years of biological evolution on earth, and its subsequent integration into the far more complex cellular machinery responsible for the complete oxidative degradation of carbohydrates during the subsequent billion years attests to its universal importance. In the next two chapters the constituents of the aerobic metabolic systems will be examined. A consideration of electron transport in the facultatively anaerobic bacterium, *E. coli,* will lead to the realization that the constituents of the electron transport chain (Chapter 7) may have evolved independently of the enzymes that catalyzed aerobic carbohydrate degradation (Chapter 6). Integration and adaptation of preexisting proteins into novel, more complex pathways undoubtedly provided the means which allowed living organisms to expand their metabolic capabilities, increase their diversity, and develop to the degrees of complexity found on earth today.

> *Religions die when they are proved to be true. Science is the record of dead religions.*
>
> —OSCAR WILDE

BIBLIOGRAPHY

Anderson, C. M., F. H. Zuckey, and T. A. Steitz, "Space-Filling Models of Kinase Clefts and Conformation Changes," *Science,* **204:** 375–380 (1979).

Becker, W. M., "Anaerobic Production of ATP," in *Biochemistry,* G. Zubay, ed., pp. 283–321, Addison-Wesley, Reading, MA (1983).

Bosca, L., and C. Corredor, "Is Phosphofructokinase the Rate-Limiting Step to Glycolysis?," *Trends in Biochemical Science,* **9:** 372–373 (1984).

Branden, C. I., and H. Eklund, "Structure and Mechanisms of Liver Alcohol Dehydrogenase, Lactate Dehydrogenase and Glyceraldehyde-3-phosphate Dehydrogenase," in *Dehydrogenases Requiring Nicotinamide Coenzymes,* J. Jeffery, ed., *Experientia Supplementum,* Birkhauser Verlag, Basel, Switzerland (1980).

De Crombrugghe, B., S. Busby, and Henri Buc, "Cyclic AMP Receptor Protein: Role in Transcription Activation," *Science,* **224:** 831–838 (1984).

Finean, J. B., R. Coleman, and R. H. Mitchell, *Membranes and Their Cellular Functions,* Blackwell, Palo Alto, CA (1984).

Florkin, M., *A History of Biochemistry. Part III. History and Identification of the Sources of Free Energy in Organisms,* Comprehensive Biochemistry, Vol. 31, Elsevier/North Holland, Amsterdam (1975).

Gancedo, C., and R. Serrano, "Energy Yielding Metabolism in Yeasts," in *The Yeast,* J. S. Harrison and A. H. Rose, eds., Academic, New York (1984).

Hers, H. G., and L. Hue, "Gluconeogenesis and Related Aspects of Glycolysis," *Annual Review of Biochemistry,* **52:** 617–653 (1983).

Jacobson, G. R., and M. H. Saier, Jr., "Biological Membranes: Transport," in *Biochemistry,* G. Zubay, ed., pp. 621–657, Addison-Wesley, Reading, MA (1983).

Jacobson, G. R., C. A. Lee, J. E., Leonard, and M. H. Saier, Jr., "Mannitol-specific Enzyme II of the Bacterial Phosphotransferase System I. Properties of the Purified Permease," *Journal of Biological Chemistry,* **258:** 10748–10756 (1983).

Jenkins, J. D., D. P. Madden, and T. L. Steck, "Association of Phosphofructokinase and Aldolase with the Membrane of the Intact Erythrocyte," *Journal of Biological Chemistry,* **259:** 9374–9378 (1984).

Kane, J. F., ed., *Multifunctional Proteins: Catalytic/Structural and Regulatory,* CRC Press, Boca Raton, FL (1983).

Konings, W. N., R. Otto, B. T. Brink, G. T. Robillard, M. G. L. Elferink, and K. J. Hellingwerf, "Relation Between the Proton Motive Force and Solute Transport in Bacteria," *Biochemical Society Transactions,* **12:** 152–154 (1984).

Lee, C. A., and M. H. Saier, Jr., "Mannitol-specific Enzyme II of the Bacterial Phosphotransferase System III. The Nucleotide Sequence of the Permease Gene," *Journal of Biological Chemistry,* **258:** 10761–10767 (1983).

Leonard, J. E., and M. H. Saier, Jr., "Mannitol-specific Enzyme II of the Bacterial Phosphotransferase System II. Reconstitution of Vectorial Transphosphorylation in Phospholipid Vesicles," *Journal of Biological Chemistry,* **258:** 10757–10760 (1983).

Morse, D. E., and B. L. Horecker, "The Mechanisms of Action of Aldolases," in *Advances in Enzymology,* F. F. Nord, ed., **31:** 125–182, Wiley-Interscience, New York (1968).

Muirhead, H., "Triosephosphate Isomerase, Pyruvate Kinase, and Other α/β-Barrel Enzymes," *Trends in Biochemical Sciences,* **8:** 326–329 (1983).

Nagradova, N. K., L. I. Ashmarina, R. A. Asryants, T. V. Cherednikova, T. O. Golovina, and V. I. Muronetz, "Glyceraldehyde-3-phosphate Dehydrogenase: The Role of Subunit Interactions in Enzyme Functioning," *Advances in Enzyme Regulation,* **19:** 171–204 (1980).

Osumi, T., and M. H. Saier, Jr., "Regulation of Lactose Permease Activity by the Phosphoenolpyruvate:Sugar Phosphotransferase System: Evidence for Direct Binding of the Glucose-specific Enzyme III to the Lactose Permease," *Proceedings of the National Academy of Sciences USA,* **79:** 1457–1461 (1982).

Reizer, J., J. Deutscher, S. Sutrina, J. Thompson, and M. H. Saier, Jr., "Regulation of Sugar Accumulation in Gram-positive Bacteria: Exclusion and Expulsion Mechanisms involving ATP-Dependent Phosphorylation of a Transport Protein," *Trends in Biochemical Science,* **10:** 32–35 (1985).

Saier, M. H., Jr., *Mechanisms and Regulation of Carbohydrate Transport in Bacteria,* Academic, New York (1985).

Saier, M. H., Jr., F. C. Grenier, C. A. Lee, and E. B. Waygood, "Evidence for the Evolutionary Relatedness of the Proteins of the Bacterial Phosphoenolpyruvate:Sugar Phosphotransferase System," *Journal of Cellular Biochemistry,* **27:** 43–56 (1985).

Saier, M. H., Jr., and G. R. Jacobson, *The Molecular Basis of Sex and Differentiation,* Springer-Verlag, New York (1984).

Saier, M. H., Jr., "The Role of the Cell Surface in Regulating the Internal Environment," in *The Bacteria, a Treatise on Structure and Function,* Vol. VII, J. R. Sokatch and L. N. Ornston, eds., pp. 167–227, Academic, New York (1979).

Strominger, J., and G. Zubay, "Structure and Synthesis of Sugars," in *Biochemistry,* G. Zubay, ed., pp. 437–467, Addison-Wesley, Reading, MA (1983).

Uyeda, K., "Phosphofructokinase," in *Advances in Enzymology,* A. Meister, ed., Vol. 48, pp. 193–244, Wiley, New York (1979).

Veneziale, C. M., ed., *The Regulation of Carbohydrate Formation and Utilization in Mammals,* University Park Press, Baltimore, MD (1981).

Walker, R., "The Molecular Biology of Enzyme Synthesis: Regulatory Mechanisms of Enzyme Adaptation," Wiley, New York (1983).

Wimmer, M. J., and I. A. Rose, "Mechanisms of Enzyme-Catalyzed Group Transfer Reactions," *Annual Review of Biochemistry,* **47**: 1031–1078 (1978).

Wood, W. A., ed., *Methods in Enzymology: Carbohydrate Metabolism* (Parts A–E), *Vol. 9* (1966); *Vol. 41* (1975); *Vol. 42* (1975); *Vol. 89* (1982); *Vol. 90* (1982), Academic, New York.

Chapter 6

Aerobic Metabolism of Carbohydrates

> *I have yet to see a problem however complicated that when you look at it the right way does not become more complicated.*
>
> —PAUL ALDESTON

In the previous chapter, we noted that the glycolytic cycle can occur in the complete absence of oxygen. The normal functioning of this cycle under anaerobic conditions requires the reoxidation of the NADH which it generates. Hence, terminal carbon metabolites such as pyruvate or acetaldehyde are reduced to lactate or ethanol, respectively.

In the presence of oxygen, the three-carbon compounds generated by glycolysis can be completely oxidized to CO_2, yielding about twenty times as much energy per glucose molecule metabolized as is possible under anaerobic conditions. The pathway for this oxidative process includes the reactions of glycolysis, the pyruvate dehydrogenase-catalyzed reaction, a reaction converting a C_3-acid to a C_4-acid, the tricarboxylic acid cycle (TCA cycle, also called the citrate or Krebs cycle), electron transport, and oxidative phosphorylation. Without any one of the constituent enzymes of any one of these processes, the efficient aerobic conversion of a glucose molecule to ATP cannot occur.

In this chapter the enzymes that allow functioning of the TCA cycle will be evaluated. It is into this cycle that carbohydrates, fatty acids, amino acids, and various other compounds all feed for the final oxidation of their metabolites. The utilization of C_2 compounds usually requires the enzymes of the glyoxalate shunt. These and other related subjects will be considered in this chapter. Chapter 7 will be devoted to the subjects of electron transport and oxidative phosphorylation.

In order for metabolites to be utilized by bacteria or eukaryotic cells, they must enter the compartment which houses the catabolic enzymes responsible for their degradation. The organelle in which substrate oxidation occurs in the eukaryotic cell is the mitochondrion. The inner membrane of this organelle contains a variety of transport systems which allow communication between the mitochondrial matrix and the cytoplasm. The entire bacterial cell is the compartment in which all corresponding reactions occur in prokaryotes. Accordingly, the plasma membranes of these cells must contain permeases which allow the uptake of extracellularly available metabolites if these substrates are to be utilized. As transport is necessarily the first step in metabolite utilization, we shall initiate our discussion of oxidative metabolism with this subject.

6.1 TRANSPORT OF METABOLIC INTERMEDIATES IN BACTERIA AND MITOCHONDRIA

Gram-negative bacteria and mitochondria possess superficially similar envelopes consisting of inner and outer membranes. In both cases the outer membranes are nonspecifically permeable to water-soluble solutes by virtue of the presence of proteinaceous, hydrophilic, transmembrane pores which allow passive passage of solutes through these membranes. By contrast, the inner membranes are permeable to certain solutes by virtue of the presence of highly stereospecific transport proteins. Bacteria such as *Salmonella typhimurium,* an intracellular parasite of animals, possess transport systems for glycolytic intermediates such as hexose phosphates, the 2- and 3-phosphoglycerates, and phosphoenolpyruvate (Table 6.1). Some of these transport systems, which function

TABLE 6.1 SOLUTE TRANSPORT SYSTEMS FOR INTERMEDIATES OF GLYCOLYSIS AND THE KREBS CYCLE IN ENTERIC BACTERIA (*ESCHERICHIA COLI* AND *SALMONELLA TYPHIMURIUM*)

Transport system	Substrates	Mechanism
Hexose-P	Glucose-1- and 6-P Fructose-1- and 6-P Mannose-1- and 6-P	H^+ symport
Dihydroxyacetone	Dihydroxyacetone	PTS
Glycerate	Glycerate	Not known
Phosphoglycerate	2-P-glycerate 3-P-glycerate P-enolpyruvate	H^+ symport
Pyruvate	Pyruvate	H^+ symport
Dicarboxylate	Succinate Fumarate Malate Oxaloacetate	H^+ symport
Tricarboxylate	Citrate *cis*-Aconitate Isocitrate	Na^+ symport
α-Ketoglutarate	α-Ketoglutarate	Not known
Dicarboxylate amino acids	Aspartate Glutamate	Several
Acetate	Acetate	Acetyl CoA synthase?
Fatty acids	Most fatty acids	Acyl CoA synthase?
P_i	P_i	Several

by H^+:solute symport (cotransport), are lacking in *E. coli,* which is an extracellular parasite of animals. Synthesis of these transport systems is only induced when the substrates are present in the extracellular medium in which the bacteria are growing. The presence of these compounds in the bacterial cytoplasm is not sufficient to induce their syntheses. This fact makes physiological sense because syntheses of these transport systems in the absence of an external source of the substrate would allow leakage of intracellular nutrients from the cell cytoplasm with no benefit to the cell. Transmembrane regulatory proteins that bind an inducer on the external surface of the cytoplasmic membrane and a DNA-binding protein on the internal surface of the membrane may mediate transcriptional regulation of the genes encoding these transport proteins.

Bacteria also possess transport systems for dihydroxyacetone and glycerate which enter glycolysis upon phosphorylation (Table 6.1). None of these transport systems are found in mitochondria since their substrates are metabolized in the cytoplasm of eukaryotic cells. However, some of these compounds can enter the matrix of the mitochondrion due to the lack of specificity of transport systems which normally function with other substrates.

Oxidizable substrates which feed into the Krebs cycle are generally transported across both bacterial and mitochondrial membranes although by different mechanisms. In bacteria they are actively accumulated by cotransport (symport) with protons or Na^+. Such active transport processes allow these substrates to be accumulated in the bacterial cytoplasm to concentrations which approach the K_M values of the enzymes which act upon them, even when their extracellular concentrations are very low. By contrast, mitochondria usually transport these compounds by *exchange facilitators* which possess low affinities for their substrates and can exchange one such substrate for another (Table 6.2). Such a mechanism is reasonable because the concentrations of these compounds are normally high, both in the mitochondrial matrix and in the cytoplasm. A sequence of exchange transport processes which reveals the coupling of these systems to each other is depicted schematically in Figure 6.1.

TABLE 6.2 SOLUTE TRANSPORT SYSTEMS IN THE INNER MITOCHONDRIAL MEMBRANE OF MANY EUKARYOTES

Transport system	Substrates
Phosphate:hydroxide antiporter	$H_2PO_4^-$; OH^-
Phosphate:malate (glutamate) antiporter	$HPO_4^=$; malate; glutamate
Pyruvate:H^+ symporter	Pyruvate
L-Glutamate:H^+ symporter	L-Glutamate
Dicarboxylate antiporter #1	$HPO_4^=$; $SO_4^=$; malonate; succinate; oxaloacetate; sulfite; thiosulfate
Dicarboxylate antiporter #2	α-ketoglutarate; L-malate; succinate
Glutamate:aspartate antiporter	Aspartate; glutamate + H^+
Tricarboxylate antiporter	Citrate; isocitrate; L-malate; succinate; phosphoenolpyruvate
Adenine nucleotide antiporter	ATP; ADP
Carnitine:acyl carnitine antiporter	Carnitine; acetylcarnitine; acylcarnitine

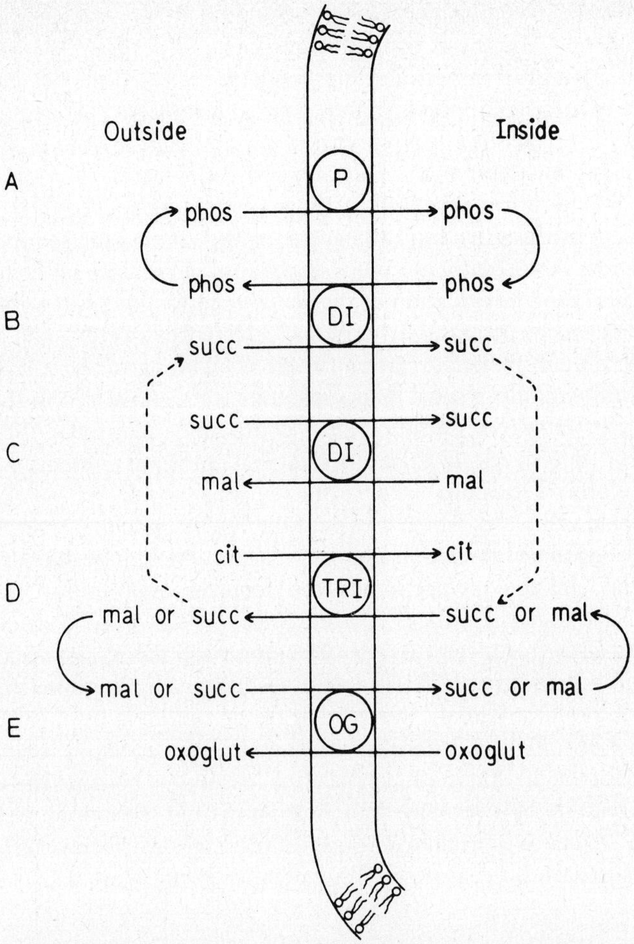

Figure 6.1 Mitochondrial transport systems for the exchange of phosphate and various Krebs cycle intermediates across the inner mitochondrial membrane. (A) The phosphate transporter; (B) the dicarboxylate antiporter #1 catalyzing phosphate/dicarboxylate antiport; (C) the dicarboxylate antiporter #1 catalyzing succinate/malate antiport; (D) the tricarboxylate antiporter catalyzing citrate/malate (or succinate) antiport; (E) the dicarboxylate antiporter #2 catalyzing α-ketoglutarate (oxoglut)/malate (or succinate) antiport. The transport systems depicted are those listed in Table 6.2. (Reproduced with permission from P. Mitchell, "Compartmentation and Communication in Living Systems. Ligand Conduction: A General Catalytic Principle in Chemical, Osmotic, and Chemiosmotic Reaction Systems, *European Journal of Biochemistry,* **95,** 1–20, 1979.)

Acetate, fatty acids, and inorganic phosphate are also transported across bacterial and mitochondrial membranes by quite different mechanisms. While bacteria do not catalyze the uptake of nucleotides, an adenine nucleotide transporter is capable of very rapidly exchanging ATP for ADP across the inner mitochondrial membrane (Table 6.2). This system keeps the energy charge of the cytoplasm in equilibrium with that of the mitochondrial matrix. While mitochondria do not readily transport the nicotinamide coenzymes, reducing equivalents can enter the mitochondrial matrix by exchange of a reduced dicarboxylate anion (aspartate or malate) for an oxidized dicarboxylate molecule (oxaloacetate). These exchange transport systems can be thought of as essential components of the Krebs cycle which bridge the spatial gap in the compartmentalized eukaryotic cell.

6.2 INTERCONVERSION OF PYRUVATE, PHOSPHOENOLPYRUVATE (PEP) AND OXALOACETATE (OA)

The key end-products of glycolysis include phosphoenolpyruvate (PEP) and pyruvate, while the two starting compounds that allow normal functioning of the Krebs cycle are oxaloacetate and acetyl CoA. Acetyl CoA is synthesized from pyruvate by the reaction catalyzed by the pyruvate dehydrogenase complex (Section 6.4). Specific enzymes catalyze the interconversion of the other three compounds as shown in Figure 6.2. The properties of these enzymes are summarized in Table 6.3. While most living organisms possess only three or four of these enzymes, a few microorganisms possess all or most of them. One such organism is *Pseudomonas citronellolis.* In such an organism the unregulated functioning of any two enzymes catalyzing opposing reactions would result in the futile expenditure of metabolic energy. Consequently, virtually all

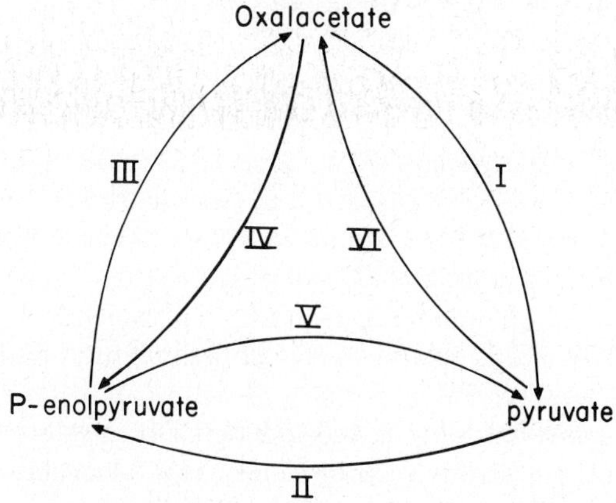

Figure 6.2 Schematic illustration of the enzymic interconversions of phosphoenolpyruvate, pyruvate, and oxaloacetate. The enzymes that catalyze each of the six interconversions are listed in Table 6.3 together with the numbered reactions shown in the figure.

TABLE 6.3 ENZYMES THAT CATALYZE THE INTERCONVERSION OF OXALOACETATE (OA), PYRUVATE (PRV), AND PHOSPHOENOLPYRUVATE (PEP)

Reaction in Figure 6.2	Trivial name	Systematic name	E.C. #	Cofactor(s)
I	OA decarboxylase	OA carboxy-lyase	4.1.1.3	Biotin + Na^+ or Mn^{++}
II	PEP synthase (prv, water dikinase)	ATP:prv, water phosphotransferase	2.7.9.2	Mn^{++}
II, V	prv, phosphate dikinase	ATP:prv, phosphate phosphotransferase	2.7.9.1	Mg^{++}
III	PEP carboxylase	Phosphate:OA carboxy-lyase (phosphorylating)	4.1.1.31	Mg^{++}; a thiol
III, IV, V	PEP carboxytransphosphorylase [PEP carboxykinase (P_2)]	Pyrophosphate:OA carboxy-lyase (transphosphorylating)	4.1.1.38	
IV	PEP carboxykinase (GTP)	GTP:OA carboxy-lyase (transphosphorylating)	4.1.1.32	Mn^{++}
V	prv kinase	ATP:prv 2-O-phosphotransferase	2.7.1.40	Mg^{++}, K^+
VI	prv carboxylase	prv:HCO_3^- ligase (ADP forming)	6.4.1.1	Biotin; Mn^{++} or Zn^{++}

of these enzymes are subject to allosteric control as indicated in Figure 6.3. In this section these enzymes, their relationships to one another, and their physiological significance in a variety of organisms will be discussed.

6.2.1 Oxaloacetate Decarboxylase

Oxaloacetate decarboxylase is not present in most eukaryotes (Table 6.3). It is found in many bacterial species, however, and is required for the anaerobic utilization of Krebs cycle intermediates such as citrate. Citrate is first cleaved to oxaloacetate and acetyl CoA in a reaction catalyzed by an ATP-dependent citrate lyase. Oxaloacetate is then decarboxylated to pyruvate and CO_2 in a reaction catalyzed by oxaloacetate decarboxylase. In some bacteria this enzyme is a membrane-bound biotin-containing enzyme which specifically requires Na^+ but not a divalent cation for activity. Other bacterial oxaloacetate decarboxylases are biotin-independent, divalent cation-dependent enzymes which exhibit cooperativity with respect to oxaloacetate binding. The latter enzymes are allosterically activated by NAD^+ and $NADP^+$ and are inhibited by acetate. The former, biotin-dependent enzymes are not regulated by these agents but are strongly inhibited by glyoxalate, oxalate and 2-oxomalonate.

Membrane-bound, Na^+-dependent oxaloacetate decarboxylase has been solubilized from the bacterial plasma membrane using detergents and has been purified free of all contaminating proteins. It has an apparent subunit molecular weight of

TABLE 6.3 *(Continued)*

Reaction catalyzed	Present in			
	Yeast, animals	*E. coli*	Pseudomonas	Propionibacteria
OA → prv + CO_2	(+)	−	+	−
prv + ATP + H_2O → PEP + AMP + P_i	−	+	+	−
prv + ATP + P_i → PEP + AMP + P_2	−	−	−	+
PEP + HCO_3^- → OA + P_i	−	+	+	−
PEP + P_i + CO_2 → OA + P_2 PEP + P_i → prv + P_2	−	−	−	+
OA + GTP → PEP + GDP + CO_2	+	+	−	−
PEP + ADP → prv + ATP	+	+	+	+
prv + HCO_3^- + ATP → OA + ADP + P_i	+	−	+	−

68,000 and may exist in the membrane in an oligomeric form. When the solubilized enzyme is reconstituted in a vesicular phospholipid membrane lacking other bacterial proteins, the addition of oxaloacetate to the extravesicular medium results in the active accumulation of Na^+ in the intravesicular space, and this accumulation is abolished by the addition of avidin, an inhibitor of biotin function. These observations suggest that oxaloacetate decarboxylation in the intact bacterial cell is coupled to the active extrusion of Na^+ from the cell. It seems that this enzyme serves two separate but tightly coupled functions, one chemical and one vectorial. The decarboxylation of oxaloacetate provides the energy for the generation of a Na^+ electrochemical gradient. The electrochemical Na^+ gradient can then be utilized to drive solute uptake or to synthesize ATP in the process termed oxidative phosphorylation. The coupling of transmembrane Na^+ movements with decarboxylation of oxaloacetate therefore allows the enzyme to interconvert cellular chemical and chemiosmotic energies. The interconversion of these two forms of energy will be discussed more fully in Chapter 7.

6.2.2 PEP Synthase

PEP synthase is present in many bacteria but is lacking from animal tissues and yeast (Table 6.3). In *E. coli,* this gluconeogenic enzyme is synthesized when the bacteria are grown on 3-carbon substrates. In *Pseudomonas citronellolis* it is synthesized constitutively. The enzyme replaces the pyruvate carboxylase–PEP carboxykinase bypass

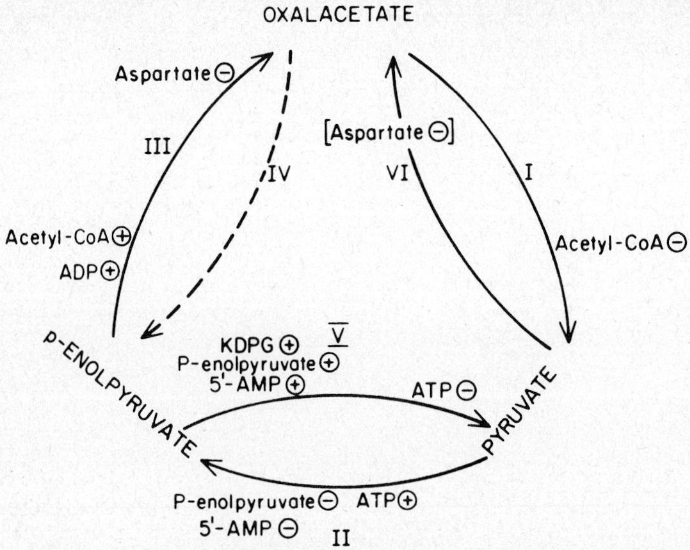

Figure 6.3 Allosteric regulation of the enzymes catalyzing the interconversion of pyruvate, phosphoenolpyruvate, and oxaloacetate in *P. citronellolis.* The allosteric effectors that inhibit (−) or activate (+) the enzyme, indicated by number, are shown. Enzymes are indicated by number as in Figure 6.2 and Table 6.3. Enzyme IV has not been detected in this organism. KDPG, 2-keto-3-deoxy-6-phosphogluconate. (Reproduced with permission from R. W. O'Brien, D. T. Chuang, B. L. Taylor, and M. F. Utter, "Novel Enzymic Machinery for the Metabolism of Oxalacetate, Phosphoenolpyruvate, and Pyruvate in *Pseudomonas citronellolis,*" *Journal of Biological Chemistry,* **252,** 1257–1263, 1977.)

used by eukaryotic cells (see Table 6.3). *E. coli* PEP synthase is a dimer of molecular weight 150,000. Some evidence suggests that the enzyme functions by a "half-of-sites" mechanism in which a histidyl residue in the enzyme is phosphorylated on the N-3 position. The reaction proceeds in two steps:

$$\mathrm{E + ATP + H_2O \rightarrow E(his)P + AMP + P_i} \tag{6.1}$$

$$\mathrm{E(his)P + pyruvate \rightarrow E + PEP} \tag{6.2}$$

The phosphoryl moiety of the phosphoenzyme is derived from the β-position of ATP, while the inorganic phosphate produced in equation (6.1) is derived from the γ-phosphoryl moiety of ATP. As indicated in Figure 6.3, PEP synthase in *Pseudomonas citronellolis* is subject to product inhibition by PEP and AMP and is activated by ATP.

In a different bacterium, *Propionibacterium shermanii* a similar enzyme, called pyruvate,phosphate dikinase, catalyzes a phosphorolytic reaction which serves the same physiological function as PEP synthase (see Table 6.3). This enzyme is also a dimer of molecular weight 150,000. Like the *E. coli* enzyme, it forms a phosphorylated enzyme intermediate in which a histidyl residue is derivatized. It may also function by a half-of-sites type mechanism. In some organisms this enzyme functions in the opposite direction, replacing pyruvate kinase. It seems clear that PEP synthase and pyruvate,phosphate dikinase have a common evolutionary ancestry.

Pyruvate, phosphate dikinase catalyzes three partial reactions, each of which occurs at a separate site on the enzyme surface. At site 1, P_2 is transferred from ATP to a histidyl residue in the protein, generating AMP as the byproduct. At site 2, P_i is converted to P_2 with the histidyl pyrophosphate serving as the phosphoryl donor. At site 3, pyruvate is phosphorylated by the phosphorylated histidyl residue, regenerating the free form of the enzyme. Oxalate is a transition-state analogue of enolpyruvate which binds only to the phosphorylated enzyme. The dikinase is the only known example of a pyrophosphorylated enzyme intermediate.

6.2.3 PEP Carboxylase

PEP carboxylase is found in plants and bacteria but not in fungi or animals. This enzyme catalyzes the carboxylation of PEP in a reaction which yields oxaloacetate. Unlike pyruvate carboxylase from animal tissues (enzyme VI in Table 6.3), PEP carboxylase does not contain biotin or depend on a nucleoside triphosphate. A concerted reaction mechanism has been proposed as shown in Figure 6.4.

PEP carboxylases from all biological sources examined appear to be subject to allosteric regulation. The *Pseudomonas* enzyme, for example, is activated by acetyl CoA and ADP and allosterically inhibited by aspartate (Figure 6.3). In *E. coli,* fructose-1,6-diphosphate, acetyl CoA, GTP, and GDP all activate the enzyme while aspartate inhibits it. In the latter bacterium, this enzyme is the only one capable of synthesizing

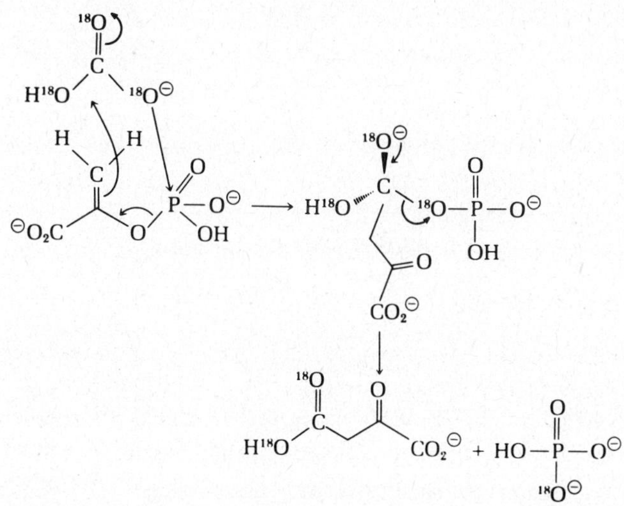

Figure 6.4 Possible mechanism for the reaction catalyzed by PEP carboxylase. [^{18}O]Bicarbonate was utilized to elucidate the reaction mechanism. The radioactive label appears in both products, oxaloacetate and inorganic phosphate, in a ratio of 2:1.

a Krebs cycle intermediate from an end-product of glycolysis. It is therefore an essential, anaplerotic enzyme.

In propionibacteria, PEP carboxytransphosphorylase replaces PEP carboxylase and/or PEP carboxykinase found in other organisms. The reaction catalyzed by this enzyme differs from that catalyzed by PEP carboxylase in at least three respects (Table 6.3). First, the enzyme acts on carbon dioxide rather than bicarbonate; second, the phosphoryl group of PEP is transferred to inorganic phosphate with the synthesis of pyrophosphate. Pyrophosphoenolpyruvate is apparently an intermediate in the reaction. And finally, in the absence of CO_2, pyruvate is generated in a reaction which is functionally analogous to the pyruvate kinase reaction (Table 6.3). PEP carboxytransphosphorylase is a tetrameric enzyme which dissociates to less active dimers and monomers.

Other enzymes in propionibacteria synthesize and utilize pyrophosphate instead of ATP. For example, phosphofructokinase in these organisms utilizes pyrophosphate instead of ATP as the phosphoryl donor, and P_2 may be generated by electron transfer during the reduction of fumarate. Proton-translocating pyrophosphatases have also been reported. Pyrophosphate can be thought of as a very primitive, perhaps the most primitive, form of high-energy phosphate available to living organisms. It may have been the evolutionary precursor of ATP. The generation of this compound during bacterial photosynthesis (the most primitive form of photosynthesis) argues in favor of this notion. It is possible that the pyrophosphate-utilizing enzymes in propionibacteria represent relics of a biological age which has largely passed.

6.2.4 PEP Carboxykinase

PEP carboxykinase together with pyruvate carboxylase (enzyme VI in Table 6.3) provides the pathway for reversal of the pyruvate kinase step during gluconeogenesis in most eukaryotic organisms. Although present in *E. coli* (Table 6.3), the enzyme is the only one of the six common pyruvate-PEP-oxaloacetate interconverting enzymes not found in *Pseudomonas citronellolis.*

The mechanism of PEP carboxykinase appears to involve concerted decarboxylation and phosphoryl group transfer as shown in Figure 6.5. Since the reaction is only slightly exergonic, and therefore fully reversible, it is not surprising that the enzyme does not appear to be subject to allosteric regulatory control.

6.2.5 Pyruvate Kinase

Pyruvate kinase is a nearly ubiquitous enzyme which has been purified and studied from numerous biological sources. In those organisms that lack the enzyme, pyruvate,phosphate dikinase seems to serve its functional role. The pyruvate kinase from many biological sources is a tetramer of four identical subunits, each of which possesses a substrate binding site as well as allosteric regulatory sites.

Mammalian pyruvate kinase (MW = 240,000) is found in three similar isozymic forms, one which predominates in muscle and brain, one in liver, and one in kidney. Each subunit in the pyruvate kinase molecule consists of three dissimilar domains which function in catalysis and regulation. While all isozymes are subject to feed-forward activation by fructose-1,6-diP and feed-back inhibition by ATP, the liver

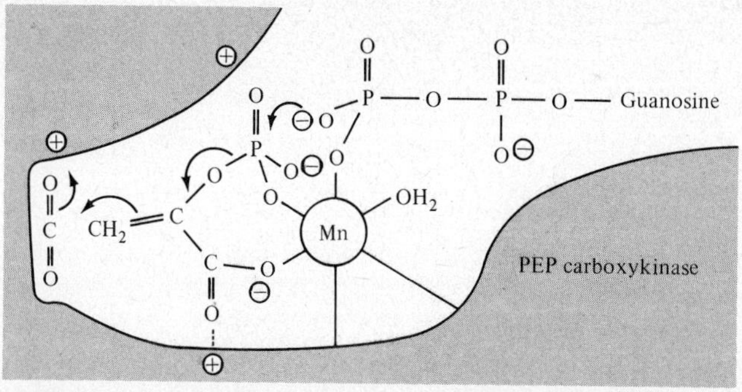

Figure 6.5 Possible mechanism for the reaction catalyzed by PEP carboxykinase. Mn^{++} is shown to function in the binding of substrates at the active site and also as an electrophilic catalyst. GDP, PEP, and CO_2 generate GTP and oxaloacetate in a single, concerted step.

enzyme is also inhibited by acetyl CoA and succinyl CoA, and is reversibly phosphorylated by a protein kinase–phosphatase system. Phosphorylation of the enzyme decreases its affinity for PEP, thereby lowering its activity. Under these conditions of enzyme phosphorylation, PEP is used primarily for glucose synthesis (gluconeogenesis). Because the protein kinase that catalyzes pyruvate kinase phosphorylation is dependent on cyclic AMP for activity, the activity of the enzyme is responsive to the plasma concentrations of glucagon and other hormones.

The mechanism of action of all known pyruvate kinases is the same. Phosphoryl transfer from PEP to ADP occurs by direct in-line phosphoryl group transfer without enzyme phosphorylation. Thus, both substrates must be present simultaneously at the active site before the reaction can occur, and the two substrate binding sites overlap to the extent that the phosphoryl moiety of PEP occupies the same site as does the γ-phosphoryl moiety of ATP. One Mg^{++} functions to bind the carboxyl group of PEP (or pyruvate) while a second Mg^{++} binds to ATP, decreasing the negative charge of the γ-phosphoryl group and thereby rendering it more susceptible to nucleophilic attack. The precise role of K^+, which is also required by the enzyme, is not known.

6.2.6 Pyruvate Carboxylase

Pyruvate carboxylase from mammalian tissues is a large tetrameric, manganese-containing, biotin-dependent enzyme (MW = 500,000) in which each of the four identical subunits contains one Mn^{++} and one covalently bound biotinyl prosthetic group. The enzyme functions by the same ATP-dependent mechanism as do most other biotin-dependent enzymes, with the carboxybiotinyl enzyme as an intermediate (Chapter 4). Pyruvate binds to the enzyme only after carboxylation of the enzyme at the expense of the high energy γ-phosphoryl bond of ATP, and a concerted reaction mechanism results in the formation of oxaloacetate (Figure 6.6). This mitochondrial enzyme provides the principal route for the synthesis of oxaloacetate from pyruvate and bicarbonate in most eukaryotic cells. Acetyl CoA is a positive effector, and in the absence of this

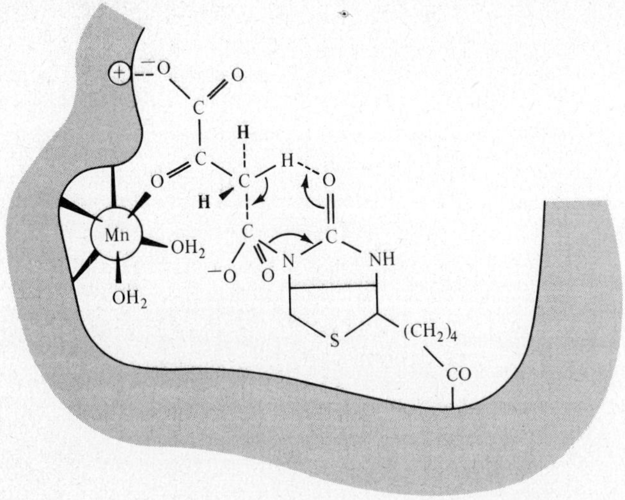

Figure 6.6 Possible mechanism for the reaction catalyzed by pyruvate carboxylase. A concerted mechanism for the transfer of the carboxyl group of *N'*-carboxybiotin to pyruvate is depicted. An active-site Mn^{++} functions to hold the substrate in correct orientation for reaction and also as an electrophilic catalyst.

agent, the enzyme is essentially inactive. ATP is a second energy-rich positive effector. A requirement of the enzyme for energy in the form of two indicators of the energy state of the mitochondrion presumably reflects its essential role in gluconeogenesis (see the next section). Although pyruvate carboxylase is lacking in *E. coli,* which carboxylates 3-carbon compounds exclusively by the biotin-independent PEP carboxylase-catalyzed reaction, many other microorganisms do possess this enzyme.

6.3 GLUCONEOGENESIS

In order for living organisms to grow at the expense of carbon and energy sources other than carbohydrates, they must be capable of synthesizing sugars from simpler starting materials. This process is called gluconeogenesis. Organisms that can synthesize sugars at the expense of C_3 compounds always possess the two enzymes that allow reversal of the glycolytic cycle (fructose-1,6-diphosphatase and glucose-6-phosphatase), and most such organisms additionally contain pyruvate carboxylase and PEP carboxykinase, PEP synthase, or pyruvate,phosphate dikinase, all of which were discussed in the preceding section (Table 6.3). Of these enzymes, only one (pyruvate carboxylase) is found in the mitochondrial matrix of a eukaryotic cell. The other gluconeogenic enzymes are found in the cell cytoplasm. The mitochondrial location of pyruvate carboxylase is of importance with respect to its allosteric regulation by acetyl CoA and ATP.

Pyruvate carboxylase plus PEP carboxykinase use two nucleoside triphosphates (ATP and GTP, respectively) to convert pyruvate to PEP in a two-step process in which oxaloacetate serves as the intermediate.

$$\text{pyruvate} + \text{ATP} + \text{GTP} \rightarrow \text{PEP} + \text{ADP} + \text{GDP} + \text{P}_i \qquad (6.3)$$

These two enzymes acting together, or PEP synthase or pyruvate,phosphate dikinase acting individually, bypass the pyruvate kinase-catalyzed conversion of PEP and ADP to pyruvate and ATP. Catalysis of gluconeogenesis from C_2 compounds (acetate and ethanol) additionally requires the two enzymes specific to the glyoxalate shunt as well as those of the Krebs cycle (see Section 6.6).

The synthesis of glucose from PEP occurs essentially by the reversal of glycolysis, where ATP and NADH are consumed rather than generated. All of the steps discussed in Chapter 5 leading from PEP to fructose-1,6-diP are reversible, and the same enzymes are therefore utilized. The conversion of fructose-1,6-diP to fructose-6-P and inorganic phosphate (reversal of the phosphofructokinase reaction), however, is catalyzed by an allosterically regulated enzyme, fructose-1,6-diphosphatase:

$$\text{fructose-1,6-diP} + H_2O \xrightarrow{\text{FDPase}} \text{fructose-6-P} + \text{P}_i \qquad (6.4)$$

The cleavage of glucose-6-P to glucose is also catalyzed by a phosphatase (glucose-6-phosphatase) which catalyzes a highly exergonic and essentially irreversible reaction:

$$\text{glucose-6-P} + H_2O \xrightarrow{\text{G6Pase}} \text{glucose} + \text{P}_i \qquad (6.5)$$

In animal tissues, AMP and fructose-2,6-diphosphate (discussed in Section 5.11), which are allosteric activators of phosphofructokinase, are allosteric inhibitors of fructose-1,6-diphosphatase. It can be seen that when ATP is limiting, glycolysis is favored, but when ATP is present in excess, gluconeogenesis occurs. The energy state of the cell therefore regulates the direction of the pathway and avoids the futile cycling of the two enzymes with the consequent hydrolysis of ATP. Such a cyclic process is also prevented by the anomeric specificities of these two enzymes: while phosphofructokinase acts on the β-anomer of fructose-6-P, fructose-1,6-diphosphatase exhibits specificity for the α-anomer. Because anomerization of the sugar is relatively slow, rapid futile cycling is prevented.

6.4 THE PYRUVATE DEHYDROGENASE COMPLEX

Associated with the matrix surface of the inner mitochondrial membrane of eukaryotes and with the cytoplasmic surface of the plasma membranes of many bacteria such as *E. coli* are found three distinct, but structurally, functionally, and evolutionarily related α-keto acid dehydrogenase complexes. These are (a) the pyruvate dehydrogenase complex, (b) the α-ketoglutarate dehydrogenase complex, and (c) the branched-chain α-keto acid dehydrogenase complex. The first of these three enzyme complexes serves as a link between glycolysis and the Krebs cycle. The second is one of the Krebs cycle enzymes, and the last of these enzymes functions in the oxidative degradation of α-keto acids derived from the branched-chain aliphatic amino acids, valine, isoleucine, and leucine.

All three of these dehydrogenase complexes catalyze essentially the same reaction with different substrates. They require the same cofactors and function by the same mechanism. The reaction catalyzed by all of them is:

$$R-\overset{O}{\overset{\|}{C}}-CO_2 + NAD^+ + CoA \rightarrow R-\overset{O}{\overset{\|}{C}}-SCoA + CO_2 + NADH \qquad (6.6)$$

Pyruvate is oxidatively decarboxylated by the pyruvate dehydrogenase complex to acetyl CoA and CO_2; α-ketoglutarate is converted by the α-ketoglutarate dehydrogenase complex to succinyl CoA and CO_2, and α-ketoisovalerate (derived from valine by transamination) is oxidized by the branched-chain α-keto acid dehydrogenase complex to isobutyryl CoA and CO_2. The five cofactors present within each of these three enzyme complexes (in order of their participation in the reaction) are: (1) thiamine pyrophosphate (TPP); (2) lipoate; (3) coenzyme A (CoA); (4) flavin adenine dinucleotide (FAD); and (5) nicotinamide adenine dinucleotide (NAD^+).

The conversion of each of the α-keto acids to its corresponding decarboxylated coenzyme A thioester involves three distinct catalytic proteins. These three enzymes within each of the three dehydrogenase complexes are designated: (a) Enzyme-1 (E1, a TPP-dependent decarboxylase which oxidatively decarboxylates the α-keto acid utilizing the lipoyl moiety in enzyme 2 as electron and acyl acceptor); (b) enzyme-2 (E2, an acyl transferase containing covalently bound lipoate which transfers the acyl derivative from reduced lipoate to coenzyme A); and (c) enzyme-3 (E3, a dehydrogenase containing tightly bound FAD which oxidizes reduced lipoate in enzyme-2 and then transfers the electrons to NAD^+). The three enzymes actually catalyze five distinct reactions as outlined in Figure 6.7. First, E1 decarboxylates the α-keto acid to produce an active aldehyde (reaction 1 in Figure 6.7). This reaction occurs as outlined in Section 4.9. Second, the active aldehyde (an α-hydroxy-derivative covalently bound

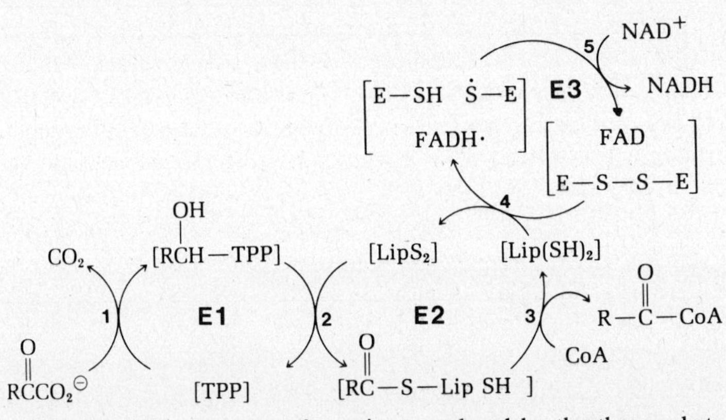

Figure 6.7 The sequence of reactions catalyzed by the three α-keto acid dehydrogenase complexes found in mitochondria and bacteria. R is a methyl group in the pyruvate dehydrogenase complex, $^{-}O_2C-(CH_2)_2-$ in the α-ketoglutarate dehydrogenase complex, and one of the branched-chain alkyl side chains of valine, isoleucine, or leucine for the branched-chain α-keto acid dehydrogenase complex. The three enzyme components of the complex are indicated E1, E2, and E3 and correspond to the α-keto acid decarboxylase, dihydrolipoyl transacetylase, and dihydrolipoyl dehydrogenase, respectively. The five reactions catalyzed by the complex are indicated 1–5. See text for details.

to TPP) is oxidized concomitant with reductive acylation of the covalently bound lipoyl moiety. In this process, the active aldehyde is effectively oxidized while the lipoyl moiety in E2 is reduced to the acyl dihydrolipoyl moiety (reaction 2). Third, the acyl group is transferred from the dihydrolipoyl moiety of E2 to coenzyme A in a reaction which requires only E2 (reaction 3). The reduced form of the lipoyl cofactor in E2 results. Fourth, E3 oxidizes the dihydrolipoyl moiety of E2, possibly by a free radical mechanism, which results in the transfer of the two hydrogen atoms from the dihydrolipoyl moiety of E2 to both FAD and a disulfide bridge (cystine) in E3 (reaction 4). This reaction regenerates the oxidized lipoyl prosthetic group of E2, preparing it for another cycle of catalysis. The two hydrogen atoms may be transferred to FAD (yielding $FADH_2$), they may be transferred to cystine in E3 (yielding two cysteine residues) or they may be individually transferred to both, yielding free radicals as illustrated in Figure 6.7. An equilibrium exists between these three forms of reduced E3. Finally, in reaction 5, a hydride ion is transferred to NAD^+, generating NADH plus a proton, and E3 is reoxidized to its native form.

Of the three α-keto acid dehydrogenase complexes, the pyruvate dehydrogenase (PDH) complex has been most extensively studied. In *E. coli* the complex has a molecular weight of about five million, and that from mammalian mitochondria is even larger. The α-keto acid dehydrogenase complexes are probably among the largest enzyme complexes found in nature.

The protein constituents of the *E. coli* pyruvate dehydrogenase complex are described in Table 6.4. The complex consists of 60 polypeptide chains of three dissimilar types. There are 24 E1 protomers (12 homodimers), 24 protomeric E2 molecules, and 12 E3 subunits (6 homodimers). The 24 E2 molecules comprise a central cubic *core* complex to which both E1 and E3 are attached. The E2 polypeptide chain contains three highly homologous repeating sequences in the N-terminal half of the protein, each of which contains a lipoyl–lysyl derivative. These three homologous sequences are separated from one another by regions of polypeptide chain which are oddly rich in alanyl and prolyl residues and are thought to be conformationally mobile. At least two of the three lipoylated segments are acetylated in the intact complex in the presence of substrate. The C-terminal half of the molecule contains the acetyltransferase active site and the binding sites for E1, E3, and other E2 subunits. Dissociation of E1 and E3 from E2 gives inactive proteins which can be reconstituted to the active complex when all three proteins are mixed at neutral pH.

TABLE 6.4 COMPONENTS OF THE *E. COLI* PYRUVATE DEHYDROGENASE COMPLEX

Enzyme	E.C. #	Coenzymes	Number of subunits per enzyme	Molecular weight		Number of subunits per complex
				Subunit	Total	
Pyruvate decarboxylase	1.2.4.1	Thiamine pyrophosphate	2	95,000	190,000	24 (12 dimers)
Dihydrolipoyl transacetylase	2.3.1.12	Lipoate, coenzyme A	24	91,000	1,700,000	24
Dihydrolipoyl dehydrogenase	1.6.4.3	FAD, NAD^+	2	56,000	112,000	12 (6 dimers)

As noted in Chapter 4, lipoate is attached to the enzyme backbone via an arm which is about 1.5 nm in length. The association of the reactive part of the lipoyl moiety with the end of this arm allows for limited mobility. The arm can potentially sweep out a circle with a radius of 1.5 nm so that the active part of the lipoyl moiety can theoretically extend for a distance of at most 3 nm. Fluorescence energy transfer experiments have shown that the average distance between TPP in E1 and FAD in E3 is about 5 nm. Since this distance exceeds the possible distance of extension allowed for by a single lipoyl–lysyl arm (3 nm), and since the end of the arm must interact with the active sites of E1, E2, and E3, at least two of the three lipoyl–lysyl moieties in each subunit of E2 are presumed to be involved. Transfer of the acyl group and the electron pair must involve at least one transfer in addition to those shown in Figure 6.7 as follows:

$$\text{(acetyldihydrolipoyl-1)-E2} + \text{(lipoyl-2)-E2} \rightarrow \text{(lipoyl-1)-E2} + \text{(acetyldihydrolipoyl-2)-E2.} \quad (6.7)$$

It is possible that each of the three lipoyl–lysyl groups in E2 functions with one of the three enzymes. This relay reaction allows the pyruvate dehydrogenase complex to overcome the problem of long distance interactions and to span the distances between sites. Some evidence indicates that the principal architectural features of the *E. coli* transacetylase are shared by the bovine heart enzyme.

In *E. coli* the activity of the pyruvate dehydrogenase complex is subject to regulatory interactions by metabolites which strictly control the supply of acetyl CoA. For example, the ratio of AMP to ATP allosterically regulates the activity of E1 (which catalyzes an essentially irreversible reaction), the ratio of coenzyme A to acetyl CoA determines the activity of E2, and the ratio of NAD^+ to NADH controls the activity of E3. As a result, a low adenylate energy charge, a low concentration of acetyl CoA, or an insufficiency of reducing power in the form of NADH all stimulate the activity of the complex to help correct the deficiency. An excess of ATP, acetyl CoA and/or NADH inhibits the enzyme complex as is required for the maintenance of homeostatic conditions. Because these effects are transmitted from one enzyme in the complex to the other two, the activities of the three enzymes are coordinated.

Like the *E. coli* pyruvate dehydrogenase complex, the mammalian enzyme is regulated by these three metabolite ratios. However, the mammalian pyruvate dehydrogenase complex is also regulated by covalent modification. In this system, the pyruvate decarboxylase component consists of an $\alpha_2\beta_2$ heterotetramer (see Table 6.5). Each α-subunit is known to possess a TPP binding site. Firmly associated with the complex are about six PDH kinase molecules, and loosely associated are about six PDH-P phosphatase molecules (Table 6.5). Each kinase molecule contains two subunits, an α-subunit (MW = 48,000) with which the catalytic activity resides, and a β-subunit (MW = 45,000) which appears to function in a regulatory capacity. The phosphatase similarly consists of a heterodimer (Table 6.5). The α-subunit (MW = 50,000) possesses phosphatase activity. While the enzyme contains tightly bound Ca^{++}, and the β-subunit (MW = 100,000) interestingly contains FAD, the function of the β-subunit remains to be established. Possibly the FAD can be reversibly reduced with regulatory consequences to the activity of the α-subunit.

TABLE 6.5 COMPONENTS OF THE BOVINE KIDNEY PYRUVATE DEHYDROGENASE COMPLEX

Enzyme	Coenzymes	Number of subunits per enzyme	Molecular weight: Subunit	Molecular weight: Total	Number of subunits per complex
Pyruvate decarboxylase	Thiamine pyrophosphate	2α	41,000	154,000	40 (20 tetramers)
		2β	36,000		40 (20 tetramers)
Dihydrolipoyl transacetylase	Lipoate, coenzyme A	60	52,000	3,100,000	60
Dihydrolipoyl dehydrogenase	FAD, NAD$^+$	2	55,000	110,000	12 (6 dimers)
Pyruvate decarboxylase kinase		1α	48,000	93,000	~6
		1β	45,000		~6
Phosphatase		1α	50,000	150,000	~6
		1β	100,000		~6

The ratio of the activities of the kinase and phosphatase is apparently influenced by the metabolite ratios discussed in the preceding paragraph. Additionally, the phosphatase requires Mg^{++} and is stimulated by Ca^{++} and by polyamines, while the kinase is inhibited by ADP and pyruvate. The kinase phosphorylates a seryl residue in one of the α-subunits of the pyruvate decarboxylase tetramer at the expense of ATP, yielding an inactive enzyme. Two further phosphoryl groups can derivatize two additional seryl residues in the same α-subunit of the decarboxylase. These additional phosphoryl groups exert no further inhibitory effect on the already inactive enzyme, but they inhibit the PDH-P phosphatase, thereby prolonging inactivation of the complex. The net effect of multiple phosphorylations is to increase the duration of the inhibitory effects of the kinase. The mammalian system is therefore subject to both allosteric regulation and covalent regulatory modifications, and sensitivity to regulatory agents is transmitted through the complex by tight subunit–subunit coupling interactions.

6.5 THE TRICARBOXYLIC ACID CYCLE

The tricarboxylic acid cycle is shown in Figure 6.8, and the eight enzymes that catalyze the various reactions are listed in Table 6.6. These eight enzymes exhibit nearly absolute specificities for their substrates and products. They are discussed individually below.

6.5.1 Citrate Synthase (The Condensing Enzyme)

Citrate synthase catalyzes a Claisen (an aldol-type) condensation of acetyl CoA with oxaloacetate. The mechanism is depicted in Figure 6.9. A basic residue in the enzyme extracts an α-proton from acetyl CoA which by virtue of thioesterification is fairly

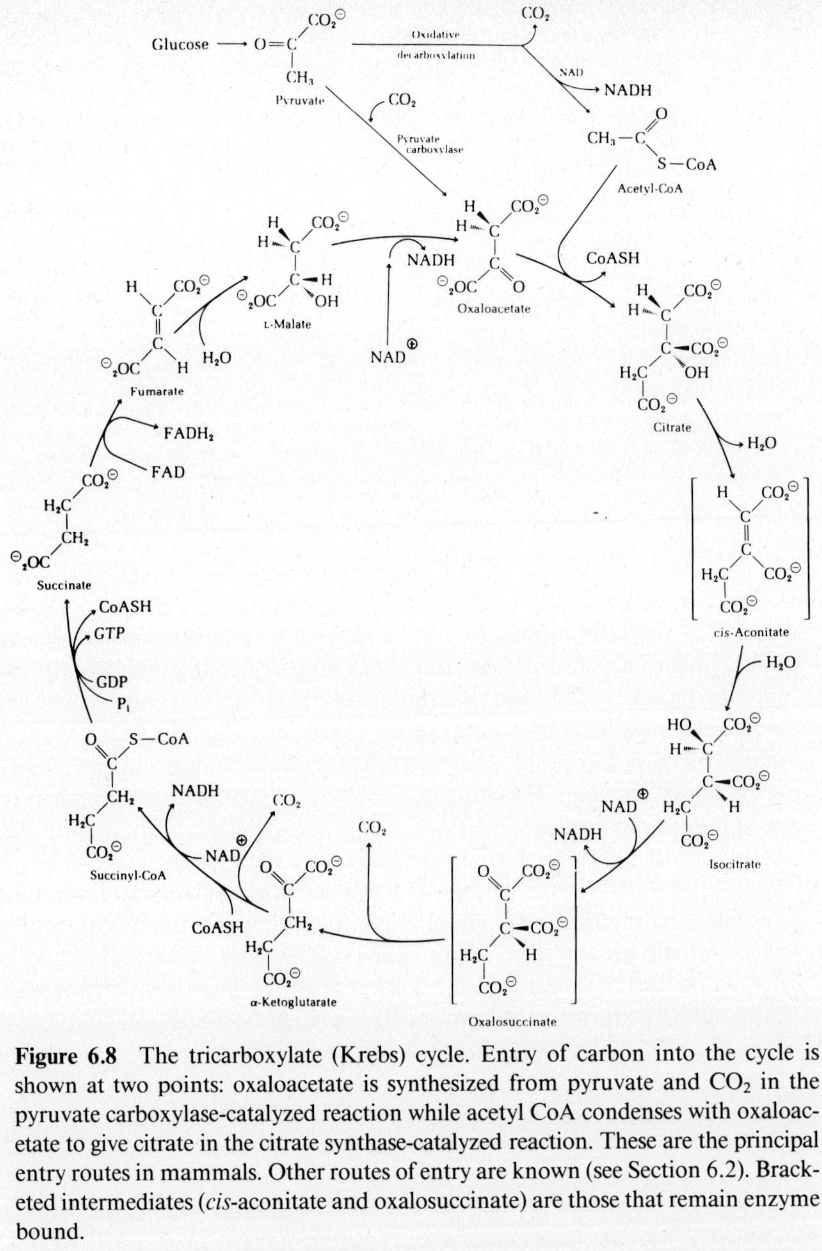

Figure 6.8 The tricarboxylate (Krebs) cycle. Entry of carbon into the cycle is shown at two points: oxaloacetate is synthesized from pyruvate and CO_2 in the pyruvate carboxylase-catalyzed reaction while acetyl CoA condenses with oxaloacetate to give citrate in the citrate synthase-catalyzed reaction. These are the principal entry routes in mammals. Other routes of entry are known (see Section 6.2). Bracketed intermediates (*cis*-aconitate and oxalosuccinate) are those that remain enzyme bound.

labile. The resultant carbanion, an excellent nucleophile, attacks the electropositive carbon atom of the keto group in oxaloacetate to give citroyl CoA (Figure 6.9). Finally, the high-energy thioester bond is hydrolyzed to give the symmetrical tricarboxylate anion, citrate, and free coenzyme A. This last step renders the process essentially irreversible. The enzyme is allosterically regulated by NADH and succinyl CoA which function as feed-back inhibitors.

TABLE 6.6 THE ENZYMES OF THE TRICARBOXYLATE CYCLE

Step	Trivial name	Systematic name	E.C. #	Cofactor(s)	Reaction catalyzed
1	Citrate synthase	Citrate oxaloacetate-lyase	4.1.3.7	Mg^{++}	Oxaloacetate + acetyl-CoA + H_2O → citrate + CoA
2	Aconitase (aconitate hydratase)	Citrate (isocitrate) hydro-lyase	4.2.1.3	Fe^{++}; thiols	Citrate → *cis*-aconitate → isocitrate
3a	Isocitrate dehydrogenase (NAD^+)	Isocitrate:NAD^+ oxidoreductase (decarboxylating)	1.1.1.41	Mn^{++}	Isocitrate + NAD^+ → α-ketoglutarate + CO_2 + NADH
3b	Isocitrate dehydrogenase ($NADP^+$)	Isocitrate:$NADP^+$ oxidoreductase (decarboxylating)	1.1.1.42	Mn^{++}	Isocitrate + $NADP^+$ → α-ketoglutarate + CO_2 + NADPH
4	α-Ketoglutarate dehydrogenase complex (3 constituent enzymes; see Table 6.7)				
5a	Succinate thiokinase (GDP forming succinyl CoA synthase)	Succinate:CoA ligase (GDP forming)	6.2.1.4	Mg^{++}	Succinyl CoA + GDP + P_i → succinate + GTP + CoA
5b	Succinate thiokinase (ADP forming succinyl CoA synthase)	Succinate:CoA ligase (ADP forming)	6.2.1.5	Mg^{++}	Succinyl CoA + ADP + P_i → succinate + ATP + CoA
6	Succinate dehydrogenase	Succinate:acceptor oxidoreductase	1.3.99.1	Fe^{++}; FAD	Succinate + acceptor → fumarate + reduced acceptor
7	Fumarase (fumarate hydrase)	L-Malate hydro-lyase	4.2.1.2	—	Fumarate + H_2O → L-malate
8	Malate dehydrogenase	L-Malate:NAD^+ dehydrogenase	1.1.1.37	—	L-Malate + NAD^+ → oxaloacetate + NADH

6.5.2 Aconitate Hydrase (Aconitase)

Aconitate hydrase catalyzes the interconversion of the symmetrical, nonoxidizable tricarboxylate anion, citrate, into isocitrate, an asymmetric, readily oxidizable tricarboxylate with two chiral centers. Isocitrate has its hydroxyl group on the 2-carbon instead of the 3-position. Water is first eliminated from citrate to yield *cis*-aconitate, a tricarboxylic acid with an unsaturation between carbon atoms 2 and 3. Subsequently, water is added back across the double bond in the opposite orientation. The substrates are held in a specific orientation on the enzyme surface with the aid of a tightly bound ferrous ion, and the OH^- and H^+ of water are removed and added trans with respect

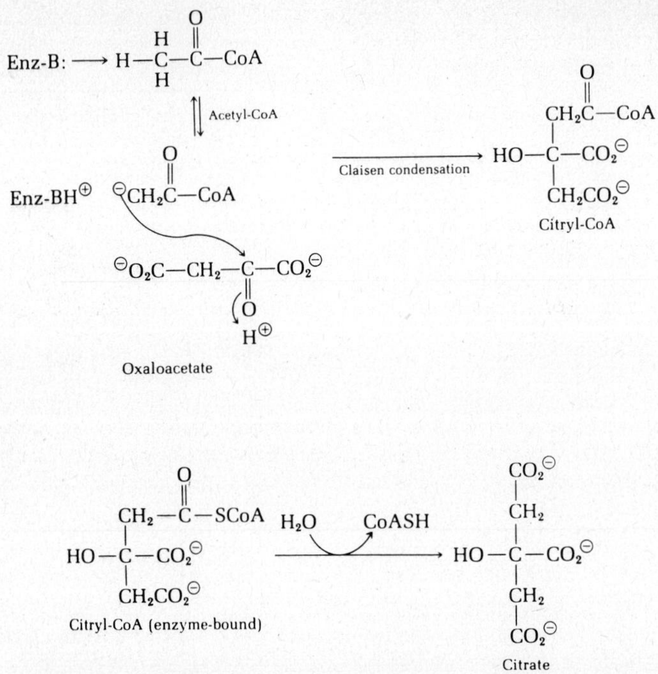

Figure 6.9 Mechanism of action of citrate synthase. A Claisen condensation (top) followed by hydrolysis of the thioester bond of citryl CoA gives rise to the product released from the enzyme surface, citrate.

to each other. This enzyme catalyzes a fully reversible reaction which is not subject to allosteric control.

6.5.3 Isocitrate Dehydrogenase

Isocitrate dehydrogenase catalyzes the oxidative decarboxylation of isocitrate in an ordered, two-step reaction sequence. First, isocitrate is oxidized with simultaneous transfer of a hydride to NAD^+, and second, oxalosuccinate, which remains tightly bound to the enzyme surface at room temperature, is decarboxylated to α-ketoglutarate.

The mammalian enzyme is a tetramer which exhibits a sigmoidal (positively cooperative) response to its substrate, isocitrate, and is allosterically regulated by adenine nucleotides. AMP and ADP activate the enzyme, lowering the K_m for isocitrate by an order of magnitude, while ATP inhibits. NADH, a product of the reaction, is also a potent inhibitor. Because decarboxylation follows dehydrogenation, the reaction catalyzed by this enzyme is essentially irreversible as expected for an allosterically regulated enzyme.

In *E. coli* the activity of this dimeric, $NADP^+$-dependent enzyme is regulated by a phosphorylation reaction catalyzed by a metabolite-sensitive isocitrate dehydrogenase-specific kinase. The phosphorylated enzyme is inactive. The extent to which

TABLE 6.7 COMPONENTS OF THE *E. COLI* α-KETOGLUTARATE DEHYDROGENASE COMPLEX

Enzyme	E.C. #	Coenzymes	Number of subunits per enzyme	Molecular weight: Subunit	Molecular weight: Total	Number of subunits per complex
α-Ketoglutarate decarboxylase	1.2.4.2	Thiamine pyrophosphate	2	95,000	190,000	12 (6 dimers)
Dihydrolipoyl transsuccinylase	2.3.1.61	Lipoate, coenzyme A	24	42,000	1,000,000	24
Dihydrolipoyl-dehydrogenase	1.6.4.3	FAD, NAD^+	2	55,000	110,000	12 (6 dimers)

the cellular enzyme population is phosphorylated determines the relative rates of catabolism (via the Krebs cycle) and anabolism (via the glyoxalate shunt) as discussed in Section 6.6.

6.5.4 α-Ketoglutarate Dehydrogenase

α-Ketoglutarate dehydrogenase is a large enzyme complex associated with the inner mitochondrial membrane which catalyzes the oxidative decarboxylation of α-ketoglutarate essentially as the pyruvate dehydrogenase complex oxidatively decarboxylates pyruvate as discussed in Section 6.4 and illustrated in figure 6.7. The composition of the α-ketoglutarate dehydrogenase complex from *E. coli* is presented in Table 6.7. The product of the five reactions catalyzed by the complex is succinyl CoA, and NAD^+ is reduced in the process (Figure 6.7). In spite of the generation of the energy-rich thioester and the endergonic reduction of NAD^+ to NADH, the decarboxylation step helps to render the process exergonic. It is therefore not surprising that this enzyme is subject to regulation by the ratio of NADH/NAD^+ and succinyl CoA/CoA. Some reports also suggest a regulatory role of the ATP/ADP ratio and Ca^{++}. In all cases, the more energetic compound of the pair is the more inhibitory.

6.5.5 Succinyl CoA Synthase (Succinate Thiokinase)

Succinyl CoA synthase couples the hydrolysis of succinyl CoA to the synthesis of GTP from GDP and inorganic phosphate in mammals or of ATP from ADP and P_i in many bacteria (Table 6.6). This process, like that catalyzed by glyceraldehyde-3-P dehydrogenase, is termed *substrate-level phosphorylation* because the formation of a high-energy pyrophosphoryl bond is coupled to a strictly chemical reaction instead of to respiratory electron transfer. It is worth noting that the formation of the initial high-energy bond in the reactions catalyzed by both glyceraldehyde-3-P dehydrogenase and α-ketoglutarate dehydrogenase involve substrate oxidation. The reaction catalyzed by succinyl CoA synthase is readily reversible, and the enzyme is not subject to allosteric regulation as expected.

The mechanism of the succinyl CoA synthase reaction appears to involve a three-step group transfer process. Inorganic phosphate first displaces the coenzyme A from the substrate with the formation of a mixed anhydride bond between succinate and phosphate. Tightly bound succinyl-P is the product:

$$\text{E} + \text{succinyl CoA} + \text{P}_i \rightarrow \text{E}\cdot\text{succinyl-P} + \text{CoA} \tag{6.8}$$

Second, the phosphoryl moiety is transferred to a histidyl residue in the protein:

$$\text{E}\cdot\text{succinyl-P} \rightarrow \text{E(his)P} + \text{succinate} \tag{6.9}$$

Third, the phosphorylated enzyme transfers its phosphoryl group directly to GDP in mammals or ADP in *E. coli* with the synthesis of GTP or ATP, respectively:

$$\text{E(his)P} + \text{G(A)DP} \rightarrow \text{E} + \text{G(A)TP}. \tag{6.10}$$

Because all three transfer reactions are reversible, the free enzyme can be phosphorylated either with a nucleoside triphosphate [Equation (6.10)] or with succinyl CoA and inorganic phosphate [Equations (6.8) and (6.9)].

The structure and mechanism of action of the *E. coli* enzyme has been studied in considerable detail. The enzyme has the subunit composition of $\alpha_2\beta_2$ with an overall molecular weight of 140,000. While the α-subunit has a molecular weight of 30,000, that of the β-subunit is 40,000. The tetrameric enzyme contains two active sites, each arranged at the interface of the α- and β-subunits. The α-subunit binds ADP or ATP and contains the active-site histidyl residue that is phosphorylated while the β-subunit binds succinate and coenzyme A. The enzyme can therefore be considered to be a *functional* homodimer where the functional unit is the α-β heterodimer.

Succinyl CoA synthase represents one of the best documented examples of an enzyme that is believed to function by a half-of-sites (alternating sites) mechanism. The evidence is as follows:

1. Only one of the two identical α-subunits was found to be phosphorylated at any one time, but both were apparently equally susceptible to phosphorylation.
2. Phosphorylation of one subunit induced a conformational change in the other which drastically decreased its susceptibility to protease digestion.
3. When an exchange reaction catalyzed by the enzyme $\{[^{18}\text{O}]\text{P}_i \rightleftharpoons \text{succinate}$; a partial reaction corresponding to equations (6.8) and (6.9)$\}$ was studied as a function of ATP concentration, the rate of [^{18}O]-exchange was found to be dependent on the ATP concentration, and this exchange reaction increased in rate more than did the ATP cleavage reaction [the partial reaction corresponding to equation (6.10)]. Variations in the coenzyme A concentration did not have a corresponding effect.
4. Succinyl CoA synthase from a mammalian tissue, known to have an α-β structure with only a single active site, showed a constant ratio of these two partial reactions as a function of GTP concentration.
5. Employing the technique of ^{31}P-nuclear magnetic resonance (NMR), it was found that the addition of succinate to the monophosphorylated *E. coli* enzyme was not sufficient to elicit the formation of succinyl-P. Addition of ATP to the already phosphorylated enzyme was required.
6. When a nonhydrolyzable analogue of ATP was used

$$\mathrm{AMP{-}O{-}\overset{O}{\underset{O^-}{P}}{-}CH_2{-}\overset{O}{\underset{O^-}{P}}{-}OH}$$

(in which the γ-phosphoryl group is linked to ADP via a methylene bridge) no phosphorylation of succinate was induced.

7. Phosphorylation of the *E. coli* enzyme with ATP at one active site was found to promote dissociation of succinyl CoA from the active site of the other functional subunit.

These experimental observations appear to establish an alternating sites-type mechanism for the *E. coli* succinyl CoA synthase. Catalysis of phosphoryl group transfer from E(his)P to succinate only occurs at one site when phosphoryl group transfer from ATP to the corresponding histidyl residue in the other subunit occurs. In other words, enzyme phosphorylation at the expense of ATP at one active site in the functionally dimeric enzyme is coupled to the dephosphorylation of the enzyme by succinate at the other active site. The fact that

$$\mathrm{AMP{-}O{-}\overset{O}{\underset{O^-}{P}}{-}CH_2{-}\overset{O}{\underset{O^-}{P}}{-}OH}$$

did not promote catalytic transfer from E(his)P to succinate argues against a simple substrate-binding-induced conformational effect. The half-of-sites phosphorylation of the enzyme is not likely to be a consequence of permanent asymmetry. Succinyl CoA synthase therefore appears to provide an example of alternating sites cooperativity.

6.5.6 Succinate Dehydrogenase

The sixth enzyme in the sequence, succinate dehydrogenase is a highly complex constituent of the inner mitochondrial membrane which functions as a constituent of the electron transport chain. The structure and function of this enzyme will be discussed in Chapter 7. As shown in Table 6.6, two adjacent hydrogen atoms on the α- and β-carbon atoms of succinate are transferred to a modified FAD molecule to generate fumarate and $FADH_2$. The deriviatized FAD molecule is covalently bound to the enzyme via a histidyl residue. The product, fumarate, contains a trans-unsaturation due to the specificity of the enzyme. While oxaloacetate inhibits the activity of succinate dehydrogenase, reduced coenzyme Q (coenzyme QH_2) has been reported to activate it. The physiological significance of this surprising observation is not known.

6.5.7 Fumarate Hydrase (Fumarase)

Fumarate hydrase catalyzes the hydration of fumarate to give L-malate. The reaction is readily reversible, and the enzyme is not subject to allosteric regulation.

6.5.8 Malate Dehydrogenase

Malate dehydrogenase oxidizes L-malate to oxaloacetate with NAD^+ as cofactor, thus completing the cycle. Although the reaction is endergonic, it is drawn in the direction of oxidation by the continuous removal of oxaloacetate in the reaction catalyzed by citrate synthase. It is not subject to regulation.

6.6 THE GLYOXALATE CYCLE

A variety of microorganisms including bacteria, protozoa, fungi, and algae can grow at the expense of 2-carbon compounds and compounds which are initially metabolized to 2-carbon fragments. These compounds include acetate, ethanol, and fatty acids. They all give rise to the same intermediate—acetyl CoA. Fatty acids are degraded to this 2-carbon derivative directly via the β-oxidation cycle (Chapter 8); ethanol is metabolized via a pathway which initially involves two oxidation steps in which electrons are transferred to NAD^+, first to give acetaldehyde and then acetate; and acetate is activated to acetyl CoA in a single step which involves the hydrolysis of ATP to AMP and pyrophosphate (Chapter 8). In the first common metabolic step involving the metabolism of these sources of carbon and energy, acetyl CoA is condensed with oxaloacetate in the citrate synthase-catalyzed reaction of the Krebs cycle to give citrate. Energy in the form of NADH and ATP can then be obtained by the oxidation of the acetyl moiety of citrate to carbon dioxide via the Krebs cycle.

Metabolism via the Krebs cycle is not sufficient for growth on acetyl CoA as a sole source of carbon because this cycle is a purely degradative pathway which alone does not allow synthesis and utilization of Krebs cycle intermediates for biosynthetic purposes. Thus, the cell must possess a molecule of oxaloacetate in order to metabolize a molecule of acetyl CoA via the Krebs cycle, and only one molecule of oxaloacetate is generated from citrate in a single turn of the cycle. In order to maintain the functioning of the cycle in the absence of an alternative source of a di- or tricarboxylic acid, no Krebs cycle intermediates can be utilized for biosynthetic or gluconeogenic purposes. The Krebs cycle alone is therefore insufficient for growth on two carbon compounds.

In order to circumvent this problem, the glyoxalate cycle, or glyoxalate bypass was invented. This cycle utilizes three steps of the Krebs cycle, those catalyzed by citrate synthase, aconitase and malate dehydrogenase, but bypasses the two oxidative steps in which CO_2 is released from isocitrate yielding a four carbon dicarboxylic acid (Figure 6.10). Instead, isocitrate is first cleaved to succinate and the two-carbon aldehydic carboxylic acid, glyoxalate ($HOC\text{-}COO^-$), in a reaction catalyzed by isocitrate lyase. Glyoxalate is then condensed with a second molecule of acetyl CoA to give L-malate. This second reaction is catalyzed by malate synthase. L-malate is then oxidized to oxaloacetate in the malate dehydrogenase-catalyzed reaction to complete the cycle. The net result of the glyoxalate bypass is the condensation of two C-2 fragments to give a C_4 compound:

$$2 \text{ acetyl CoA} + NAD^+ \rightarrow \text{succinate} + NADH + H^+ + 2 \text{ CoA} \qquad (6.11)$$

Because the glyoxalate cycle replenishes TCA cycle intermediates used for biosynthetic purposes, it is called an *anaplerotic* pathway. In eukaryotic microorganisms such as yeast, all five enzymes of the glyoxalate cycle are found in the cell cytoplasm. Thus, different isozymes of citrate synthase, aconitase, and malate dehydrogenase with dif-

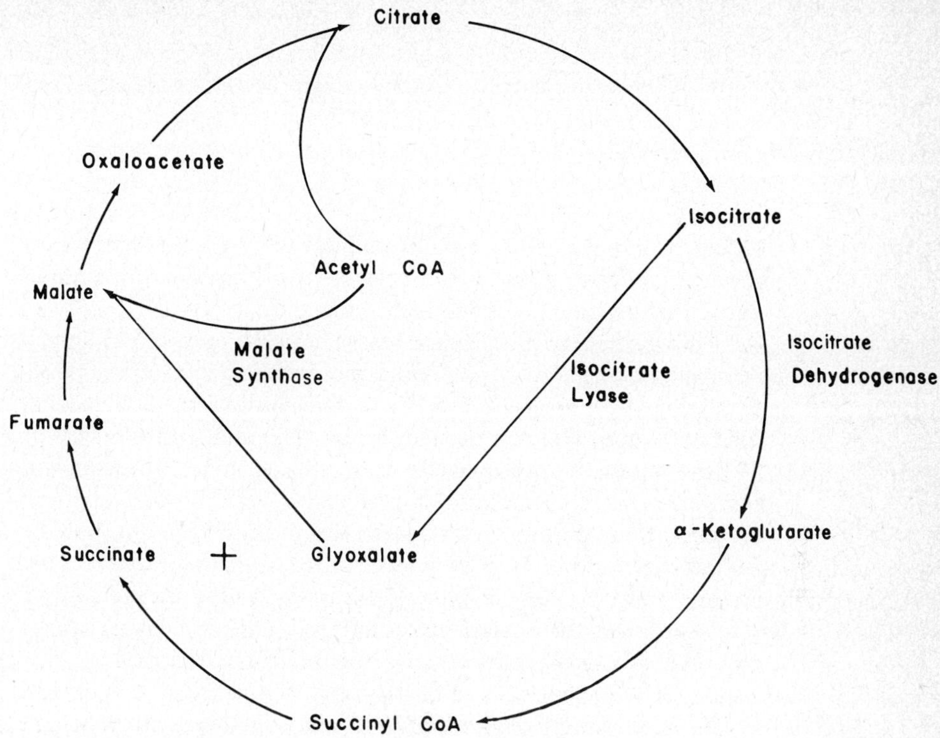

Figure 6.10 Abbreviated, schematized version of the Krebs cycle (outer circle) and the glyoxalate shunt (center). Only the unique enzymes of the shunt (isocitrate lyase and malate synthase) as well as the key regulatory enzyme controlling carbon flow through the two pathways (isocitrate dehydrogenase) are shown. (Reproduced with permission from M. H. Saier, *Mechanisms and Regulation of Carbohydrate Transport in Bacteria,* Academic, New York, 1985.)

ferent cellular locations catalyze the reactions of the Krebs cycle and the glyoxalate cycle. In plants the five enzymes of the glyoxalate cycle are housed in a distinct organelle called a *glyoxysome.*

In order for growth on a C-2 compound to occur at the maximal rate, both the glyoxalate and TCA cycles must function, and, moreover, the relative amounts of carbon that are utilized for catabolic purposes via the TCA cycle versus anabolic purposes via the glyoxalate cycle must be finely regulated. In all microorganisms capable of growth on C-2 compounds, the flow of carbon is regulated by controlling the activity of the branch point enzyme, isocitrate dehydrogenase. In eukaryotic organisms that contain an oligomeric NAD^+-dependent isocitrate dehydrogenase, the enzyme is allosterically regulated by the ratios of $[NAD^+]/[NADH]$ and [ADP]/[ATP]. While NAD^+, AMP, and ADP stimulate its activity, NADH and ATP inhibit. In *E. coli* and many other bacteria, the enzyme utilizes $NADP^+$ instead of NAD^+ and is not subject to allosteric regulation. It is controlled by reversible, covalent modification.

Synthesis of the enzymes specific to the glyoxalate pathway, isocitrate lyase and malate synthase, is induced in *E. coli* by growth on acetate. Competition between isocitrate lyase and isocitrate dehydrogenase determines the relative activities of the two pathways. Even under conditions that result in maximal induction of isocitrate lyase, isocitrate dehydrogenase has a greater V_{max} and lower K_m than the lyase. In order to increase the flow of carbon through the glyoxalate cycle, isocitrate dehydrogenase is inactivated by phosphorylation of a seryl residue in the protein.

E. coli $NADP^+$-dependent isocitrate dehydrogenase is a dimeric enzyme with a molecular weight of 100,000 consisting of two identical subunits. Each subunit can be phosphorylated by isocitrate dehydrogenase kinase on a single seryl residue, and the doubly phosphorylated dimeric enzyme is totally inactive. Cleavage of the phosphoryl moiety from the modified enzyme by isocitrate dehydrogenase-P phosphatase results in the restoration of full enzymatic activity.

The isocitrate dehydrogenase kinase has been purified to homogeneity. It consists of a single polypeptide chain with a molecular weight of 66,000. Surprisingly, this polypeptide chain exhibits both kinase and phosphatase activities. The kinase shows hyperbolic responses to its two substrates, ATP and isocitrate dehydrogenase.

The kinase and phosphatase appear to be subject to reciprocal allosteric regulation. Allosteric agents that inhibit the kinase generally activate the phosphatase and vice versa. For example, ATP and ADP inhibit the kinase, but the phosphatase is essentially inactive in their absence. Further, isocitrate, oxaloacetate, phosphoenolpyruvate, and pyruvate all activate the phosphatase by increasing the V_{max} in the presence of ADP, but these agents inhibit the kinase. The kinase–phosphatase complex, rather than isocitrate dehydrogenase therefore appears to be subject to metabolite-sensitive allosteric control. The availability of an excess of ADP, a Krebs cycle intermediate (isocitrate or oxaloacetate), or a glycolytic intermediate (PEP or pyruvate) inhibits the kinase and activates the phosphatase so that isocitrate dehydrogenase is not phosphorylated, and carbon flow proceeds through the Krebs cycle for catabolic purposes and the generation of reducing power. When the levels of the Krebs cycle and glycolytic intermediates are low, however, the kinase is relieved from inhibition, and the phosphatase is less active. Consequently, isocitrate dehydrogenase is phosphorylated and inactivated so that carbon flows through the glyoxalate shunt with a net synthesis of Krebs cycle and glycolytic intermediates. Oxaloacetate and isocitrate can be thought of as feedback inhibitors signaling the sufficiency of Krebs cycle intermediates, while PEP and pyruvate are the corresponding glycolytic intermediates which signal a sufficiency of these compounds. In this way the kinase–phosphatase is able to maintain a balance between the activities of the two cyclic pathways of C-2 metabolism, supplying quite precisely the biosynthetic and energy requirements of the cell. Displacement of the site of allosteric regulation from the target enzyme, isocitrate dehydrogenase, to the kinase–phosphatase complex presumably allows greater sensitivity to fluctuations in the concentrations of cytoplasmic metabolites. Similar cascade-type regulatory mechanisms have been noted for two other crucial metabolic processes, synthesis and hydrolysis of the glycolytic regulatory molecule, fructose-2,6-diphosphate (Chapter 5) and adenylylation and deadenylylation of glutamine synthase, the enzyme responsible for the fixation of ammonia into organic nitrogen (Chapter 9). In each of these cases, a metabolite-sensitive enzyme complex catalyzes both the forward and the reverse reactions. Presumably the incorporation of both catalytic activities in a single enzyme complex facilitates coordination of the reciprocal control of opposing activities and minimizes wasteful energy expenditure in cyclic processes.

6.7 OVERVIEW OF REGULATION IN AN AMPHIBOLIC PATHWAY

Numerous biosynthetic (anabolic) and degradative (catabolic) pathways are subject to regulation due to sensitivity of one or more of the constituent enzymes to inhibition and/or stimulation by cellular metabolites. In the case of an anabolic sequence, the regulatory metabolite is frequently the end-product of the pathway, and the enzyme that is sensitive to feedback control is the one that initiates the chemical transformation sequence. A variety of basic homeostatic negative regulatory mechanisms have been demonstrated, including single metabolite feedback, cooperative feedback, concerted feedback, and cumulative feedback (see Chapter 3). By contrast, strictly degradative sequences are generally not subject to end-product inhibition but exhibit sensitivity to regulation by compounds that serve as indicators of the energy state of the cell. Such indicators are frequently inorganic phosphate, pyrophosphate, or adenine nucleotides. These compounds signal the availability of the ultimate products of energy metabolism common to the diverse catabolic channels. These same regulatory constraints appear to be superimposed on *amphibolic* pathways, metabolic sequences which fulfill both anabolic and catabolic functions in the cell.

The glycolytic scheme and the citric acid cycle can be thought of as a continuous sequence of metabolic reactions consisting of pathway segments in which a physiologically irreversible reaction is followed by one or more reversible reactions (Figure 6.11). Each of the enzymes catalyzing an irreversible reaction is generally subject to negative allosteric feedback regulation by a product generated later in the reaction scheme. Four documented examples of this behavior in *E. coli* are phosphofructokinase, which is inhibited by phosphoenolpyruvate; phosphoenolpyruvate carboxylase, which is inhibited by aspartate and other dicarboxylic acids; pyruvate decarboxylase (the first of the three constituent enzymes of the pyruvate dehydrogenase multienzyme complex), which is subject to inhibition by acetyl CoA and other metabolites; and citrate synthase, which is inhibited by α-ketoglutarate (Figure 6.11). In each case, the inhibitory response can be considered analogous to classic end-product control, even though the products are utilized further for catabolic as well as anabolic purposes.

In dealing with the same metabolic pathway, it has been found that a metabolite generated early in the sequence may activate an enzyme which catalyzes a reaction further along in the sequence. As for the enzymes that are subject to end-product inhibition, precursor-activated enzymes usually catalyze essentially irreversible reactions. For example, in *E. coli* both phosphoenolpyruvate carboxylase and pyruvate kinase are activated by fructose-1,6-diphosphate (Figure 6.11).

In addition to end-product and precursor control, allosteric enzymes that catalyze irreversible reactions in amphibolic pathways may be subject to control by compounds that serve as indicators of the cellular energy level. As for catabolic pathways, the compounds that usually function in this capacity are AMP, ADP, ATP, pyrophosphate, and inorganic phosphate. However, since other purine and pyrimidine nucleotides may be in equilibrium with the adenine nucleotides by means of nucleoside kinases, the former compounds may also serve as indicators of cellular energy availability. Examples of energy-sensitive enzymes represented in Figure 6.11 include phosphofructokinase, which is activated by ADP and GDP; one of the two pyruvate kinases in *E. coli,* which is activated by AMP; and the pyruvate decarboxylase component of

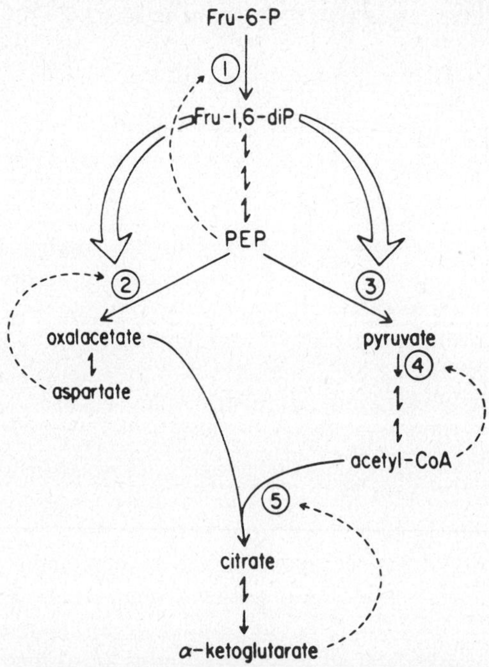

Figure 6.11 Partial reaction sequences and regulation of glycolysis and the Krebs cycle in *E. coli.* Single-headed solid arrows (⟶) indicate reactions that are essentially irreversible under physiological conditions. Reversible reactions are indicated by double-headed arrows (⇌). End-product feed-back inhibition is indicated by dashed arrows (--→), while precursor activation is indicated by solid double-lined arrows (⟹). The enzymes indicated by number are (1) phosphofructokinase (EC 2.7.1.11); (2) phosphoenolpyruvate carboxylase (EC 4.1.1.31); (3) pyruvate kinase (EC 2.7.1.40). (4) pyruvate decarboxylase (EC 1.2.4.1), and (5) citrate synthase (EC 4.1.3.7). Abbreviations: Fru-6-P, fructose 6-phosphate; Fru-1,6-P, fructose-1,6-diphosphate; PEP, phosphoenolpyruvate. (Reproduced with permission from M. H. Saier, Jr., "The Role of the Cell Surface in Regulating the Internal Environment," in *The Bacteria,* Vol. VII, pp. 167–227 Academic, New York, 1979.)

the pyruvate dehydrogenase complex, which is activated by AMP and GDP. In view of these and other observations, it has been suggested that the ratio of the cellular concentrations of purine nucleotides may be an important parameter in determining the activities of enzymes that consume or produce ATP.

The above discussion illustrates the intricacies of regulatory interactions that control metabolic pathways in bacteria. However, the situation is known to be far more complex; interacting feed-back and feed-forward loops of diverging and converging channels require the operation of additional allosteric controls. It has been shown, for example, that phosphoenolpyruvate carboxylase is activated by acetyl CoA as well as by fructose-1,6-diphosphate, and that enzymes of the citric acid cycle are subject to negative allosteric control by NADH. The relative activities of the tricarboxylate and glyoxalate cycles are controlled by covalent modification of isocitrate dehydrogenase as discussed in the preceding section. These interactions serve to integrate each of the segments of amphibolic pathways with the various catabolic and anabolic sequences. They prevent the wasteful production of excessive amounts of specific metabolites while ensuring that these compounds will be supplied in amounts sufficient to provide for the needs of the cell. They allow the maintenance of homeostasis under widely varying physiological conditions.

6.8 THE PENTOSE PHOSPHATE PATHWAY (PPP)

Living organisms are frequently capable of metabolizing a single carbon source via more than one pathway. Many bacteria, for example, can metabolize glucose via at least three pathways. The pentose phosphate pathway (the hexose monophosphate shunt) provides one alternative to glycolysis and the Krebs cycle. Functioning of the pathway requires oxygen or another terminal electron acceptor and can result in the complete oxidation of a glucose molecule to carbon dioxide. The amount of energy theoretically derived from glucose oxidation by this pathway is comparable to that obtained via glycolysis and the Krebs cycle. Why then did a second aerobic pathway for glucose metabolism evolve?

The pathway is shown in outline form in Figure 6.12. There are five advantages conferred upon a cell that is capable of metabolizing sugars via the pentose phosphate pathway. First, this pathway, which occurs in the cytoplasm of a eukaryotic cell rather than in the mitochondrial matrix, generates NADPH instead of NADH, and the former cofactor is the principal reduced pyridine nucleotide used for biosynthetic purposes. Second, ribose-5-P can be generated from glucose-6-P via this pathway, and this pentose phosphate is required for nucleic acid biosynthesis. Third, the pentose phosphate pathway allows the metabolism of trioses, tetroses, pentoses, hexoses, and heptoses, while only trioses and hexoses feed into the glycolytic pathway. Fourth, this pathways allows interconversion of C_3, C_4, C_5, C_6, and C_7 sugars. Thus, the pathway is more versatile than glycolysis. Finally, the dark reaction of photosynthesis, which allows synthesis of glucose from carbon dioxide, utilizes some of the enzymes of the pentose phosphate pathway. These considerations provide clear evolutionary pressure for the maintenance of a second carbohydrate metabolic pathway in a living cell.

The pentose phosphate pathway can be divided into two phases: the oxidative phase and the interconversion phase. Three enzymes catalyze the oxidative phase while four PPP-specific enzymes plus some of the enzymes of gluconeogenesis catalyze the interconversion phase. We shall consider the oxidative phase first.

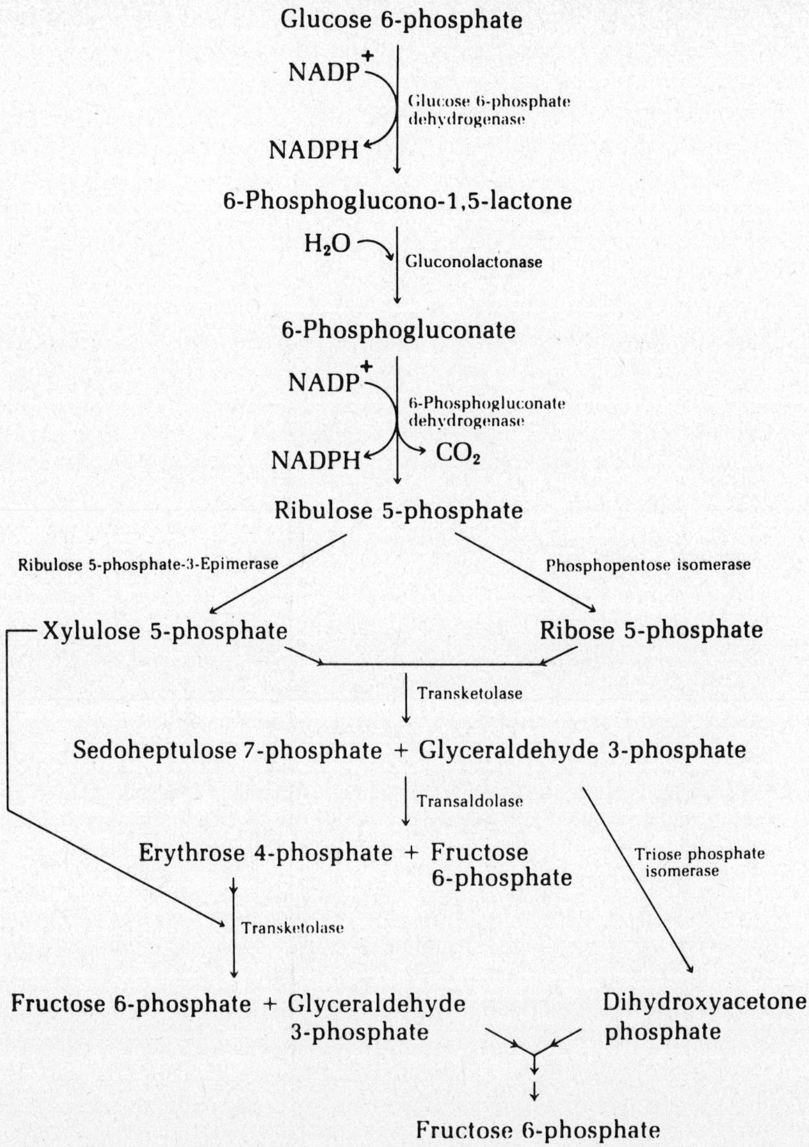

Figure 6.12 The pentose phosphate pathway showing all enzymes, substrates, intermediates, and products.

6.8.1 The Oxidative Phase

Glucose-6-P dehydrogenase catalyzes the transfer of a hydride from the one position of β-D-glucopyranosyl-6-P to $NADP^+$ yielding 6-phosphoglucono-1,5-lactone and NADPH. Gluconolactonase then hydrolyzes the lactone ring with water yielding 6-phosphogluconate. This acid is oxidized and decarboxylated to ribulose-5-phosphate in the process catalyzed by 6-phosphogluconate dehydrogenase. NADPH and CO_2 are generated as by-products of this third reaction.

Mammalian glucose-6-P dehydrogenase is strongly inhibited by NADPH, the product of the reaction, as well as by acyl CoA derivatives such as stearoyl CoA (C_{18}), palmitoyl CoA (C_{16}), and myristoyl CoA (C_{14}). The active enzyme is a dimer, and these fatty acyl derivatives cause it to dissociate to the inactive monomers. Regulation of the PPP by fatty acyl CoA derivatives is reasonable from a physiological standpoint. These derivatives are the end-products of the fatty acid biosynthetic pathway, and one of the principal uses of NADPH, generated by the PPP, is fatty acid biosynthesis (see Chapter 8). Inhibition of the pathway by the end-products of fatty acid biosynthesis is therefore an example of feedback inhibition by an indirect consequence of the activity of the PPP.

6.8.2 The Interconversion Phase

Two enzymes interconvert three different pentose phosphates. Phosphopentose isomerase interconverts ribulose-5-P and ribose-5-P, thus catalyzing the interconversion of a ketopentose phosphate and an aldopentose phosphate. The mechanism is strictly analogous to those catalyzed by glucose-6-P isomerase and triose-P isomerase discussed in Chapter 5. Phosphopentose-3-epimerase catalyzes the epimerization of the 3-hydroxyl in ribulose-5-P yielding xylulose-5-P. The hydroxyl group that changes orientation is adjacent to the activating keto group, and the 2,3-enediol logically serves as an intermediate. Thus, the first of two steps in this enzyme-catalyzed reaction involve a keto-enol tautomerization analogous to that catalyzed by the glycolytic enzyme, enolase.

Remaining interconversion steps function to allow six pentoses to rearrange their carbon skeletons to generate five hexoses so that the cycle can repeat itself. Of these remaining interconversion steps, three are specific to the PPP and are catalyzed by two interesting enzymes, transketolase and transaldolase. The former enzyme catalyzes two of the three requisite interconversions (Figure 6.12). The first step involves conversion of four C_5 sugar phosphates (two xylulose-5-phosphates and two ribose-5-phosphates) to two C_7 sugar phosphates (sedoheptulose-7-P) and two triose-3-phosphates (glyceraldehyde-3-P) (Figure 6.13). Transketolase catalyzes this reaction (Figure 6.12). Then the three top carbon atoms of C_7 (sedoheptulose-7-P) are transferred to C_3 (glyceraldehyde-3-P), yielding two molecules of C_6 (fructose-6-P). The product remaining from the bottom part of C_7 is a C_4 sugar phosphate, erythrose-4-P (Figure 6.13). This reaction is catalyzed by transaldolase (Figure 6.12). Finally, in the last interconversion reaction, the top two carbons of the two C_5 sugar phosphates, xylulose-5-P, are transferred to the remaining C_4 sugar phosphates yielding 2 molecules of a C_6 sugar phosphate, fructose-6-P. The by-products of this transketolase-catalyzed reaction are 2 molecules of glyceraldehyde-3-P [C_3 in Figure 6.13(a)]. These, then, can undergo reverse glycolysis to yield one fructose-6-P molecule. The five fructose-6-P molecules produced can be converted to five glucose-6-P molecules in the phosphoglucoisomerase-catalyzed reaction. Thus, from six pentose phosphates, derived from glucose-6-P by oxidative decarboxylation, we have obtained five hexose-phosphates. The overall reaction for one complete cycle of the PPP carried out on six molecules of glucose-6-P is:

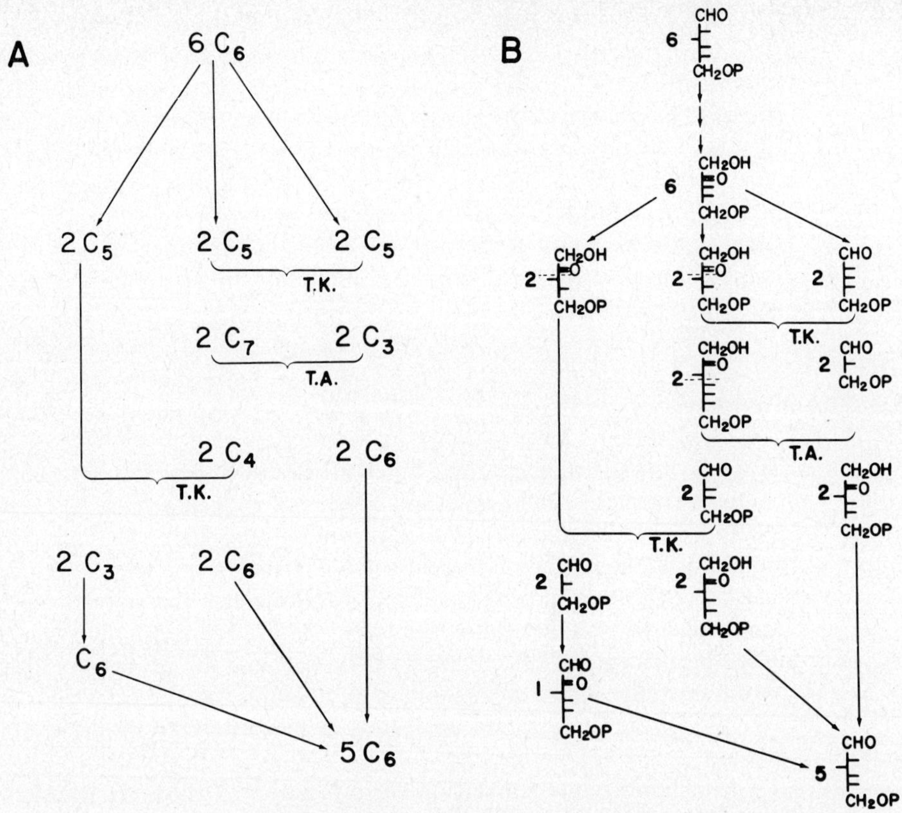

Figure 6.13 The interconversion phase of the pentose phosphate pathway illustrating the flow of carbon through the pathway. (A) Only the number of carbons in the sugars are indicated. (B) The structures of the sugars are shown. Abbreviations: T.K.: transketolase; T.A.: transaldolase.

$$6 \text{ glucose-6-P} + 12 \text{ NADP}^+ + 6 \text{ H}_2\text{O} \rightarrow 5 \text{ glucose-6-P} + 12 \text{ NADPH} + 12 \text{ H}^+ + 6 \text{ CO}_2 + \text{P}_i \quad (6.12)$$

or $$\text{glucose-6-P} + 12 \text{ NADP}^+ + 6 \text{ H}_2\text{O} \rightarrow 6 \text{ CO}_2 + 12 \text{ NADPH} + 12 \text{ H}^+ + \text{P}_i \quad (6.13)$$

The mechanisms of action of transketolase and transaldolase are well established. Transketolase is a TPP-dependent enzyme, and TPP initially serves a function similar to that in pyruvate decarboxylase (Section 4.3). The carbanion of TPP attacks the carbonyl carbon of xylulose-5-P, producing an adduct that cleaves to give a glycol-TPP carbanion and glyceraldehyde. The glycol-TPP carbanion can then attack the carbonyl carbon of either ribose-5-P to give sedoheptulose-7-P or erythrose-4-P to give fructose-6-P (Figure 6.13). The mechanism of this reaction is detailed in Figure 6.14.

As noted above, transaldolase catalyzes the transfer of the three carbon fragment

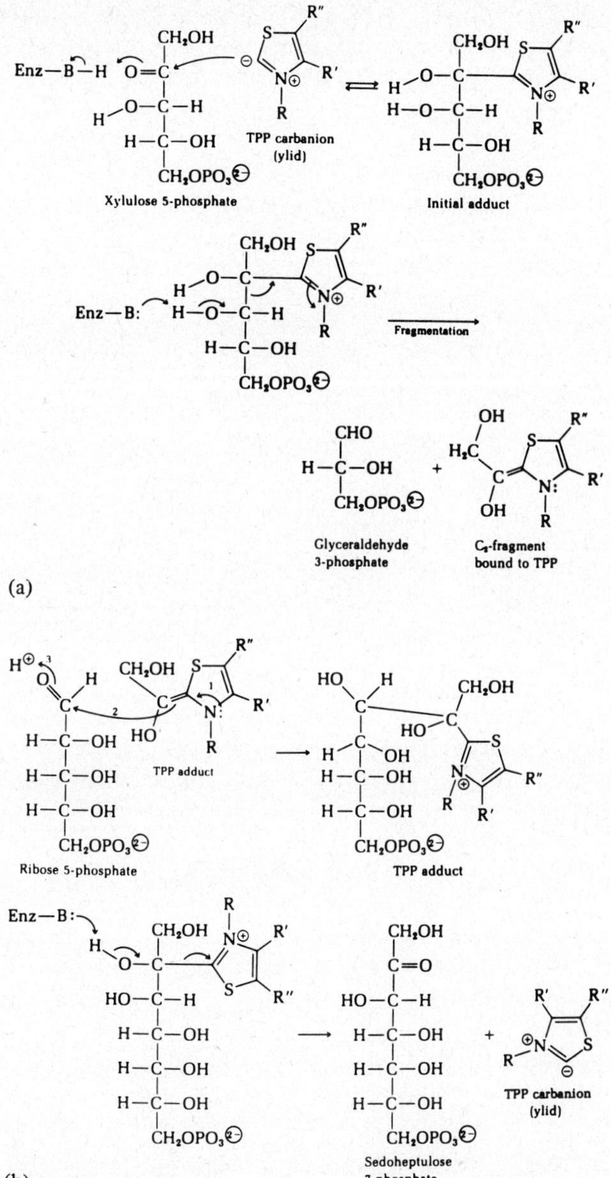

Figure 6.14 Mechanism of action of transketolase. (a) The initial step in the reaction catalyzed by transketolase is formation of a C_2 fragment that is bound to thiamine pyrophosphate. Glyceraldehyde 3-phosphate is produced in this step. (b) The second step in transketolase catalysis is nucleophilic attack of the C_2-adduct of TPP upon the carbonyl carbon of ribose 5-phosphate. The product is sedoheptulose 7-phosphate.

from the top of sedoheptulose-7-P to glyceraldehyde-3-P, yielding fructose-6-P. The mechanism of this enzyme-catalyzed reaction is essentially the same as that catalyzed by aldolase discussed in Chapter 4. Sedoheptulose forms a Schiff's base with the ϵ-amino group of a lysyl residue in the enzyme. Cleavage releases erythrose-4-P leaving a 3-carbon fragment covalently bound to the enzyme. Aldol condensation of the 3-carbon fragment with glyceraldehyde-3-P and hydrolysis of the Schiff's base linkage between the enzyme and product yields fructose-6-P.

> *Unless all existence is a medium of revelation, no particular revelation is possible.*
>
> —WILLIAM TEMPLE

BIBLIOGRAPHY

Becker, W. M., "Aerobic Production of ATP: The TCA Cycle," *Biochemistry,* G. Zubay, ed., pp. 323–361, Addison-Wesley, Reading, MA (1983).

Bild, G. S., C. A. Janson, and P. D. Boyer, "Subunit Interaction during Catalysis. ATP Modulation of Catalytic Steps in the Succinyl-CoA Synthetase Reaction," *Journal of Biological Chemistry,* **255:** 8109–8115, 1980.

Damuni, Z., M. L. Merryfield, J. S. Humphreys, and L. J. Reed, "Purification and Properties of Branched-chain α-keto Acid Dehydrogenase Phosphatase from Bovine Kidney," Proceedings of the National Academy of Science USA, **81:** 4335–4338, 1984.

Florkin, M., "The Pentose Phosphate Cycle," Ch. 55 in *A History of Biochemistry. Part V. The Unraveling of Biosynthetic Pathways,* Comprehensive Biochemistry, Vol. 33A, Elsevier/North Holland, Amsterdam (1979).

Florkin, M., "CO_2 Fixation in Heterotrophs. Gluconeogenesis," Ch. 57 in *A History of Biochemistry. Part V. The Unraveling of Biosynthetic Pathways,* Comprehensive Biochemistry, Vol. 33A, Elsevier/North Holland, Amsterdam (1979).

Florkin, M., *A History of Biochemistry. Part III. History and Identification of the Sources of Free Energy in Organisms,* Comprehensive Biochemistry, Vol. 31, Elsevier/North Holland, Amsterdam (1975).

Grivell, L. A., "Mitochondrial DNA," *Scientific American,* **248:** 78–89 (1983).

Hers, H. G., and L. Hue, "Gluconeogenesis and Related Aspects of Glycolysis," Annual Review of Biochemistry, **52:** 617–653 (1983).

Jacobson, G. R., and M. H. Saier, Jr., "Biological Membranes: Transport," in *Biochemistry,* G. Zubay, ed., pp. 621–657, Addison-Wesley, Reading, MA (1983).

Krebs, E. G., and J. A. Beavo, "Phosphorylation–Dephosphorylation of Enzymes," *Annual Review of Biochemistry,* **48:** 923–959 (1979).

O'Brien, R. W., D. T. Chuang, B. L. Taylor, and M. F. Utter, "Novel Enzymic Machinery for the Metabolism of Oxalacetate, Phosphoenolpyruvate, and Pyruvate in *Pseudomonas citronellolis,*" *Journal of Biological Chemistry,* **252:** 1257–1263 (1977).

Packman, L. C., G. Hale, and R. N. Perham, "Repeating Functional Domains in the Pyruvate Dehydrogenase Multienzyme Complex of *Escherichia coli,*" *The EMBO Journal,* **3:** 1315–1319 (1983).

Reed, L. J., and F. H. Pettit, "Phosphorylation and Dephosphorylation of Pyruvate Dehydrogenase," *Cold Spring Harbor Conferences on Cell Proliferation, Protein Phosphorylation,* **8:** 701–711, Cold Spring Harbor Laboratory, 1981.

Saier, M. H., Jr., *Mechanisms and Regulation of Carbohydrate Transport in Bacteria,* Academic, New York (1985).

Stepp, L. R., F. H. Pettit, S. J. Yeaman, and L. J. Reed, "Purification and Properties of Pyruvate Dehydrogenase Kinase from Bovine Kidney," Journal of Biological Chemistry, **258:** 9454–9458, 1983.

Teague, W. M., F. H. Pettit, T. Wu, S. R. Silberman, and L. J. Reed, "Purification and Properties of Pyruvate Dehydrogenase Phosphatase from Bovine Heart and Kidney," *Biochemistry,* **21:** 5585–5592, 1982.

Veneziale, C. M., ed., *The Regulation of Carbohydrate Formation and Utilization in Mammals,* University Park Press, Baltimore, MD (1981).

Chapter 7

Electron Transport and Oxidative Phosphorylation

> *In chemiosmotic reaction systems, the pathways of specific ligand conduction are spatially oriented through anisotropic enzyme and catalytic carrier complexes in which the reactions of chemical group transfer occur as vectorial diffusion processes of group translocation down gradients of group potential that represent real spatially directed fields of chemical force. Thus, it is easier to explain biochemistry in terms of transport than it is to explain transport in terms of biochemistry.*
>
> —PETER MITCHELL

In the previous chapter we saw that the oxidative degradation of carbohydrates results in the generation of reducing power in the form of NAD(P)H and $FADH_2$. Oxidation of glucose to CO_2 yields twelve reducing equivalents, twelve electron pairs transferred to the nicotinamide and flavin coenzymes, or two electron pairs per carbon atom oxidized to CO_2. In Chapter 8 we shall see that fatty acid oxidation yields three reducing equivalents per alkyl carbon atom oxidized, one more than for a carbon atom of glucose, because the fatty acid exists in a lower state of oxidation than does glucose. These reducing equivalents can be converted to the common energy currency of the cell, ATP, in two coupled processes termed *electron transport* and *oxidative phosphorylation.* In electron transport, the reduced coenzymes feed their electrons into the membranous electron transport chain of the mitochondrion or the bacterial cell, and as electrons are passed from one constituent of the chain to another, protons are extruded from the organelle or cell, generating a proton electrochemical gradient. The ultimate electron acceptor in this exergonic process is molecular oxygen which is reduced to water. The reentry of protons back into the organelle or cell, down their electrochemical gradient, is then coupled to the endergonic synthesis of ATP in the process referred to as oxidative phosphorylation. This process is mediated by the proton-translocating ATP synthase or ATPase.

There are, therefore, three interconvertible, but nonequivalent forms of cellular energy: electrical energy (stored in the form of reducing equivalents), chemiosmotic energy (stored in the form of ion gradients), and chemical energy (stored in the form of ATP and other high-energy phosphate compounds). All three forms of energy are absolutely required for life. The dissipation of any one of these energy forms ultimately results in loss of viability. It is the electron transport chain that interconverts electrical and chemiosmotic energy, and the reversible proton-translocating ATP synthase that interconverts chemical and chemiosmotic energy. In the first four sections of this chapter the four complexes of the mitochondrial electron transport chain will be discussed and analyzed. In Section 7.5, multiple electron transport chains of *E. coli* will be examined. Section 7.6 will be concerned with the proton-translocating ATP synthase that catalyzes oxidative phosphorylation. Finally, the membrane-associated, proton-translocating NADH/$NADP^+$ transhydrogenase will be considered in Section 7.7.

The electron transport chain of the mammalian mitochondrion is shown in Figure 7.1. This chain accomplishes the sequential passage of electrons from the initial electron donor (NADH or succinate in Figure 7.1) to the terminal electron acceptor, molecular oxygen. Twenty intermediate electron carriers are shown in the figure, although more may exist. The electron transfer chain is divided into four respiratory complexes or electron transport assemblies. These four complexes were physically separated from one another years ago following solubilization from the membrane using detergents and salt fractionation. Their identities and properties are summarized in Table 7.1.

The first of these assemblies, complex I, called NADH:coenzyme Q reductase, oxidizes NADH and reduces ubiquinone, also called coenzyme Q. This assembly consists of several protein carriers. One such carrier, a flavoprotein, contains FMN as its prosthetic group, and this cofactor probably functions by a free radical mechanism to split the electron pair derived from NADH into two free electrons which are then transferred sequentially to several iron–sulfur centers within the complex. One of these iron–sulfur centers probably reduces ubiquinone. Protons are vectorially translocated across the membrane from the internal compartment of the organelle or cell to the external milieu in a process tightly coupled to the flow of electrons through the complex.

Complex II, also called succinate:coenzyme Q reductase, consists of a flavoprotein

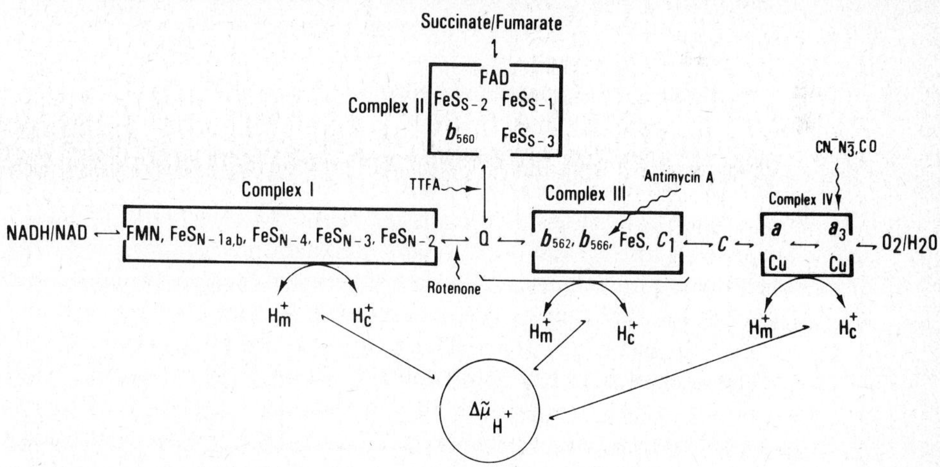

Figure 7.1 Proposed sequence of electron flow within the mitochondrial electron transport chain. The figure reveals the constituents of the four respiratory assemblies, I–IV, which can be physically separated following membrane disruption with detergents. H^+ denotes a protein from the matrix of the mitochondrion (*m*) being extruded to the cell cytoplasm (*c*) as an electron passes through the respiratory complex. $\Delta\mu_{H^+}$ denotes the proton electrochemical gradient. ⟿ denotes an inhibitor of electron flow. Other abbreviations are as presented in the text. (Courtesy of Dr. Y. Hatefi, Scripps Research Foundation, La Jolla, California)

TABLE 7.1 COMPONENTS AND PROPERTIES OF THE FOUR ELECTRON TRANSPORT ASSEMBLIES THAT COMPRISE THE ELECTRON TRANSFER CHAIN IN BOVINE HEART MUSCLE MITOCHONDRIA

Complex	Name	Electron flow is coupled to H^+ efflux	Approximate MW	Number of dissimilar protein constituents	Prosthetic groups	Oligomeric structure
I	NADH:coenzyme Q reductase	Yes	800,000	25	1 FMN ≥4 Fe-S centers CoQ	Monomeric
II	Succinate:coenzyme Q reductase	No	130,000	4	1 FAD 3 Fe-S centers 1 cytochrome b_{560} CoQ	Monomeric
III	Coenzyme QH_2: cytochrome *c* reductase	Yes	500,000	10	2 cytochrome *b* 1 Fe-S center 1 cytochrome c_1	Dimeric
IV	Cytochrome *c* oxidase	Yes	300,000	12	1 cytochrome *a* 1 Cu_A 1 cytochrome a_3 1 Cu_B	Dimeric

which contains covalently bound FAD and several iron–sulfur centers. One of the iron–sulfur centers or a *b*-type cytochrome found in this complex probably reduces ubiquinone. As for the NADH:coenzyme Q reductase, the flavin coenzyme, in this case FAD, probably functions to split the electron pair obtained from succinate into two free electrons which are transferred sequentially to several iron–sulfur proteins and then to the mobile ubiquinone. Electron flow through complex II is not coupled to transmembrane proton transport.

Complex III, coenzyme QH_2:cytochrome *c* reductase, accepts electrons from reduced ubiquinone (which also can function by a free radical mechanism), and these unpaired electrons are transferred first, to two *b*-type cytochromes, then possibly via coenzyme Q to an iron–sulfur protein found exclusively in complex III, subsequently to cytochrome c_1, and finally to the peripheral membrane protein constituent of the electron transfer chain, cytochrome *c*. Proton extrusion from the eukaryotic organelle is coupled to the flow of electrons through complex III.

Finally, complex IV, cytochrome *c* oxidase, accepts electrons from cytochrome *c*, reducing cytochrome *a*, a reducible copper atom called Cu_A, cytochrome a_3, and a second copper atom, called Cu_B. Four distinct prosthetic groups are therefore essential, protein-bound constituents of complex IV. Molecular oxygen is reduced to water in the final step catalyzed by this complex, and protons are vectorally transported across the membrane.

The sequence of electron flow has been revealed in part by the use of specific inhibitors. Thus, in the presence of an efficient electron donor and acceptor, an inhibitor of a particular electron carrier will leave any carrier above the point of inhibition in the reduced state, while any carrier below that point will be oxidized. The oxidation state of a carrier can be determined by spectroscopic means since the prosthetic groups of many of these proteins absorb in the visible and ultraviolet regions of the spectrum and show different spectral properties when reduced and oxidized. Other carriers such as the iron–sulfur proteins can be visualized by alternative spectroscopic techniques such as electron paramagnetic resonance (EPR). The sites of action of several inhibitors of electron flow are illustrated in Figure 7.1. These include rotenone, which inhibits electron flow from complex I to ubiquinone; antimycin A, which exerts its effect within complex III; and cyanide, which blocks electron flow through complex IV.

The energetics of electron flow through the mitochondrial electron transport chain are schematically approximated by the diagram in Figure 7.2. As shown, the chain can be thought of as a series of electron carriers arranged in accord with their natural affinities for electrons. It is worth noting that this order, based on the standard reduction potentials of the carriers, corresponds to the known order of the carriers in the chain shown in Figure 7.1. It is probable that the specificity of each electron

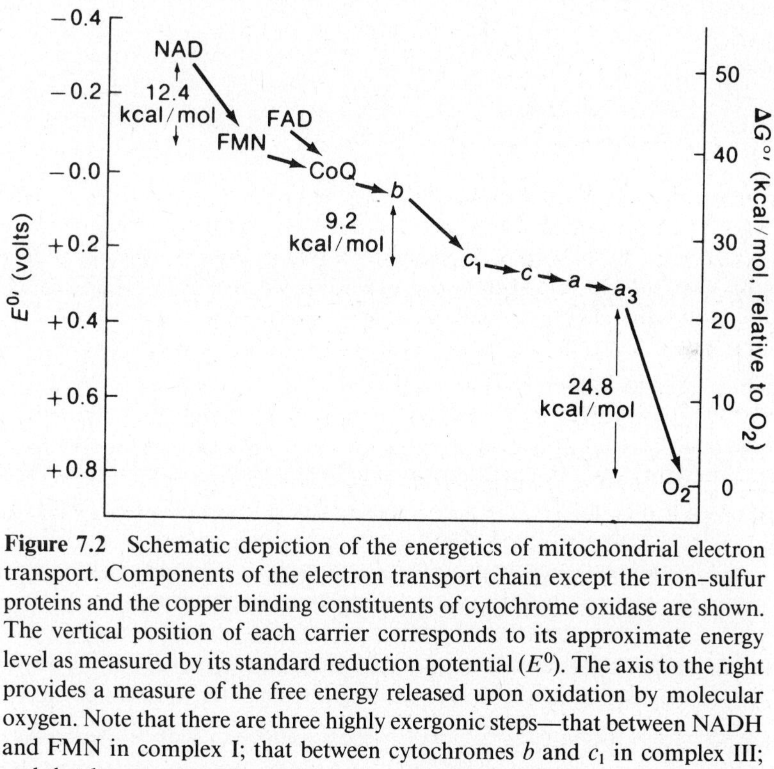

Figure 7.2 Schematic depiction of the energetics of mitochondrial electron transport. Components of the electron transport chain except the iron–sulfur proteins and the copper binding constituents of cytochrome oxidase are shown. The vertical position of each carrier corresponds to its approximate energy level as measured by its standard reduction potential (E^0). The axis to the right provides a measure of the free energy released upon oxidation by molecular oxygen. Note that there are three highly exergonic steps—that between NADH and FMN in complex I; that between cytochromes *b* and c_1 in complex III; and that between cytochrome a_3 and oxygen in complex IV. It has been suggested that these three steps may correspond to the three proton-translocating coupling sites of oxidative phosphorylation, but this possibility has not been established. (Reproduced with permission from W. M. Becker, "Aerobic Production of ATP: Electron Transport," in *Biochemistry,* G. Zubay, ed., Addison Wesley, Reading, MA, 1983.)

transfer step is determined by the catalytic properties of each carrier protein, but the specificities of these carriers were determined during evolutionary history in part by the natural tendencies of electrons to flow to progressively lower energy states.

7.1 NADH:COENZYME Q REDUCTASE (MITOCHONDRIAL RESPIRATORY COMPLEX I)

Complex I was first isolated and has been most extensively studied from bovine heart muscle mitochondria. The reconstituted complex catalyzes the electron transport-dependent transmembrane transport of protons across artificial membranes. The functional relationships of the many protein constituents of the complex are still poorly defined, and the nature of the energy-coupling process, by which electron flow is linked to the transmembrane flux of protons, is unknown.

Complex I has an aggregate molecular weight of about 800,000. It has been reported to consist of about 25 distinct polypeptide chains, each present in about equimolar amounts. The subunit molecular weights range from about 9,000 to about 75,000. The complex contains a single FMN-containing protein and at least four, and possibly as many as eight, distinct iron–sulfur centers. Stoichiometric analyses indicate that there are about 20 molecules of iron and acid-labile sulfide per molecule of FMN, and a single FMN molecule is present per enzyme complex monomer. Coenzyme Q is also present within the isolated complex, possibly bound to a coenzyme Q-binding protein.

Of the four principal iron–sulfur centers within complex I which undergo rapid redox reactions, one, designated N_1, is binuclear, containing two iron and two acid-labile sulfides. The other three (N_2, N_3, and N_4) are tetranuclear, each containing four nonheme iron atoms as well as four acid-labile sulfides. The structures of bi- and tetranuclear iron–sulfur centers are illustrated in Figure 4.23. These four Fe-S centers account for fourteen of the twenty nonheme iron atoms found in complex I. The proposed constituents of the electron transport chain of complex I are shown in Figure 7.3. Electrons are thought to pass from NADH to FMN, and then to the four different iron–sulfur centers, N-1, N-4, N-3, and N-2, possibly in this sequence. Reduced N-2 may effect the reduction of coenzyme Q.

The overall structure proposed for complex I is unique to lipoprotein complexes. On the basis of solubilization and reconstitution experiments, it has been suggested that the complex consists of a sheath of small hydrophobic proteins which interact with an annulus of membrane phospholipids. These hydrophobic proteins are assumed to anchor several catalytic, water-soluble proteins to the internal portion of the complex.

Complex I

$$\text{NADH/NAD} \longleftrightarrow \left[\text{FMN, FeS}_{N-1a,b}\text{, FeS}_{N-4}\text{, FeS}_{N-3}\text{, FeS}_{N-2}\right] \longleftrightarrow \text{Q}$$

Figure 7.3 Proposed electron transfer components within respiratory complex I of the mammalian mitochondrial transfer chain. It should be noted that the kinetic sequence of electron transfer within Complex I is not established.

Thus, none of these internal proteins are in direct contact with the phospholipid bilayer. The largest of these proteins, of about 75,000 daltons, has been shown to traverse the membrane. This large internal protein of the complex as well as a 50,000-dalton internal protein may bear the FMN and Fe-S prosthetic groups.

7.2 SUCCINATE:COENZYME Q REDUCTASE (MITOCHONDRIAL RESPIRATORY COMPLEX II)

Bovine heart mitochondrial complex II is a well-defined entity which has been purified and analyzed in some detail. It has a molecular weight of about 130,000 and contains four major polypeptide chains present in about equimolar amounts with apparent molecular weights of 70,000, 27,000, 16,000, and 14,000 (Table 7.2). It contains a single FAD molecule, a single cytochrome (cytochrome b_{560}), and about eight nonheme iron atoms as well as eight acid-labile sulfides. The two large polypeptide chains are the subunits of succinate dehydrogenase that can be released together from the membrane in a water-soluble form. The two smaller subunits form a separable hydrophobic moiety of the complex which contains the cytochrome b_{560} heme (Table 7.2). Presumably, the smaller moiety binds succinate dehydrogenase to the membrane.

Compositional analyses of the two separated subunits of succinate dehydrogenase have shown that each contains about four nonheme iron atoms and four acid-labile sulfides. Based in part on analogies with the *E. coli* succinate dehydrogenase (Section 7.5.2), it has been suggested that the smaller subunit contains two binuclear [2Fe-2S] clusters (designated S-1 and S-2), while the larger subunit contains a single tetranuclear [4Fe-4S] cluster (designated S-3). However, these possibilities have not been thoroughly established, and the presence of a three-iron cluster has been suggested.

The heterodimeric, water-soluble succinate dehydrogenase catalyzes the oxidation of succinate with artificial dyes serving as electron acceptors. The hydrophobic moiety of complex II, however, containing cytochrome b_{560}, is essential for the reconstitution of intact succinate:coenzyme Q reductase activity. Moreover, a *b*-type cytochrome has been found associated with complex II preparations from fungi (*Neurospora*) and bacteria (*E. coli* and *B. subtilis*). Mutants of *B. subtilis* that cannot synthesize heme do not contain a functional succinate:coenzyme Q reductase, and the succinate de-

TABLE 7.2 PROPOSED COMPOSITION OF BOVINE HEART MUSCLE MITOCHONDRIAL COMPLEX II

Protein complex or protein subunit	MW	Proposed prosthetic groups
Intact complex	130,000	
Hydrophilic moiety (succinate dehydrogenase)	100,000	
Large subunit	70,000	1 FAD; 1 [4Fe-4S] (S3)
Small subunit	27,000	2 [2Fe-2S] (S1 and S2)[a]
Hydrophobic moiety (cytochrome b_{560})	30,000	
Large subunit	16,000	1 cytochrome b_{560}
Small subunit	14,000	1 coenzyme Q binding site

[a] The presence of a three-iron center is supported by some recent experiments.

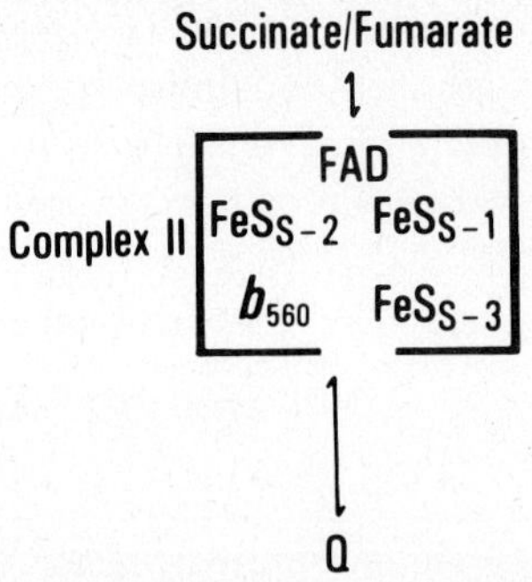

Figure 7.4 Scheme showing the transfer of electrons through respiratory complex II of the mammalian mitochondrial electron transfer chain. The figure does not imply a specific sequence of electron flow.

hydrogenase is no longer membrane-bound. These results serve to implicate cytochrome b_{560} as an essential constituent of complex II which may serve as the membrane attachment site for succinate dehydrogenase as well as an electron carrier. It is not yet established that cytochrome b_{560} is an essential electron transfer constituent of complex II. It has been suggested that one of the two small hydrophobic polypeptide chains carries the heme group while the other is a coenzyme Q binding protein. A possible additional function of the hydrophobic moiety of complex II is proper interaction with complex III. A proposed scheme for the passage of electrons through respiratory complex II is shown in Figure 7.4, but the order of electron transfer through the three iron–sulfur centers of the complex is not known.

7.3 COENZYME QH_2:CYTOCHROME *c* REDUCTASE (MITOCHONDRIAL RESPIRATORY COMPLEX III)

Respiratory complexes III and IV from bovine mitochondria are superficially similar. These multisubunit enzymes are each composed of about twelve polypeptide chains, some of which are encoded by mitochondrial genes and some by nuclear genes. Both complexes traverse the inner mitochondrial membrane, have high molecular weights, are present in the membrane as dimeric species, and have been proposed to function by half-of-sites mechanisms.

The subunits of bovine heart muscle complex III, their proposed functional identities, and their molecular weights are summarized in Table 7.3. One molecule of each of the eleven polypeptide chains appears to be present in each monomeric complex. These proteins have been identified as two "core" proteins of unknown function (subunits I and II), cytochrome *b* (subunit III which contains two heme groups, b_{566} and b_{562}), cytochrome c_1 (subunit IV), and the single iron–sulfur protein of complex III (subunit V). Presumed functions of some of the smaller subunits are also indicated in the table. The sum of the subunit molecular weights agrees with the empirically determined complex molecular weight (240,000). The molecular weight calculated from hydrodynamic measurements (about 420,000) suggests that the complex is present in the membrane as a dimer. The monomeric complex is elongated, traversing the inner mitochondrial membrane, and protruding far into the aqueous phases on both sides of the membrane. The overall length is about 150 Å.

The details of electron transfer through the complex coupled to proton extrusion are far from established. Both in the native mitochondrial membrane and in recon-

TABLE 7.3 SUBUNIT COMPOSITION OF COENZYME QH_2:CYTOCHROME *c* REDUCTASE ISOLATED FROM BOVINE HEART MUSCLE MITOCHONDRIA

Subunit	Proposed identity, function, or association[a]	MW (kD)
I	Core protein I	45.5
II	Core protein II	44
III	Cytochrome *b*	42
IV	Cytochrome c_1	31
V	Rieske's Fe_2S_2 protein	24
VI	Forms the Q_i center	13.3
VII	Associated with I and II	9.5
VIII	Cytochrome *c* hinge protein (associated with IV)	9.2
IX	Forms the Q_o center (associated with III)	8.0
X	Associated with IV	7.2
XI	Associated with V	6.4

[a] A single copy of each subunit is proposed to be present in the monomeric coenzyme QH_2:cytochrome *c* reductase.

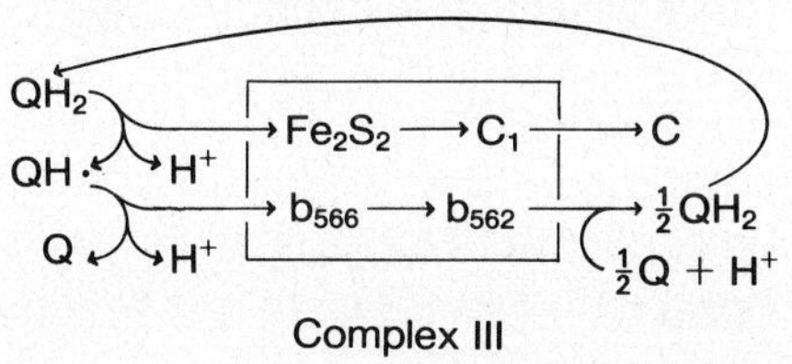

Figure 7.5 Scheme showing the constituent prosthetic groups in respiratory complex III of the mammalian mitochondrial electron transfer chain. The figure illustrates one form of the Q cycle and a possible pathway of electron flow through the complex. Two protons are extruded from the mitochondrion per electron pair that passes through the complex from coenzyme QH_2 to cytochrome *c*, but the step coupled to proton extrusion has not been identified. QH_2: ubiquinol (reduced coenzyme Q); QH·: the free radical semiquinone; Q: ubiquinone (oxidized coenzyme Q).

stituted liposomes, coenzyme QH_2:cytochrome *c* reductase catalyzes transmembrane proton translocation, but how proton transport is coupled to electron flow is not known. Figure 7.5 illustrates one proposal for the passage of electrons from coenzyme QH_2 through complex III to cytochrome *c*. This figure illustrates one version of the Q cycle. QH_2 functions by a free radical mechanism to reduce the iron–sulfur center in complex III, which then passes its electron on to cytochrome c_1 and cytochrome *c*. The latter two proteins are localized to the cytoplasmic surface of the mitochondrion. The semiquinone free radical (QH·) may then pass its free electron sequentially to each of the two *b* cytochromes and to oxidized ubiquinone so that the reduced coenzyme Q generated can cycle back, as shown in Figure 7.5, to repeat the process.

Two coenzyme Q binding sites (Q_i and Q_o, respectively) are believed to be localized to the inner and outer surfaces of the mitochondrial inner membrane. Subunits VI and IX may, in part, comprise these binding sites (Table 7.3). Two spatially distinct quinone binding sites in complex III may be important to the vectorial proton translocation process. Whether or not the dimeric structure of coenzyme QH_2:cytochrome *c* reductase is of functional importance has yet to be ascertained.

7.4 CYTOCHROME *c* OXIDASE (MITOCHONDRIAL RESPIRATORY COMPLEX IV)

Purified cytochrome oxidase (complex IV), like coenzyme QH_2:cytochrome *c* reductase, consists of multiple subunits regardless of the biological source. The most complex of these, from mammalian tissues, consists of up to twelve subunits as indicated in Table 7.4. The enzyme from bovine heart is among the best characterized since the amino acid sequences of most of the subunits are known. Of the subunits listed in the table, the largest of these, subunits I, II, and III, are the only ones that have been associated with specific functions. The yeast enzyme consists of seven or eight subunits that are similar in many respects to those of the mammalian complex. However, several of the smaller subunits found in the mammalian enzyme are absent from yeast cytochrome oxidase. Cytochrome oxidases from several aerobic bacteria consist of two or possibly three subunits, but these enzymes are unfortunately relatively poorly characterized. The two or three subunits of the bacterial enzymes possibly correspond in function to subunits I, II, and III of the eukaryotic enzyme complex.

In all of the eukaryotic enzyme complexes, two heme *a* groups and two copper atoms are found per monomer of 150,000 molecular weight. The two copper atoms are associated with subunit II, while one of the heme *a* molecules is probably associated with subunit I; the other is associated with subunit II. The amino acid sequence of subunit II shows sequence homology with three other copper binding proteins. Cytochrome *c* appears to interact with subunits II and III.

TABLE 7.4 SUBUNIT COMPOSITION OF BOVINE HEART MUSCLE CYTOCHROME *c* OXIDASE[a]

Subunit	Apparent MW (kD) (from SDS gel electrophoresis)	Actual MW (kD)
I	45	56.1
II	27.5	26.0
III	26	29.9
IV	18	17.2
V	10.7	12.4
VI	9.5	10.7
VII	8.0	10.0
VIII	7.5	8.5
IX	5.1	5.5
X	4.9	4.9
XI	4.7	
XII	4.3	

[a] Actual molecular weight (MW) values for subunits I, II, and III were calculated from mitochondrial DNA sequence data. Molecular weight values for the other subunits were calculated from amino acid sequence data. The functional significance of some of the smaller subunits is questionable. A single copy of each subunit is proposed to be present in the monomeric cytochrome oxidase complex.

The transport of protons through the enzyme complex is thought to occur via subunit III for two reasons. First, if the enzyme complex is depleted of subunit III, the rate of respiration is normal, but protons are not pumped across the membrane. Second, dicyclohexylcarbodiimide (DCCD), which blocks proton translocation through the proton-translocating ATPase as discussed in Section 7.6, also reacts specifically with subunit III and blocks proton transport in reconstituted cytochrome oxidase vesicles. The amino acid sequence of the DCCD-binding site is similar to that of the *c* subunit in the F_0F_1 ATPase: it consists of a hydrophobic stretch of amino acids interrupted by a single DCCD-sensitive glutamyl residue. The functions of the remaining subunits in the mammalian oxidase (IV–VIII in Table 7.4) are not known. They have been postulated to function (a) in regulation, (b) in the coupling of electron flow to (or uncoupling of electron flow from) proton transport under specific conditions, or (c) in the insertion and/or assembly of the complex. It is interesting to note that in many eukaryotes, while subunits I, II, and III are encoded by the mitochondrial genome, the other subunits are encoded by nuclear genes and are synthesized on cytoplasmic ribosomes.

The structure of the monomeric cytochrome oxidase has been partially elucidated using physical techniques. The complex is shaped like a skewed "Y" with a transmembrane length of 110 Å. The two arms of the "Y" are 55 Å long, and their centers are separated by about 40 Å. The stem of the "Y" projects about 50 Å into the aqueous phase on the cytoplasmic (external) side of the mitochondrion, while the two arms of the "Y" project about 20 Å into the matrix. The approximate structure of the monomer is shown in Figure 7.6. While subunits I and VI appear to be largely embedded in the membrane, subunits II and III are exposed to the external surface where they interact with cytochrome *c*, and subunits IV and VII are exposed to the matrix surface. Subunit III, which is of particular interest in view of its proposed proton transport function, very likely contains seven transmembrane α-helices. These α-helices contain many hydroxylic amino acyl residues which might conceivably function as part of a transmembrane hydrogen-bonded structure which, in conjunction with the DCCD-sensitive glutamyl residue, could serve as the transmembrane proton channel.

Cytochrome oxidase probably exists in the mitochondrial membrane as a dimer (MW = 300,000) with a symmetry axis perpendicular to the plane of the membrane. That this is a functional dimer was first suggested from studies that showed that covalent chemical cross-linking of cytochrome *c* to the enzyme blocked electron transfer maximally when one cytochrome *c* was bound per dimer. It was suggested that the small cytochrome *c* molecule sits in the crevice between subunit II of one oxidase monomer and subunit III of the other.

Oxidation of reduced heme *a* by O_2 occurs in two kinetically distinct phases with different temperature dependencies. This result and other kinetic and structural observations have led to the suggestion that the two structurally similar cytochrome *a* molecules in the dimeric cytochrome oxidase function by a half-of-sites (alternating sites; anticooperativity; reciprocal interaction; flip-flop)-type mechanism. Since the same proposal has been made for complex III of the respiratory chain and for the proton-translocating ATPase, it is possible that such mechanisms are a general characteristic of certain chemiosmotically coupled energy-transducing systems.

As noted previously, all cytochrome oxidase monomers studied to date contain

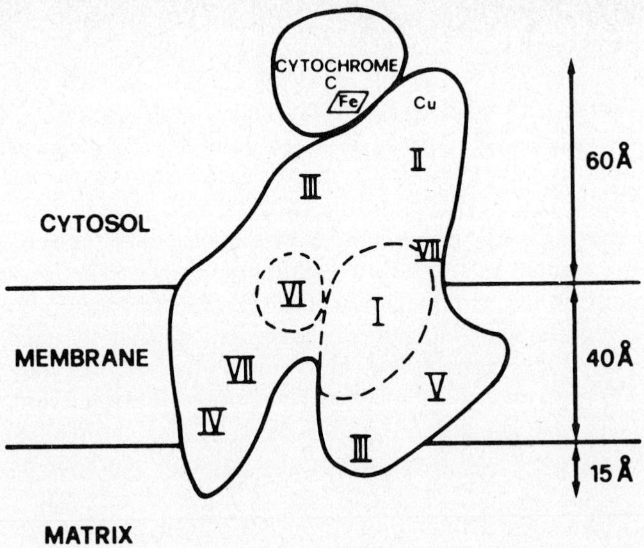

Figure 7.6 An approximate sketch of the three-dimensional structure of the cytochrome oxidase monomer in the inner mitochondrial membrane. The approximate locations of the individual subunits I–VIII listed in Table 7.4 are shown, as is the interaction site with cytochrome *c*. The functional unit is probably a dimeric structure which has been proposed to function by a *half-of-sites* type mechanism. (Reproduced with permission from A. Azzi, "Cytochrome *c* Oxidase. Towards a Clarification of its Structure, Interactions, and Mechanisms," *Biochimica Biophysica Acta,* **594:** 231–252, 1980.)

two hemes (a and a_3) and two copper atoms (Cu_A and Cu_B) per monomer. Electrons are first donated to the oxidase by cytochrome c with the a-type cytochrome serving as the primary acceptor. Cu_A appears to be in rapid redox equilibrium with heme a. Because proton transport appears to be linked to the electron transfer step involving cytochromes c and a, it has been suggested that subunit II contains heme a and Cu_A, and that the proton channel of subunit III is in close proximity. They may function as a unit by an unspecified mechanism.

From the heme a-Cu_A center, electrons are transferred to the second reactive center in the monomer, the O_2 reduction center consisting of cytochrome a_3 and Cu_B. Heme a_3 may be bound to subunit I while Cu_B is bound to a nearby domain of subunit II. It is known that heme a_3 and Cu_B are closely associated both physically and functionally. The two metals (Fe^{++} and Cu^{+}) form a binuclear center that cooperatively catalyzes O_2 reduction to water. These two metal atoms are probably no more than 7 Å apart. Electron transfer through the complex may therefore occur as shown in Figure 7.7.

A specific mechanism for the reduction of molecular oxygen, based on many independent experimental observations, has been proposed (Figure 7.8). Since a one-electron reduction step converting O_2 to O_2^- is very unfavorable energetically, O_2 re-

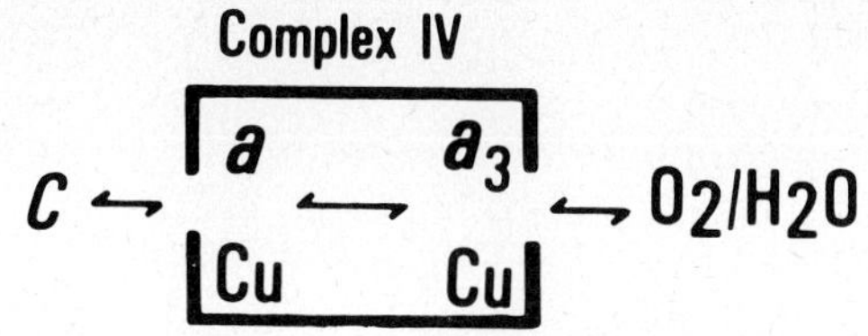

Figure 7.7 Scheme showing the proposed transfer of electrons through respiratory complex IV of the mammalian mitochondrial electron transfer chain.

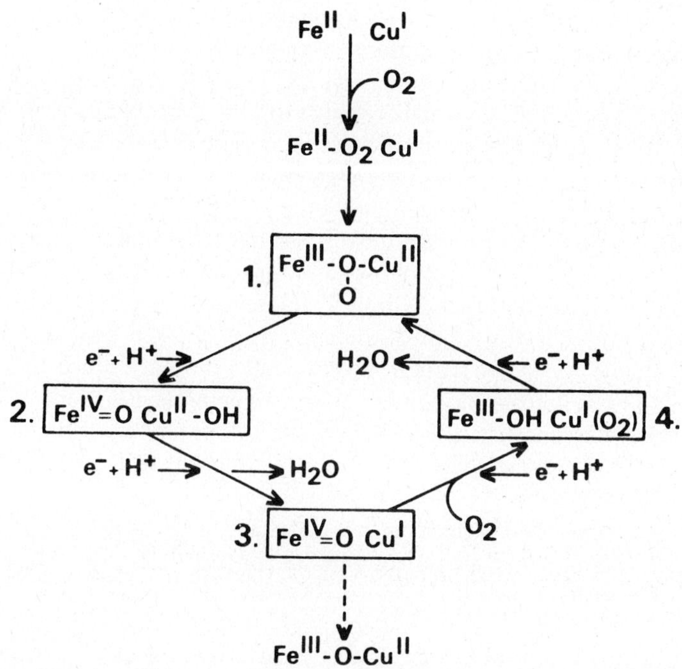

Figure 7.8 Proposed catalytic cycle for the reduction of molecular oxygen to water. Fe and Cu denote the heme iron in heme a_3 and Cu_B, respectively. It is suggested that all intermediates of oxygen reduction form complexes with the two metals, with a single electron being fed into this complex from the heme *a*-Cu_A center at each of the four steps shown between intermediates 1 and 2, 2 and 3, 3 and 4, and 4 and 1. (Reproduced with permission from M. Wikstrom, K. Krab, and M. Saraste, "Proton-Translocating Cytochrome Complexes," in *Annual Review of Biochemistry,* **50:** 623–655, 1981.)

duction is proposed to start by a concerted two-electron transfer yielding bound peroxide (structure 1 in Figure 7.8). The next proposed intermediate is a "ferryl" iron derivative of the a_3Cu_B center (structure 2 in Figure 7.8). Subsequently, two successive one-electron transfers, each accompanied by protonation of the intermediates (structures 3 and 4), result in the release of one water molecule (in the step between intermediates 2 and 3). The regeneration of the initial metal-bound peroxide intermediate shown in structure 1 of Figure 7.8, occurs with the final electron transfer to structure 4 and the release of the second water molecule to the medium.

7.5 RESPIRATORY CHAINS OF *E. coli*

The respiratory chain in mammalian mitochondria has been found to be complex in terms of the number of its protein constituents but highly specialized with respect to the allowable electron donors and acceptors. Thus, NADH and succinate serve as effective electron donors, each donating electrons to its respective dehydrogenase complex (respiratory complex I or II), while a single acceptor, molecular oxygen, can be reduced as a result of the activity of a single oxidase complex, the linear sequence of electron carriers comprising respiratory complexes III and IV. In *E. coli,* the situation appears to be both simpler and more complex. The individual dehydrogenases consist of fewer proteins than in mammalian mitochondria, but there are far more of them. Moreover, there are several terminal electron acceptors, each of which is reduced by a distinct reductase. Figure 7.9 presents a schematic and simplified view of this situation. In addition to the dehydrogenases that oxidize NADH and succinate (found in both bacteria and eukaryotic mitochondria), other quite distinct integral membrane dehydrogenases oxidize α-glycerol phosphate, formate, both D- and L-lactate, certain D- and L-amino acids, molecular hydrogen, and several other potential electron donors. Moreover, there are at least four distinct terminal electron transfer chains, one that reduces fumarate, one that reduces nitrate, and two that reduce molecular oxygen (Figure 7.9). Two quinones, ubiquinone and menaquinone, function as electron carriers linking the dehydrogenases to the reductases. While this link can sometimes be provided by only one or the other of these two quinones, some electron transport chains appear to function with either.

As noted above, each electron transfer chain, responsible for the oxidation of a single electron donor by a single acceptor, is simpler in *E. coli* than in mammalian mitochondria, but the total number of electron carriers in *E. coli* exceeds those in eukaryotes. For example, there are in excess of a dozen primary dehydrogenases, many distinct iron–sulfur centers, at least eight cytochromes, two different quinones

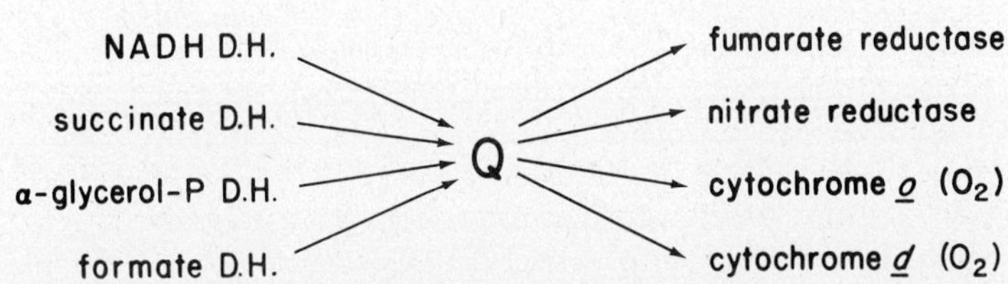

Figure 7.9 Electron flow through the various electron transfer chains of *E. coli.* The figure depicts four dehydrogenases which accept electrons from primary electron donors and pass these electrons to a quinone (Q), either ubiquinone or menaquinone. The electrons are subsequently passed through the different reductase complexes to the terminal electron acceptors. Some of the dehydrogenases and all of the reductases are multicomponent complexes in the membrane containing several essential electron carriers. A few of the dehydrogenases appear to consist of a single protein which passes its electrons directly to coenzyme Q. Many dehydrogenases in addition to those shown in the figure have been characterized in *E. coli.*

and probably five terminal reductases in *E. coli.* This bacterium possesses far greater metabolic versatility than any eukaryote, allowing electron transfer under many conditions inconsistent with life in higher organisms including strictly anaerobic conditions. This fact may have allowed the evolution of electron transport chains in prokaryotes long before the introduction of molecular oxygen on earth.

A number of the respiratory complexes from *E. coli* have been purified and studied. A few of the better characterized systems will be described below.

7.5.1 NADH Dehydrogenase

A single gene (designated *ndh*) encodes the respiratory NADH dehydrogenase. This gene has been cloned, sequenced, and amplified, and the amplified protein has been purified to homogeneity. The enzyme is a single polypeptide chain (MW = 47,300) containing tightly bound FAD, lipid, and one ubiquinone molecule per molecule of dehydrogenase. The protein has an overall polarity of 43%, typical of soluble proteins, but it possesses hydrophobic regions which may dictate its association with the membrane. It is not known if this protein functions in conjunction with [Fe-S]-containing subunits.

7.5.2 Succinate Dehydrogenase

The *sdh* operon (*sdhCDAB*) encoding the four protein constituents of the succinate dehydrogenase complex has been cloned and sequenced. Moreover, the complex has been purified by several investigators. These studies have shown that the enzyme consists of a flavoprotein subunit (*sdhA;* MW = 64,300) containing covalently bound FAD and possibly an [Fe_4-S_4] center, an iron–sulfur protein (*sdhB;* MW = 26,000) containing two [Fe_2-S_2] centers, and two hydrophobic "anchor" subunits (*sdhC;* MW = 14,200; and *sdhD;* MW = 12,800). A *b*-type cytochrome has also been found in association with the purified complex which has a total molecular weight of about 150,000. Each of the subunits of the system are thought to be present in equimolar amounts. The striking similarity between the *E. coli* and mammalian dehydrogenase complexes is worthy of note. Moreover, the structural similarities with the *E. coli* fumarate reductase suggest that these two enzyme complexes evolved from a common ancestral operon. Fumarate reductase will be discussed in Section 7.5.5.

7.5.3 L-Glycerol-3-Phosphate Dehydrogenase

Two dehydrogenases catalyze the oxidation of α-glycerol phosphate to dihydroxyacetone phosphate. The *aerobic* enzyme can function with nitrate or oxygen but not fumarate as the terminal electron acceptor, while the *anaerobic* enzyme functions with fumarate or nitrate but not oxygen as the electron acceptor. Both enzymes are membrane-bound flavoproteins (MW = 80,000) which transfer electrons to the electron transfer chain. They are distinct from a soluble biosynthetic enzyme which catalyzes the NAD(P)H-dependent reduction of dihydroxyacetonephosphate for phospholipid biosynthetic purposes.

7.5.4 Formate Dehydrogenase

This enzyme has been purified and studied in considerable detail. It contains a molybdenum cofactor, [Fe-S] centers, a cytochrome b_{550}, and covalently bound selenium. It consists of three subunits: α (MW = 110,000); β (MW = 32,000), and γ (MW = 20,000). The stoichiometries of these subunits in the intact complex may be $\alpha_2\beta_2\gamma_4$. In all of these respects the complex resembles nitrate reductase suggesting a close evolutionary relationship between these two catalytic systems. The dehydrogenase appears to pump two protons per electron pair transferred from formate to quinone.

7.5.5 Fumarate Reductase

As noted in Section 7.5.2, the succinate–fumarate couple can be utilized as either oxidant or reductant for the *E. coli* respiratory chain. The forward and reverse reactions are catalyzed by distinct but related enzymes, succinate dehydrogenase and fumarate reductase, respectively. Properties of the latter enzyme are summarized in Table 7.5 while those of the former enzyme were presented in Section 7.5.2. Both enzymes consist of four polypeptide chains, a flavoprotein of about 69,000 molecular weight containing covalently bound FAD {[8 α-*N*(3)-histidyl]FAD}, an iron–sulfur protein of about 27,000 molecular weight, and two anchor proteins of about 14,000 and 13,000 molecular weights. When the anchor proteins are not made the two larger polypeptide constituents of the fumarate reductase complex appear in the cytoplasmic fraction. The flavoprotein subunit may contain an iron–sulfur center of the [Fe_4-S_4]-type while the 27,000 molecular weight subunit possibly contains two [Fe_2-S_2] centers. The same composition is likely for the succinate dehydrogenase complexes of *E. coli* and mammalian mitochondria.

In spite of the structural similarities between fumarate reductase and succinate dehydrogenase, the two enzymes are easily distinguishable. First, succinate dehydrogenase is induced aerobically and repressed under anaerobic conditions, while fumarate reductase is repressed by O_2 and NO_3^- but expressed anaerobically in the presence of fumarate. Second, fumarate reductase has higher affinity for fumarate than succinate, while the converse is true for succinate dehydrogenase. Third, the four genes encoding the fumarate reductase complex comprise an operon (*frdABCD*) which maps at 93 min. on the *E. coli* chromosome, while the *sdh* operon, encoding the four proteins of the succinate dehydrogenase complex, maps at about 16 min. These two operons must

TABLE 7.5 SUBUNIT COMPOSITION OF FUMARATE REDUCTASE FROM *E. COLI*

frd gene	Subunit	MW	Stoichiometry	Probable prosthetic groups
A	Flavo, Fe-S protein	66,052	1	[8 α-*N*(3)-histidyl]-FAD and $[Fe_4S_4]_1$
B	Fe-S protein	27,092	1	$[Fe_2S_2]_2$[a]
C	Anchor protein$_1$	15,000	1	(cytochrome *b*?)
D	Anchor protein$_2$	14,000	1	

[a] The presence of a three-iron center is supported by some recent experiments.

have arisen by duplication of a single precursor operon, possibly as a result of a chromosomal duplication event as discussed in Section 5.10.

7.5.6 Nitrate Reductase

This terminal electron acceptor reduces nitrate to nitrite, which is excreted from the bacterial cell into the growth medium. The reductase consists of three subunits, α (MW = 150,000), β (MW = 60,000), and γ (MW = 20,000). The molecular weight value of the intact complex (500,000) implies a stoichiometry of $\alpha_2\beta_2\gamma_4$.

The α-subunit is thought to provide the active site of the enzyme and probably contains the nitrate-binding site, $FMNH_2$, and the molybdenum-complexed cofactor shown in Figure 7.10. The complex contains several distinct iron–sulfur centers including at least two dissimilar [Fe_2-S_2] centers and one [Fe_4-S_4] center, and the β-subunit is a likely site for at least some of these prosthetic groups. The γ-subunit has been shown to be a *b*-type cytochrome. While the α- and β-subunits are localized to the cytoplasmic side of the membrane, the γ-subunit is exposed to the periplasmic side. Thus, the complex spans the membrane. It is interesting to note that while four protons (or their equivalent) are believed to be extruded from the bacterial cell when formate reduces either nitrate or oxygen, and two protons (or their equivalent) are probably extruded when succinate reduces one of these electron acceptors, neither the nitrate reductase complex nor one of the *E. coli* cytochrome oxidase complexes (to be discussed next) appears to function as a proton pump.

7.5.7 Cytochrome Oxidase

E. coli appears to contain two (and possibly three) cytochrome-containing electron transfer chains which function as terminal oxidases to reduce molecular oxygen. The major functional oxidase in *E. coli* is a cyanide- and carbon monoxide-sensitive *b*-type cytochrome called cytochrome *o* (for oxidase). The alternative major oxidase, a cytochrome that is more resistant than cytochrome *o* to cyanide and carbon mon-

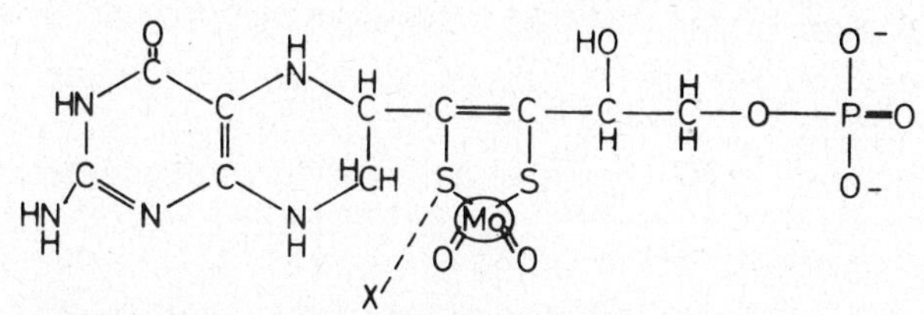

Figure 7.10 Structure of the molybdenum-containing cofactor required for normal functioning of the formate dehydrogenase and nitrate reductase complexes in the cytoplasmic membrane of *E. coli.* Synthesis of the cofactor and its insertion into the enzymes are thought to be multistep, enzyme-catalyzed processes, but the details of these steps are not yet known. (Reproduced with permission from W. J. Ingledew and R. K. Poole, "The Respiratory Chain of *Escherichia coli*," *Microbiological Reviews,* **48:** 222–271, 1984.)

oxide, is called cytochrome *d*. Synthesis of the latter system is induced under conditions of low oxygen tension, and it possesses tenfold higher affinity for O_2 than cytochrome *o*. The third (minor) oxidase has been tentatively identified as cytochrome a_1, but it is poorly characterized.

The cytochrome *o* and cytochrome *d* complexes have been separated from one another and purified to near homogeneity. Analyses of the former preparation by one group of investigators revealed the presence of equimolar amounts of two polypeptide chains with apparent molecular weights of 55,000 and 33,000. A second group of investigators identified these two proteins as well as two smaller polypeptide chains (molecular weights equal to 21,000 and 14,000). It is not yet clear whether the two smaller proteins represent loosely associated components of the complex or contaminating proteins.

Spectral characteristics of the two-polypeptide cytochrome *o* complex demonstrated the presence of cytochrome b_{562} as well as cytochrome *o*. Approximately two heme groups and two copper atoms were present per molecule of oxidase. Detectable nonheme iron, ubiquinone, and menaquinone were reported to be absent.

The cytochrome *o* oxidase preparations were reconstituted in artificial phospholipid vesicular systems called proteoliposomes. In the presence of molecular oxygen and an appropriate electron donor, such as reduced ubiquinone, both the purified two-polypeptide cytochrome *o* oxidase and the four-polypeptide cytochrome *o* oxidase preparations generated a proton electrochemical gradient (interior negative and alkaline). Studies with the latter preparation led to the suggestion that this potential gradient was not due to proton transport across the membrane. Instead, the membrane potential was thought to result from vectorial electron flow from the outer surface of the membrane to the inner surface while the pH gradient was thought to result from the nonvectorial consumption and release of protons at the inner and outer surfaces of the membrane, respectively. Because of the unique nature of this proposal, it should be considered tentative until confirmed.

Following purification, the cytochrome *d* complex was found to be composed of equimolar amounts of two polypeptide chains with apparent molecular weights of 51,000 and 26,000. Spectral characteristics indicated the presence of a cytochrome b_{558} as well as cytochrome *d*. The two heme molecules were present in equimolar amounts, one molecule of each per molecule of the two-polypeptide complex.

Like the cytochrome *o* complex, the purified cytochrome *d* complex generated a membrane potential when allowed to transfer electrons from an electron donor to oxygen following reconstitution in a vesicular phospholipid membrane. Thus, it appears that there is a coupling site in each of the two terminal oxidases. The proposed arrangement of cytochromes in the terminal portion of the *E. coli* respiratory chain is therefore:

$$\text{cyt } b_{556} \rightarrow \text{Q} \begin{cases} \nearrow \text{cyt } b_{562} \rightarrow \text{cyt } o \rightarrow O_2 \text{ (low affinity)} \\ \searrow \text{cyt } b_{558} \rightarrow \text{cyt } d \rightarrow O_2 \text{ (high affinity)} \end{cases}$$

In view of the similarities of the two terminal oxidases, it would not be surprising if they shared a common evolutionary ancestor.

7.6 PROTON-TRANSLOCATING ATP SYNTHASES (ATPases) IN OXIDATIVE PHOSPHORYLATION

The reversible synthesis of ATP in response to a proton electrochemical gradient is catalyzed by the proton-translocating ATP synthase (named for the forward reaction) or ATPase (named for the reverse reaction). The enzymes found in bacteria, mitochondria, and chloroplasts are actually protein complexes which consist of eight dissimilar subunits in bacteria and chloroplasts and ten or more subunits in eukaryotic mitochondria. These subunits function in concert to couple the exergonic flux of protons down their electrochemical gradient with the endergonic synthesis of ATP from ADP and inorganic phosphate. They also catalyze the reverse reaction: the endergonic flux of protons up their electrochemical gradient in a process driven by the exergonic hydrolysis of ATP.

The proton electrochemical gradient is also called the proton motive force, or pmf. At least in some bacteria, and probably in all cells and organelles which synthesize ATP in response to a proton motive force, the ATP synthetic rate is observed to be a sigmoidal function of the pmf. A certain threshold value of the pmf is required before significant ATP synthesis is observed. This fact suggests the involvement of more than one proton in the synthesis of each ATP molecule, the involvement of cooperative subunit interactions in the coupling of H^+ influx to ATP synthesis, or both. As will be seen later in this section, cooperativity with respect to adenine nucleotide binding to the ATPase active site moiety is well established for the ATPases from several prokaryotic and eukaryotic sources.

The ATP synthases from two bacterial species, a thermophilic Gram-positive *Bacillus* species and *E. coli,* have been extensively studied. Each of the ATP synthases has been solubilized, dissociated into its constituent subunits, and reconstituted in an artificial membrane. In addition, the *E. coli* enzyme has been examined employing a combination of genetic approaches. Because the genes encoding all of the subunits of the *E. coli* ATPase have been cloned and sequenced, many structural aspects of this system have been elucidated.

In *E. coli,* a single operon, a single genetic unit of transcription, encodes all of the subunits of the ATP synthase (Figure 7.11). Three of these subunits are found together as a complex embedded in the phospholipid bilayer of the cytoplasmic membrane. They are called the a, b, and c subunits, and comprise the so-called F_0 moiety of the ATP synthase. The remaining five known subunits form a peripheral membrane complex, designated F_1, which in the bacterial cell is associated with the F_0 moiety of the synthase. These five water-soluble subunits are designated α, β, γ, δ and, ϵ. The intact ATP synthase is sometimes called the F_0F_1 complex. Some of the properties of the protein subunits of the *Bacillus* and *E. coli* ATPases are presented in Tables 7.6 and 7.7, respectively.

Biochemical studies comparing the structures and modes of action of the ATPases of *E. coli, Bacillus,* mitochondria, and chloroplasts, have provided compelling evidence for analogous structural elements and mechanisms. Thus, the F_1 moieties of all of these ATPases consist of the same five dissimilar subunits, probably in the same stoichiometries. The F_0 moieties also exhibit structural similarities, all possessing similar c subunits which contain an essential glutamyl or aspartyl residue. When these residues

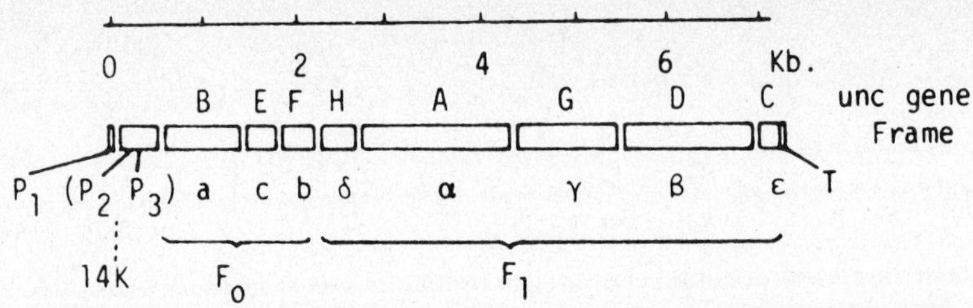

Figure 7.11 Arrangement of genes in the *unc* (uncoupled) operon of *E. coli* which encodes the eight subunits of the proton-translocating ATP synthase. The figure shows the positions and relative sizes of the structural genes (designated *uncA-H*) which encode subunits a, b, and c of the F_0 moiety as well as subunits α–ϵ which comprise the F_1 moiety of the synthase. Sequencing of the *unc* operon revealed an additional reading frame for a protein of 14,000 daltons (14K), but the function of this protein is not known. Three possible promoters P_1, P_2, and P_3 may control transcription of the *unc* operon, but only one of these (P_1) has been shown to be active in *in vitro* transcription experiments. A typical terminator region (T) was found to hybridize with the promoter sequence (P_1). The scale in kilobases (Kb) is also shown. (Reproduced with permission from M. Futai and H. Kanazawa, "Structure and Function of Proton-Translocating Adenosine Triphosphatase (F_0F_1): Biochemical and Molecular Biological Approaches, *Microbiological Reviews,* **47:** 285–312, 1983.)

are derivatized by the reagent, dicyclohexylcarbodiimide (DCCD), the F_0 complex is inactivated. The inactivated F_0 channel is incapable of catalyzing proton translocation across the membrane, and the intact F_0F_1 ATPase is no longer capable of catalyzing rapid ATP hydrolysis. For this reason, subunit c is sometimes called the DCCD-binding protein or proteolipid. Incorporation of one covalent DCCD molecule per F_0 complex has been reported to be sufficient to completely inhibit proton transport. If this observation is correct, it provides independent evidence for the involvement of cooperative subunit interactions in the normal functioning of the proton-translocating ATP synthase.

Studies on the pH profile of proton translocation through the F_0 moiety of the ATPase have led to the suggestion that the carboxyl group of the DCCD-sensitive residue to subunit c comprises a monoprotic H^+ binding site within the H^+ channel. Interestingly, the pKa of this residue is near neutrality, presumably because of its localization within a hydrophobic environment of the phospholipid bilayer.

Each of the small c subunits from all organisms appears to consist of two membrane-embedded antiparallel α-helicies. A β-turn on the cytoplasmic side of the bacterial membrane separates these two helicies, and both the N- and C-termini of the protein are exposed on the external face of the membrane. The DCCD-sensitive glutamyl or aspartyl residue is in the middle of one of these two helicies. Several studies with the eukaryotic and thermophilic ATPases suggest that the F_0 channel consists of an oligomeric arrangement of c subunits with the most likely arrangement being a hexamer (Table 7.6). However, it should be noted that a stoichiometry of ten c subunits per ATPase molecule has been reported for the *E. coli* enzyme (Table 7.7). The stoichiometric differences reported for the *Bacillus* and *E. coli* enzymes probably reflect dif-

TABLE 7.6 PROPERTIES OF THE PROTEIN CONSTITUENTS OF THE F_0F_1 COMPLEX OF THE THERMOPHILIC BACTERIUM, *BACILLUS* PS_3

Complex	Protein subunit	Approximate MW	Probable stoichiometries	Demonstrable catalytic function(s) in reconstitution experiments	Presumed functional unit
F_1	α	56,000	3	Stimulates ATPase activity of β-subunit	
	β	53,000	3	Possesses active site for ADP and ATP binding	ATP-dependent proton "pump" (α, β, γ)
	γ	32,000	1	Stimulates ATPase activity of β-subunit; functions with δ and ϵ to regulate H^+ transport by F_0	"Gate", regulating proton transport in the channel (γ, δ, ϵ)
	δ	16,000	1		
	ϵ	11,000	1	Required for binding of F_1 to F_0 (δ, ϵ, b)	
F_0	b	14,000	3		
	a	30,000	1	Transmembrane proton translocation (b, a, c)	"Channel", through which protons traverse the membrane
	c	6,000	6		

ferences in experimental approaches rather than a fundamental difference in the oligomeric structure of the F_0 complexes.

While the function of the a subunit in F_0 is not known, it is highly hydrophobic and may pass through the membrane in α-helical array as many as seven times. It might comprise part of the H^+ channel (Table 7.6). The two hydrophilic b subunits, however, are largely localized to the cytoplasmic surface, being embedded in the membrane only at their N-termini. Disruption of the C-terminal part of the b subunits prevents proper binding of F_1 to F_0, renders the ATPase function of F_1 in the reconstituted F_0F_1 complex insensitive to DCCD inhibition, and prevents proper coupling between ATP synthesis and H^+ flux. The F_0 moiety of the mitochondrial ATPase appears to contain the same three subunits as well as two additional subunits not found in the bacterial enzyme complex.

Based on these results and the results of reconstitution studies with limited combinations of the subunits of the bacterial ATPases, the functions of proton channel, proton gate, and proton pump (ATPase) have been assigned to the different subunits of the F_0F_1 complex as summarized in Table 7.6. The most likely structural arrangement of the subunits in the intact F_0F_1 complex is shown in Figure 7.12.

The F_1 moiety of the ATP synthase of many organisms is easily released from the membrane and purified by conventional means. From all sources, the subunit composition appears to be the same: $\alpha_3\beta_3\gamma\delta\epsilon$ (Tables 7.6 and 7.7). This result alone

TABLE 7.7 PROPERTIES OF SUBUNITS OF THE H^+-TRANSLOCATING ATP SYNTHASE (F_0F_1) OF *E. COLI*[a]

Subunit	MW	Number of amino acid residues	Stoichiometries	Polarity
F_1				
α	55,259	513	3	0.43
β	50,117	459	3	0.44
γ	31,414	287	1	0.46
δ	19,303	177	1	0.44
ϵ	14,914	138	1	0.44
F_0				
b	17,244	156	2	0.48
a	30,275	271	1	0.32
c	8,246	79	10 (6?)	0.23
14K	14,087	130		0.25

[a] The molecular weight values and numbers of amino acyl residues were determined from the gene sequences. Polarity (hydropathy) analyses (summarized above) revealed that all subunits except for the a and c subunits of F_0 exhibit the properties of typical soluble proteins. Consequently, only the a and c subunits are likely to be largely embedded within the membrane. The properties of the 14K protein were deduced from the nucleotide sequence of the *unc* operon (see Figure 7.11). This protein has not yet been identified, and its function is unknown.

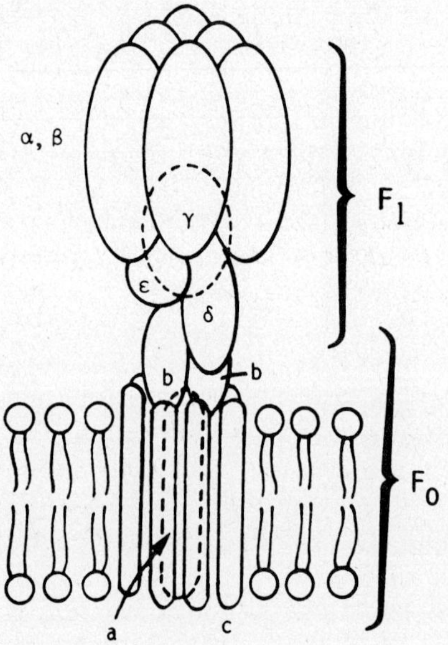

Figure 7.12 Proposed structure of the proton-translocating F_0F_1 ATP synthase from *E. coli.* The model shown is based on reconstitution experiments, subunit stoichiometries, predicted secondary structures, and subunit interactions. The subunits are not drawn to scale. The presence of the a and c subunits within the membrane corresponds to predictions based on the polarity (hydropathy) analysis recorded in Table 7.7. Subunits γ, δ and ϵ of F_1, and the two b-subunits of F_0 are shown to bind the $\alpha_3\beta_3$ hexamer of F_1 to the ac_6 heptamer of F_0. (Reproduced with permission from M. Futai and H. Kanazawa, "Structure and Function of Proton-Translocating Adenosine Triphosphatase (F_0F_1): Biochemical and Molecular Biological Approaches," *Microbiological Reviews,* **47:** 285–312, 1983.)

suggests common structural elements and evolutionary origins for these molecules. Amino acyl sequence analyses have confirmed this conclusion. For example, the amino acyl sequences of the β-subunits of bovine mitochondrial F_1, of maize chloroplast F_1, and of *E. coli* F_1, were found to be 70% homologous. Although the other subunits exhibited less homology, these results provide firm evidence for a close evolutionary relationship between the prokaryotic and eukaryotic organellar proteins. Sequence analyses of the *E. coli* enzyme have also revealed that the α- and β-chains exhibit substantial sequence homology, suggesting a common evolutionary ancestry for these two subunits.

While reconstituted ATPase activity depends on the presence of the α-, β-, and γ-subunits of F_1, the δ- and ϵ-subunits appear to function as the stalk, attaching the hexagonal F_1 to F_0. They also inhibit the free flux of protons through F_0. Both the α- and β-subunits possess adenine nucleotide binding sites, and some evidence indicates that the β-subunit is the catalytic subunit. For example, reconstitution of ATPase activity from the F_1 component of the *Bacillus* ATPase can be demonstrated when either the β- and γ-subunits are mixed, or when the α-, β-, and δ- subunits are mixed. Further, treatment of F_1 with reagents against specific amino acyl residues indicate that 1 mole each of highly reactive arginyl, tyrosyl, and glutamyl or aspartyl residues, all within each β-subunit, is essential for catalytic activity. Several lysyl residues also appear to be required. Substrate protection experiments indicate that the arginyl residue binds inorganic phosphate to the active site, the reactive side-chain carboxyl group participates in Mg^{++} binding, and the lysyl and tyrosyl residues function in ADP binding. A speculative model for the binding and synthesis of substrates and products at the active site of the β-subunit is shown in Figure 7.13. It is interesting to note that analogous studies of the adenine nucleotide binding site of pyruvate kinase have led to the proposal of a similar active site for this enzyme.

The catalytic process of ATP synthesis or hydrolysis probably does not involve the formation of a phosphoenzyme intermediate. A concerted mechanism in which ATP is the first covalent derivative of both ADP and P_i has been suggested. At low ATP concentrations, F_1 catalyzes $H_2O^{18} \rightleftharpoons HPO_4^=$ exchange under conditions of steady-state ATP hydrolysis. Surprisingly, this exchange reaction is not observed at high ATP concentrations. These observations have led to the suggestion that ATP hydrolysis at the catalytic site involves cooperative interactions between different active sites within the oligomeric F_1. There appear to be up to six adenine nucleotide binding sites in F_1.

Cooperativity of substrate hydrolysis has been demonstrated with both mammalian and *E. coli* F_1. High-affinity substrate binding at the first catalytic site is accompanied by very slow hydrolysis. However, the apparent binding affinity of the first site decreases several orders of magnitude, and the rate of hydrolysis increases twentyfold when a second site is occupied with substrate. An *alternating sites* mechanism has been proposed in which the second, low-affinity site is converted to a high-affinity site when the products of hydrolysis, ADP and P_i, are released from the first site. Only when ATP is bound at both sites is rapid ATP hydrolysis observed. When studied over a wide range of ATP concentrations, the kinetic data can be interpreted in terms of three interacting sites, but not in terms of two or three independently functioning active sites.

Several investigators have measured the equilibrium constant for the reaction: ATP $\rightarrow$ ADP + P_i associated with the first, high-affinity binding site. The K_{eq} was found to be near 1, showing that ATP synthesis from ADP and P_i can occur on the enzyme surface without the input of metabolic energy. In fact, synthesis of ATP by isolated F_1 has been demonstrated, proving that energy in the form of a proton flux is not required for ATP synthesis at the F_1 active site. The results support a proposal

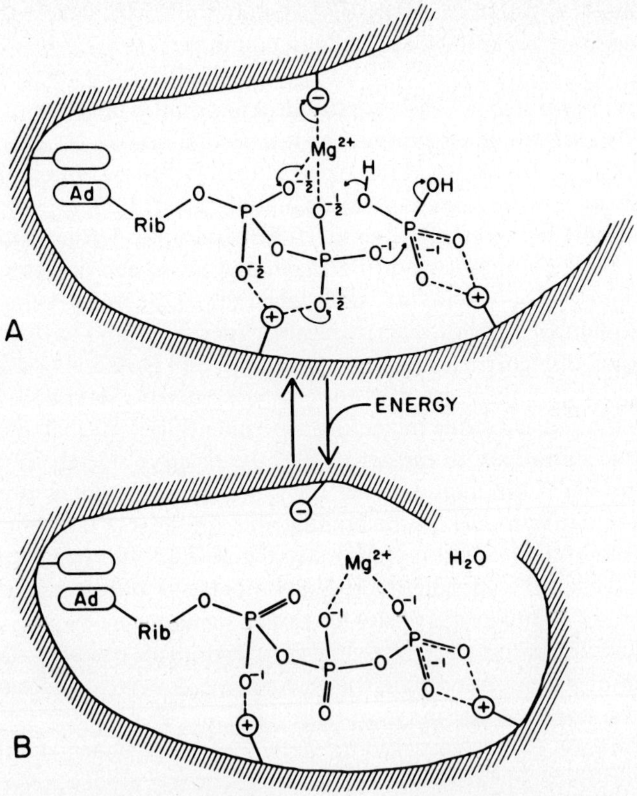

Figure 7.13 A speculative scheme for ATP synthesis at the catalytic site of the β-subunit of the F_1 component of the proton-translocating ATPase. (Reproduced with permission from R. L. Cross, "The Mechanism and Regulation of ATP Synthesis by F_1-ATPases," *Annual Review of Biochemistry,* **50,** 681–714, 1981.)

that energy input in the form of a proton flux through the ATP synthase functions to alter the ATP binding affinity rather than to promote ATP synthesis. One possibility is that energy effects release of ATP, previously synthesized from ADP and P_i at the F_1 active site. The energy responsible for ATP synthesis is presumably provided by compensatory conformational changes in the protein which accompany substrate binding. It should be noted, however, that the conformational change induced by site–site cooperativity in the F_1 moiety has not yet been shown to be related to the conformational change which is induced by ATP-driven proton pumping in the intact F_0F_1 complex. Only when such a relationship is demonstrated will the results provide clear evidence for the proposed indirect, conformational mechanism for the coupling of ATP synthesis to proton movement.

The question of the principal mechanism(s) responsible for the regulation of the activity of the proton-translocating ATP synthase remains largely unanswered. However, some studies suggest that regulation of F_1 from mitochondria is mediated by heat-stable, low molecular weight inhibitory proteins of 8,000–13,000 daltons. The inhibitors appear to bind to the β-subunit of F_1 and inhibit binding of inorganic phosphate. The inhibitory effect of one such protein from rat liver mitochondria is reversed by the Ca^{++}-binding protein, calmodulin (see Section 3.8). It is possible that some of the inhibitors bind to F_1 only under conditions of energy depletion so that they prevent the wasteful hydrolysis of ATP when the proton electrochemical gradient is insufficient for ATP synthesis. Consistent with this physiological function, MgATP may be required for its binding to F_1. Other proposed mechanisms of regulation involve reversible sulfhydryl oxidation and small molecule ligand binding. These possibilities will undoubtedly be the subject of intensive investigations in the near future.

7.7 MEMBRANE-BOUND, PROTON-TRANSLOCATING TRANSHYDROGENASES

Associated with the inner mitochondrial membranes of eukaryotes and the cytoplasmic membranes of bacteria are related proton-translocating transhydrogenases (E.C.1.6.1.1) which catalyze the following reaction:

$$NADH + NADP^+ + H^+(out) \rightleftharpoons NAD^+ + NADPH + H^+(in) \qquad (7.1)$$

The integral membrane transhydrogenase catalyzes hydride exchange between the pyridine nucleotide couples $NADH/NAD^+$ and $NADPH/NADP^+$ in a process that is coupled to the translocation of one or possibly two protons across the membrane. The principal function of the reaction seems to be to generate NADPH for anabolic purposes. Input of energy in the form of a membrane potential drives the reaction to the right when protons flow down their electrochemical gradient into the mitochondrion or the bacterial cell.

The active site of the energy-linked transhydrogenase from mitochondria faces the mitochondrial matrix. Hydride transfer apparently occurs directly from the A-position of NADH to the B-position of $NADP^+$. A ternary complex between NADH, $NADP^+$ and enzyme occurs with NADH bound to one discrete site and $NADP^+$ presumably bound to an adjacent site on the surface of the enzyme. The enzyme-catalyzed reaction shows sequential kinetics, and inhibitors that compete for binding with NAD^+ or NADH are noncompetitive with respect to $NADP^+$ or NADPH. These results argue in favor of an enzyme active site with two distinct substrate binding sites, one specific for NAD^+ and NADH, the other specific for $NADP^+$ and NADPH.

The mechanistic details by which hydride transfer is coupled to transmembrane proton transport have not been elucidated. However, the transhydrogenase from bovine heart mitochondria has been purified, and its proton-translocating transhydrogenase activity has been reconstituted in a vesicular proteoliposome membrane. The purified, reconstituted protein is a dimer of two apparently identical polypeptide chains (MW = 110,000). The proton translocation function of the enzyme is irreversibly inhibited by dicyclohexylcarbodiimide (DCCD), the same reagent that blocks proton translocation through the proton-translocating ATPase and cytochrome oxidase complexes. Under conditions that abolish proton transport, transhydrogenation is inhibited only 30% by this reagent. It seems that DCCD must derivatize an H^+-binding domain which is localized outside the transhydrogenase active site.

The model depicted in Figure 7.14 is consistent with the evidence presently available concerning proton-translocating transhydrogenases. NADH and $NADP^+$ must be simultaneously bound to the active site of the enzyme with one nicotinamide ring on top of the other (π-stacking?) in order for reaction to occur. The binding of these two pyridine nucleotides at their respective sites induces a conformational change (transition *a* in Figure 7.14) which causes a basic residue (B_1) on the external surface of the enzyme to undergo a shift in pK_a value. A proton from the external medium consequently binds to B_1. Hydride shift from NADH to $NADP^+$ is accompanied by a second conformational change (transition *b*) which causes the proton to pass from (B_1) to the DCCD-sensitive carboxyl group (B_2) and then to a third residue localized to the inner surface of the membrane (B_3). Dissociation of the two pyridine nucleotides from the active site is accompanied by H^+ release into the internal milieu (transition *c* in Figure 7.14). Because the enzyme is a homodimer, a possible half-of-sites-type

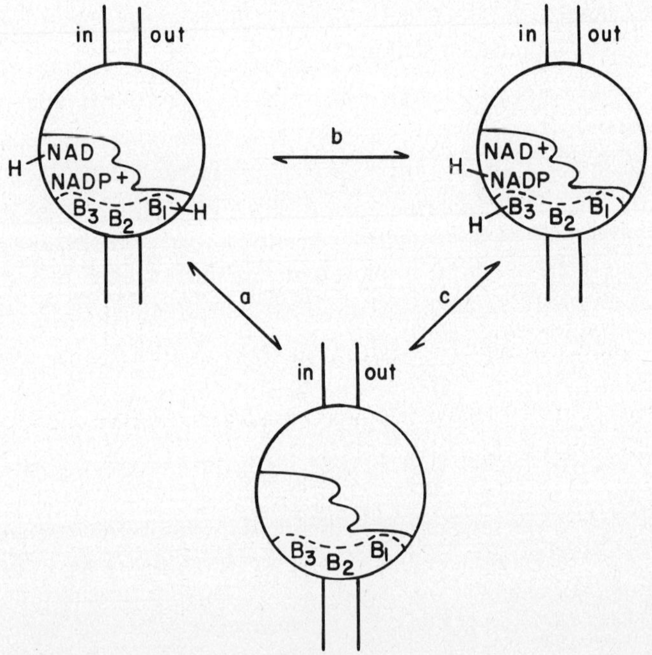

Figure 7.14 Schematic depiction of a plausible mechanism for the vectorial oxidoreduction reaction catalyzed by the proton-translocating transhydrogenase of mammalian mitochondria. The figure illustrates the three conformational transitions (a, b, and c) which are presumed to accompany substrate binding, hydride transfer, and product dissociation, respectively. These three transitions are suggested to promote proton association at B_1, proton-translocation from B_1 to B_2 and B_3, and dissociation of the proton from B_3, respectively. While B_1 and B_3 are hypothetical basic residues in the transhydrogenase, B_2 may be the DCCD-sensitive β- or γ-carboxyl group of an aspartyl or glutamyl residue in the enzyme.

mechanism for this reaction must be considered. Indeed, recent work has shown that when one mole of dicyclohexylcarbodiimide (DCCD) is covalently incorporated into the dimeric enzyme, activity is completely lost. Quantitative inactivation of the enzyme was also observed when a reactive NAD^+ analogue, *para*-fluorosulfonylbenzoyladenosine, was covalently incorporated into the transhydrogenase. Because this reagent proved fully effective when only one-half of the active sites were derivatized, a half-of-sites mechanism was implied. It should be kept in mind that several alternatives to the proposed mechanism shown in Figure 7.14 are equally plausible.

Comparison of the proton-translocating transhydrogenases with the proton-translocating mitochondrial or bacterial respiratory complexes reveals that of these complexes, the transhydrogenase is by far the most simple biochemical system for investigating proton-coupled electron transfer. It may prove to be an ideal model system for the elucidation of the mechanism by which the coupling of a vectorial process to electron flow is accomplished.

> *Evolution, like the tinker, does not produce innovations from scratch. It works on what already exists, transforming a system to give it a new function or combining several systems to produce a more complex one.*
>
> —*F. Jacob*

BIBLIOGRAPHY

Amzel, L. M., and P. L. Pedersen, "Proton ATPases: Structure and Mechanism," *Annual Review of Biochemistry* **52:** 801–824 (1983).

Azzi, A., "Cytochrome *c* Oxidase: Towards a Clarification of its Structure, Interactions and Mechanism," *Biochimica et Biophysica Acta,* **594:** 231–252 (1980).

Becker, W. M., "Aerobic Production of ATP: Electron Transport," *Biochemistry,* G. Zubay, ed., pp. 363–407, Addison-Wesley, Reading, MA (1983).

Bolis, C. L., E. J. M. Helmreich, and H. Passow, eds., *Information and Energy Transduction in Biological Membranes,* Proceedings of the International Conference on Biological Membranes Held in Crans-sur-Sierre (Valais), Switzerland, June, 1983, A. R. Liss, New York (1984).

Chock, P. B., S. G. Rhee, and E. R. Stadtman, "Interconvertible Enzyme Cascades in Cellular Regulation," *Annual Review of Biochemistry,* **49:** 813–843 (1980).

Cross, R. L., "The Mechanism and Regulation of ATP Synthesis by F_1-ATPases," *Annual Review of Biochemistry,* **50:** 681–714 (1981).

Ferguson, S. J., and M. C. Sorgato, "Proton Electrochemical Gradients and Energy-Transduction Processes," *Annual Review of Biochemistry,* **51:** 185–217 (1982).

Fisher, R. R., and S. R. Earle, "Membrane-Bound Pyridine Dinucleotide Transhydrogenase," in *The Pyridine Nucleotide Coenzymes,* J. Everse, B. Henderson, and K. You, eds., Academic, New York (1982).

Futai, M., and H. Kanazawa, "Structure and Function of Proton-Translocating Adenosine Triphosphatase (F_0F_1): Biochemical and Molecular Biological Approaches," *Microbiological Reviews,* **47:** 285–312 (1983).

Hatefi, Y., "The Mitochondrial Electron Transport and Oxidative Phosphorylation System," *Annual Review of Biochemistry,* **54:** 1015–1069 (1985).

Higuti, T., "Conformational Coupling in H^+-pumps and ATP Synthesis—Its Analysis with Anisotropic Inhibitors of Energy Transduction in Oxidative Phosphorylation," *Molecular and Cellular Biochemistry,* **61:** 37–61 (1984).

Hinkle, P. C., and R. E. McCarty, "How Cells Make ATP," *Scientific American,* **238:** 104–123 (1978).

Ingledew, W. J., and R. K. Poole, "The Respiratory Chains of *Escherichia coli,*" *Microbiological Reviews,* **48:** 222–271 (1984).

Kinoshita, N., T. Unemoto, and H. Kobayashi, "Proton Motive Force Is Not Obligatory for Growth of *Escherichia coli,*" *Journal of Bacteriology,* **160:** 1074–1077 (1984).

Kita, K., K. Konishi, and Y. Anraku, "Terminal Oxidases of *Escherichia coli* Aerobic Respiratory Chain. I. Purification and Properties of Cytochrome b_{562}–*o* Complex from Cells in the Early Exponential Phase of Aerobic Growth," *Journal of Biological Chemistry,* **259:** 3368–3374 (1984).

Kita, K., K. Konishi, and Y. Anraku, "Terminal Oxidases of *Escherichia coli* Aerobic Respiratory Chain. II. Purification and Properties of Cytochrome b_{558}–*d* Complex from Cells Grown with Limited Oxygen and Evidence of Branched Electron-Carrying Systems," *Journal of Biological Chemistry,* **259:** 3375–3381 (1984).

Lever, A. B. P., and H. B. Gray, eds., *Iron Porphyrins,* Addison-Wesley, Reading, MA (1983).

Matsushita, K., L. Patel, and H. R. Kaback, "Cytochrome *o*-Type Oxidase from *Escherichia coli.* Characterization of the Enzyme and Mechanism of Electrochemical Proton Gradient Generation," *Biochemistry,* **23:** 4703–4714 (1984).

Milazzo, G., and M. Blank, eds., *Bioelectrochemistry I: Biological Redox Reactions,* Plenum, New York (1983).

Mitchell, P., "Compartmentation and Communication in Living Systems. Ligand Conduction: a General Catalytic Principle in Chemical, Osmotic and Chemiosmotic Reaction Systems," The Ninth Sir Hans Krebs Lecture, *European Journal of Biochemistry,* **95:** 1–20 (1979).

Phelps, D. C., and Y. Hatefi, "Interaction of Purified Nicotinamidenucleotide Transhydrogenase with Dicyclohexylcarbodiimide," *Biochemistry,* **23:** 4475–4480 (1984).

Racker, E. *A New Look at Mechanisms of Bioenergetics,* Academic, New York (1976).

Saier, M. H., Jr., *Mechanisms and Regulation of Carbohydrate Transport in Bacteria,* Academic, New York (1985).

Saier, M. H., Jr., and C. D. Stiles, *Molecular Dynamics in Biological Membranes,* Heidelberg Science Library 22, Springer-Verlag, New York (1975).

Spiro, T. G., ed., *Copper Proteins,* Wiley, New York (1981).

Spiro, T. G., ed., *Iron–Sulfur Proteins,* Wiley, New York (1982).

Walker, J. E., M. Saraste, and N. J. Gay, "The *unc* Operon: Nucleotide Sequence, Regulation, and Structure of ATP-synthase," *Biochimica et Biophysica Acta,* **768:** 164–200 (1984).

Weiner, J. H., B. D. Lemire, R. W. Jones, W. F. Anderson, and D. G. Scraba, "A Model for the Structure of Fumarate Reductase in the Cytoplasmic Membrane of *Escherichia coli,*" *Journal of Cellular Biochemistry,* **24:** 207–216 (1984).

Chapter 8

Fatty Acid Oxidation and Biosynthesis

> *Seek simplicity but distrust it.*
>
> —A. N. WHITEHEAD

Fatty acids, the energy-rich hydrophobic constituents of triglycerides and phospholipids, represent one of the major classes of macromolecular building blocks of all living cells. The majority of these acids are long, straight-chained hydrocarbons terminated with a single carboxyl group. The most common are even-numbered, having 16 or 18 carbons. Branched-chain fatty acids and those containing an odd number of carbons are found only infrequently in nature. This fact reflects their mode of biosynthesis which in turn is related to the mechanism of their degradation.

Fatty acids are synthesized from acetate by the sequential addition of C_2 units to the carboxy terminal end of the growing hydrocarbon chain:

$$R{-}CO_2^- + CH_3{-}CO_2^- \rightarrow R{-}CH_2{-}CH_2{-}CO_2^- \qquad (8.1)$$

In a conceptually similar, but reversed, process, fatty acids are degraded by the sequential removal of C_2 units from the carboxy terminal end of the shrinking hydrocarbon chain:

$$R{-}CH_2{-}CH_2{-}CO_2^- \rightarrow R{-}CO_2^- + CH_3{-}CO_2^- \qquad (8.2)$$

On the basis of this information alone, one process appears to be the reverse of the other. In principle this is true, but in detail, the biosynthetic and degradative processes are very different. In this chapter we shall first compare the two processes and then examine each one in detail. The comparison will allow us to evaluate the differences between a strictly anabolic process and a closely related process which serves a strictly catabolic role.

8.1 COMPARATIVE CHARACTERISTICS OF FATTY ACID DEGRADATION AND BIOSYNTHESIS

As noted above, fatty acid oxidation and biosynthesis are superficially similar, resulting from the removal from or addition to the hydrocarbon chain of a two-carbon fragment. The two processes differ in the following fundamental respects.

(1) The oxidative and biosynthetic enzymes are distinct, and in the compartmentalized eukaryotic cell they are found in different intracellular locations. While the biosynthetic machinery is found in the cytoplasm, the enzymes of fatty acid oxidation are localized to the mitochondrial matrix.

(2) The type of acyl group carrier differs for the two processes. Coenzyme A serves as the acyl carrier for the oxidative process, but the biosynthetic process utilizes a small protein called acyl carrier protein (ACP). While this difference might appear to be major, both molecules contain the same active moiety to which the acyl group is attached, and this moiety is derived from the vitamin, pantothenate. Functionally, therefore, coenzyme A and ACP are equivalent.

(3) The form in which the two-carbon fragment is added to or removed from the fatty acyl chain differs for the two processes: acetyl CoA is cleaved from the hydrocarbon chain after oxidation of the β-carbon, but malonyl CoA is utilized as the C_2-donor for biosynthetic purposes. Decarboxylation of malonyl CoA provides the energy for bond formation.

(4) Both processes function with β-hydroxy acyl intermediates, but the stereoisomeric configuration of the β-hydroxyl groups differ. The D-isomer is formed during biosynthesis while the L-isomer is formed during degradation.

(5) Both the oxidative and biosynthetic processes involve a redox reaction in which a β-keto acid and a β-hydroxy acid are interconverted. While the oxidative process utilizes NAD^+ as the electron acceptor for β-hydroxyacyl CoA dehydrogenation, NADPH is used for the reduction of the β-ketoacyl-ACP derivative.

(6) Both processes catalyze the interconversion of a saturated acyl derivative and a trans Δ^2 enoyl derivative of the acid. While the oxidative enzyme utilizes FAD as the electron acceptor, NADPH serves as the electron donor for the biosynthetic process.

(7) Finally, as might be expected, the two processes respond quite differently to regulatory metabolites in the cell. Citrate activates the biosynthetic process by activating the enzyme complex which synthesizes malonyl CoA, and this enzyme requires bicarbonate as substrate. Neither compound regulates β-oxidation. The oxidative and biosynthetic processes are illustrated in Figures 8.1 and 8.2, respectively.

8.2 β-OXIDATION OF FATTY ACIDS

E. coli can utilize fatty acids as sole sources of carbon for growth. The presence of exogenous long-chain fatty acids induces expression of the *fad* (*f*atty *a*cid *d*egradation) regulon provided that glucose or another catabolite repressing carbohydrate is not

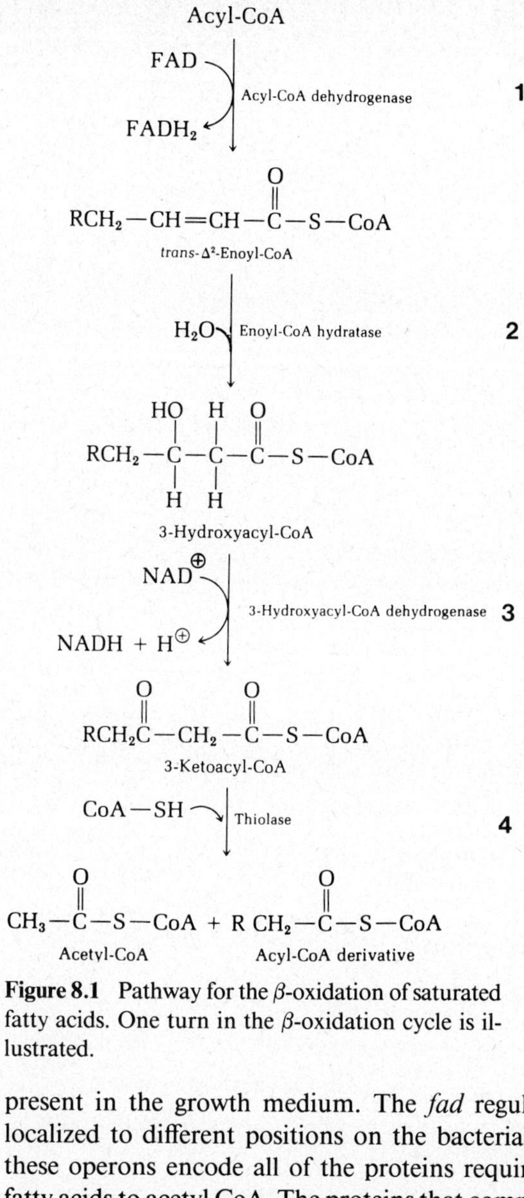

Figure 8.1 Pathway for the β-oxidation of saturated fatty acids. One turn in the β-oxidation cycle is illustrated.

present in the growth medium. The *fad* regulon includes several distinct operons localized to different positions on the bacterial chromosome, and the genes within these operons encode all of the proteins required for the degradation of exogenous fatty acids to acetyl CoA. The proteins that comprise the fatty acid degradation system, some of their properties, and the designations of the structural genes that encode these proteins in *E. coli,* are summarized in Table 8.1. A repressor protein (encoded by the *fadR* gene) and the cyclic AMP receptor protein (encoded by the *crp* gene) render transcription of the regulon responsive to the presence of cytoplasmic fatty acyl derivatives and to cytoplasmic concentrations of cyclic AMP, respectively. Since carbohydrates regulate cellular cyclic AMP concentrations, catabolite repression is at least in part mediated by cyclic AMP and its receptor protein.

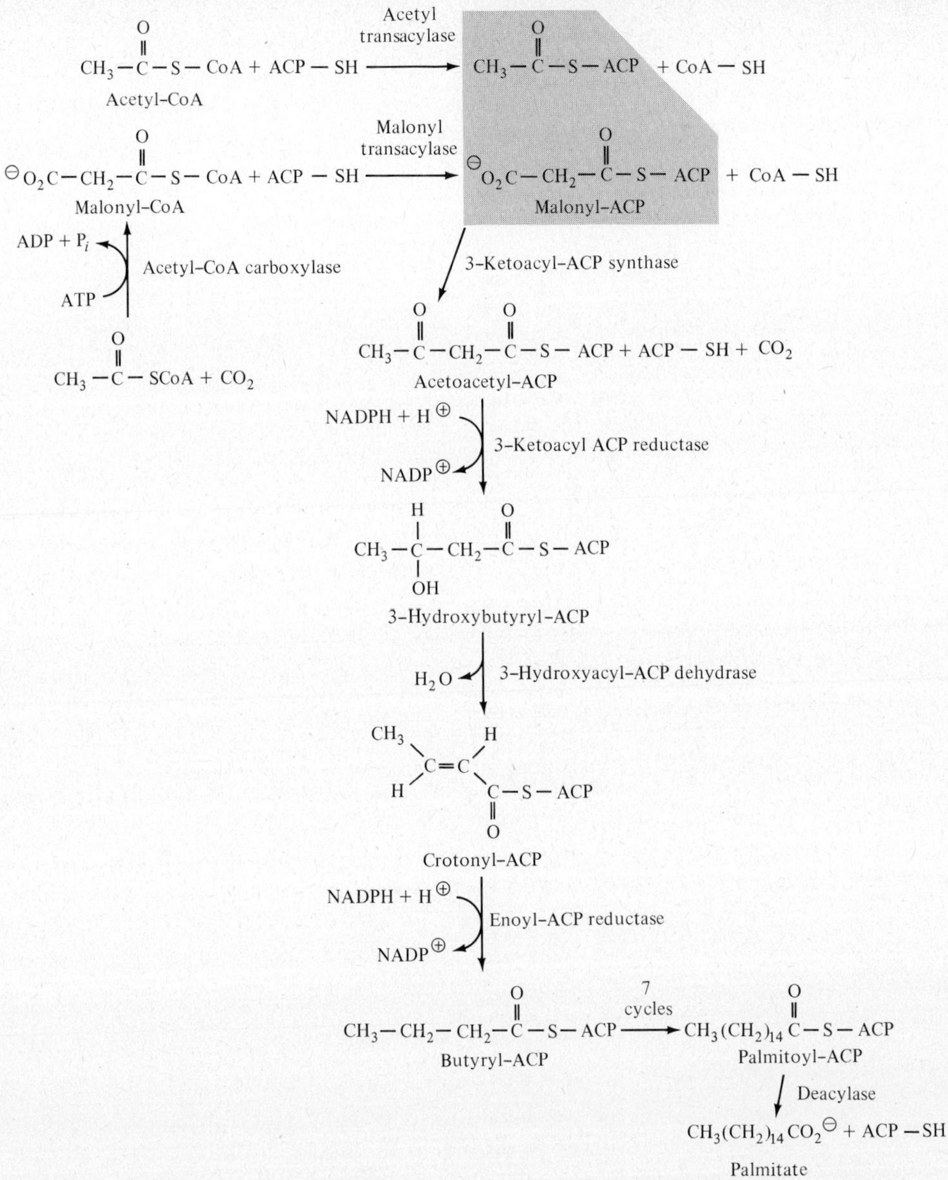

Figure 8.2 Pathway for the biosynthesis of straight-chain, saturated fatty acids. Reactions responsible for the addition of one C-2 unit to the growing fatty acid chain are illustrated.

Entry of fatty acids into the cell cytoplasm appears to be mediated by *porin* proteins (which allow passage across the outer membrane of the *E. coli* envelope), as well as an integral cytoplasmic membrane protein with an approximate molecular weight of 43,000 daltons (which transports the fatty acid across the inner membrane). The latter protein is the product of the *fadL* gene. The mechanism of its action is unknown.

TABLE 8.1 PROPERTIES OF ENZYMES RESPONSIBLE FOR FATTY ACID DEGRADATION IN *ESCHERICHIA COLI*

			Molecular weight	
Enzyme activity	E.C. #	Gene	Subunit	Complex
Fatty acid transporter		*fadL*	43,000	?
Acyl CoA synthase	6.2.1.3	*fadD*	47,000	130,000
Acyl CoA dehydrogenase	1.3.99.3	*fadE*	?	?
Enoyl CoA hydratase	4.2.1.17	*fadB*	78,000	240,000
3-Hydroxyacyl CoA dehydrogenase	1.1.1.35	*fadB*	78,000	240,000
3-Ketoacyl CoA thiolase	2.3.1.16	*fadA*	42,000	240,000
3-Hydroxyacyl CoA epimerase	5.1.2.3	*fadB*	78,000	240,000
cis Δ^2-trans Δ^2 enoyl CoA isomerase	5.3.3.3	*fadB*	78,000	240,000

A single acyl CoA synthase, with broad substrate specificity for the fatty acid substrate, is responsible for synthesizing fatty acyl CoA derivatives from free fatty acids in *E. coli.* This enzyme, encoded by the *fadD* gene, is loosely associated with the inner surface of the cytoplasmic membrane and may function to derivatize fatty acids with coenzyme A as they dissociate from the *fadL* encoded transporter. The coupled process of transport and thioesterification, mediated by the *fadL* and *fadD* gene products, has been termed *vectorial thioesterification* by analogy with *vectorial phosphorylation* mediated by the bacterial phosphotransferase system (Chapter 5).

The first metabolic enzyme catalyzing degradation of the acyl CoA derivative is acyl CoA dehydrogenase, the product of the *fadE* gene. This poorly characterized enzyme, presumed to function with FAD as its redox cofactor, gives rise to an α,β-trans-unsaturated acyl CoA derivative (reaction 1 in Figure 8.1). All remaining catalytic activities responsible for the conversion of an acyl CoA derivative to acetyl CoA are associated with a single multifunctional enzyme complex with a net molecular weight of 240,000. This complex consists of a heterotetramer of $\alpha_2\beta_2$ structure. The α subunit (MW = 78,000; encoded by the *fadB* gene) catalyzes both the hydration of the α,β-unsaturated acyl CoA derivative (reaction 2 in Figure 8.1) and the subsequent dehydrogenation of the resultant β-hydroxy acyl CoA derivative to the β-keto acyl CoA derivative (reaction 3 in Figure 8.1). The former reaction can be catalyzed by a distinct soluble enzyme as well as the $\alpha_2\beta_2$ tetramer. The dehydrogenation reaction occurs with NAD^+ as the electron acceptor.

The fourth and last reaction depicted in Figure 8.1, cleavage of the β-keto thioester to acetyl CoA and an acyl CoA derivative of two fewer carbon atoms than the starting compound, is catalyzed by 3-ketoacyl CoA thiolase. This enzyme activity resides with the β-subunit of the heterotetramer (MW = 42,000, encoded by the *fadA* gene). However, two such enzymes are present in *E. coli,* one of which is specific for short-chain fatty acyl derivatives, the other which acts on long-chain fatty acyl derivatives. Only the latter enzyme is present in the $\alpha_2\beta_2$ tetramer. The other thiolase is a distinct soluble enzyme encoded by a separate gene.

Two additional catalytic activities of the complex have been identified which may be associated with the α-subunit. These two activities are an isomerization reaction which interconverts trans Δ^2 enoyl CoA derivatives and the corresponding cis Δ^3

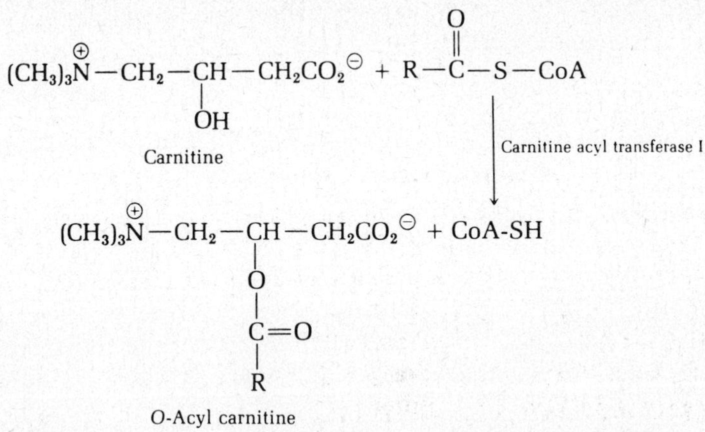

Figure 8.3 Acylation of carnitine in the carnitine acyl transferase-catalyzed reaction. This reaction allows fatty acyl groups to cross the mitochondrial membrane (see text).

derivative (a reaction that allows oxidative degradation of naturally occurring unsaturated fatty acids) and an epimerization reaction interconverting the D- and L-isomers of 3-hydroxyacyl CoA (a reaction that allows utilization of naturally occurring D-hydroxy fatty acids).

In eukaryotes, the thioesters of fatty acids are synthesized by acyl CoA synthases in the cytoplasm, while all subsequent oxidative steps occur in the mitochondrial matrix. Consequently, a derivative of the fatty acid must cross the inner mitochondrial membrane. The membrane is impermeable to acyl CoA derivatives, so an interconversion process is required. The long-chain fatty acyl group is transferred from coenzyme A to carnitine in a reaction catalyzed by carnitine-acyl transferase I, localized to the outer surface of the inner mitochondrial membrane. The reaction catalyzed by this enzyme is shown in Figure 8.3. Subsequently, acyl carnitine is transported into the mitochondrion in exchange for free carnitine. The acyl carnitine–carnitine antiporter catalyzes this vectorial reaction (see Table 6.2). Finally, carnitine acyl transferase II, localized to the inner surface of the inner mitochondrial membrane, transfers the acyl group to a free coenzyme A molecule, releasing a free carnitine molecule which can exchange into the cytoplasm for another acyl carnitine molecule.

At least three acyl CoA synthases in mammals and as many in bacteria catalyze the acylation of coenzyme A. One is specific for acetate, a second functions with short-chain fatty acids (C_4 to C_{12}) and uses GTP as activating nucleoside triphosphate (NTP), and a third acts on long-chain fatty acids. The reaction catalyzed by each of these enzymes is essentially the same:

$$\mathrm{R{-}C}\begin{matrix}\mathrm{//O} \\ \\ \mathrm{\backslash O^-}\end{matrix} + \mathrm{CoA} + \mathrm{NTP} \rightarrow \mathrm{R{-}C}\begin{matrix}\mathrm{//O} \\ \\ \mathrm{\backslash CoA}\end{matrix} + \mathrm{NMP} + \mathrm{P_2} \qquad (8.3)$$

The mechanism is shown in Figure 8.4. It should be noted that cleavage of both phosphoanhydride bonds of the nucleoside triphosphate provides the driving force for this reaction, rendering it essentially irreversible.

Acyl CoA dehydrogenases act on an acyl CoA derivative as shown in reaction 1 of Figure 8.1, converting it to trans Δ^2-enoyl CoA. FAD is reduced in the process. At least three such dehydrogenases are known in mitochondria, and these differ with respect to their specificities for fatty acyl CoAs of different chain lengths. An additional dehydrogenase, termed the *electron-transferring flavoprotein,* oxidizes the acyl CoA dehydrogenases, transferring the electrons to the electron transport chain.

Enoyl-CoA hydratase stereospecifically adds water across the 2,3-double bond of trans-enoyl CoA in a process that is analogous to the hydration of fumarate in the TCA cycle (Chapter 6). Only a single such protein is known in mitochondria. The L- (or *S*-) isomer of hydroxyacyl CoA is produced. L-β-hydroxyacyl CoA dehydrogenase subsequently oxidizes the L-hydroxyacyl CoA derivative to 3-ketoacyl CoA by an NAD^+-dependent dehydrogenase (reaction 3 of Figure 8.1). A single such enzyme has been identified in mitochondria. Finally, β-ketothiolases (also called thiolases) catalyze a Claisen cleavage, thereby completing a cycle of β-oxidation. Two such enzymes are known, one of which is specific for acetoacetyl CoA. It is worth noting that per turn

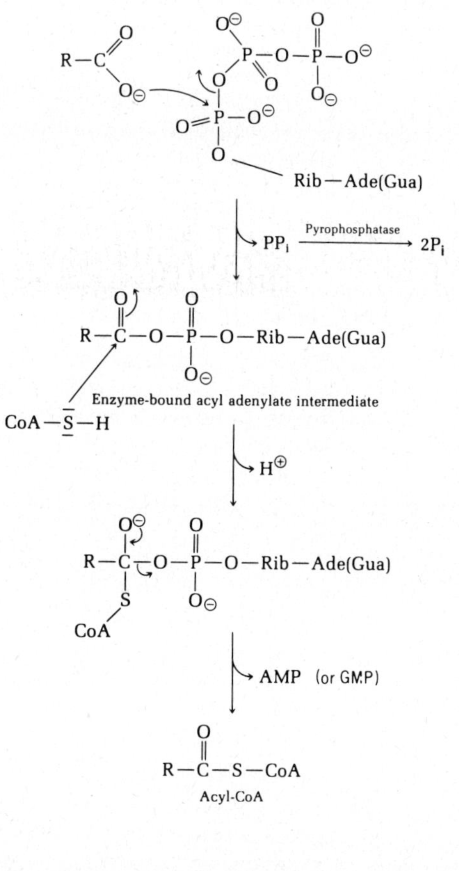

Figure 8.4 Mechanism of acyl CoA synthase. The enzyme-bound acyl adenylate intermediate is a highly reactive mixed anhydride. AMP is a good leaving group which is displaced by the sulfhydryl group of coenzyme A.

of the β-oxidation cycle, one $FADH_2$ and one NADH are generated. These reduced coenzymes normally feed into the electron transfer chain to generate five moles of ATP by oxidative phosphorylation (Chapter 7). Acetyl CoA can, of course, be oxidized via the TCA cycle.

8.3 INITIATION OF FATTY ACID BIOSYNTHESIS: ACETYL CoA CARBOXYLASE

The pathway for fatty acid biosynthesis shown in Figure 8.2 is apparently the same for all living organisms. The major differences between the catabolic and anabolic pathways shown in Figures 8.1 and 8.2 were elaborated in Section 8.1. The first step involves the synthesis of malonyl CoA from acetyl CoA. This reaction is catalyzed by acetyl CoA carboxylase. Subsequently, both malonyl CoA and acetyl CoA are transferred to the fatty acid synthase where they are condensed and reduced.

The *E. coli* fatty acid synthase consists of the acyl carrier protein (ACP) and at least six distinct enzymes. By contrast, the yeast enzyme consists of two dissimilar subunits, A and B, each of which is multifunctional and is encoded by a separate gene. Since the prosthetic group, phosphopantetheine, is probably covalently bound to the A subunit (Figure 8.5), there is no distinct acyl carrier protein. The mammalian fatty acid synthase complex consists of two copies of a single polypeptide chain, each of which possesses all of the requisite catalytic activities as well as covalently bound phosphopantetheine.

Acetyl CoA carboxylase catalyzes the first essential reaction specific to fatty acid biosynthesis, and this reaction is essentially irreversible. It is therefore not surprising that it is subject to regulation in virtually all living organisms. The enzyme contains biotin covalently linked to the ε-amino group of a lysyl residue in the protein (see Chapter 4). Bicarbonate is first transferred to the coenzyme in a reaction which requires ATP hydrolysis as discussed in Section 4.9, and, subsequently, the carboxyl group is

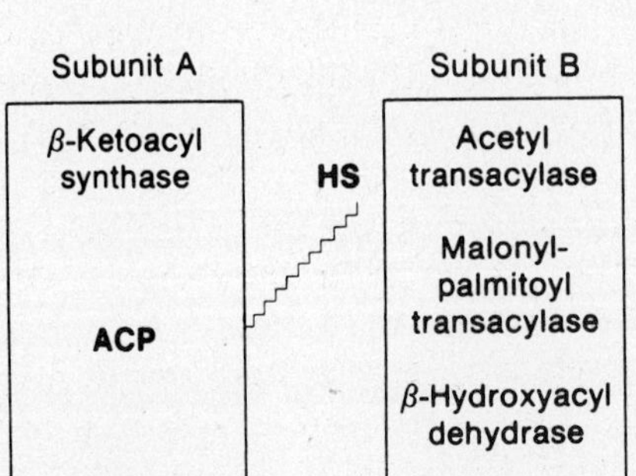

Figure 8.5 Schematic depiction of the yeast fatty acid synthase complex. The complex consists of two large polypeptide chains, A and B, containing at least 6 enzyme activities. The acyl carrier protein (ACP) segment is associated with subunit A. The pantetheine molecule is linked to the hydroxyl group of a seryl residue in the protein via a phosphodiester linkage. The sulfhydryl group at the end of this "arm," of 1.5 nm length, is the site of thioesterification by acetyl, malonyl, or acyl groups. It presumably interacts with all active sites within the complex. (Reproduced with permission from "Metabolism of Fatty Acids and Triglycerols," in *Biochemistry,* G. Zubay, ed., Addison-Wesley, Reading, MA, 1983.)

transferred to acetyl CoA. The reaction mechanism is analogous to that catalyzed by pyruvate carboxylase (Chapter 6).

The acetyl CoA carboxylase from *E. coli* has been extensively characterized. The enzyme consists of three protein components. First, the biotin carboxyl carrier protein (BCCP) has a molecular weight of 22,500 and contains covalently bound biotin. Second, biotin carboxylase has a molecular weight of 100,000 and consists of a homodimer, each subunit of which has a molecular weight of 50,000. Finally, a carboxyltransferase has a molecular weight of 130,000 and is an $\alpha_2\beta_2$ heterotetramer. The two dissimilar subunits have molecular weights of 35,000 and 30,000. Because in *E. coli* virtually all of the fatty acids synthesized are incorporated into membrane phospholipids, the carboxyltransferase is regulated by guanine nucleotides that coordinate fatty acid synthesis with phospholipid synthesis as well as with growth and cell division. The pathways for the biosynthesis of the principal phospholipids are illustrated in Figure 8.6.

While the carboxylation of the biotinyl prosthetic group in BCCP is catalyzed by the biotin carboxylase, transfer of the carboxyl group from the cofactor to acetyl CoA is catalyzed by the carboxyltransferase. Thus, carboxy biotin in BCCP must interact with two separate active sites. This is possible by virtue of the swinging-arm characteristic of the enzyme-bound cofactor. The mechanism of this second reaction is shown in Figure 8.7.

The enzyme has been purified from several mammalian sources. The enzyme from rat liver consists of a dimer of 460,000 molecular weight. Each of the two subunits contains a single biotinyl residue. The dimeric enzyme is inactive unless incubated with citrate which causes the protein to polymerize to an active form containing 10 to 20 dimers. Malonyl CoA and palmitoyl CoA deactivate and depolymerize the enzyme. The responsiveness of the mammalian carboxyl transferases to energy sources presumably reflects the role of fatty acid biosynthesis in the synthesis of fat, a principal energy storage compound in these organisms.

8.4 FATTY ACID SYNTHASES IN DIVERSE ORGANISMS

Although the fatty acid synthases from various organisms catalyze the same reactions by the same mechanisms, they exhibit marked structural differences. It was once thought that the *E. coli* enzymes existed in the intact bacterial cell as a loosely associated complex containing the acyl carrier protein (ACP) and the several constituent enzymes. More recent work showing that several of these enzymes exist in isomeric forms renders this possibility less likely. The enzymes catalyzing saturated fatty acid synthesis are shown in Figure 8.2. These proteins have been separated, purified, and studied individually.

E. coli ACP is a protein of 77 amino acyl residues with a single phosphopantetheyl residue covalently bound to serine residue-36. It can be acetylated or malonylated by transfer of one of these two acyl groups from acetyl CoA or malonyl CoA, respectively. The enzymes catalyzing these two reactions are acetyl CoA:ACP transacylase and malonyl CoA:ACP transacylase, respectively. The acetyl group is transferred from ACP to a thiol group in the third enzyme of the system, β-keto acyl-ACP synthase I. This enzyme is a dimer (MW = 80,000) of two identical subunits (MW = 40,000,

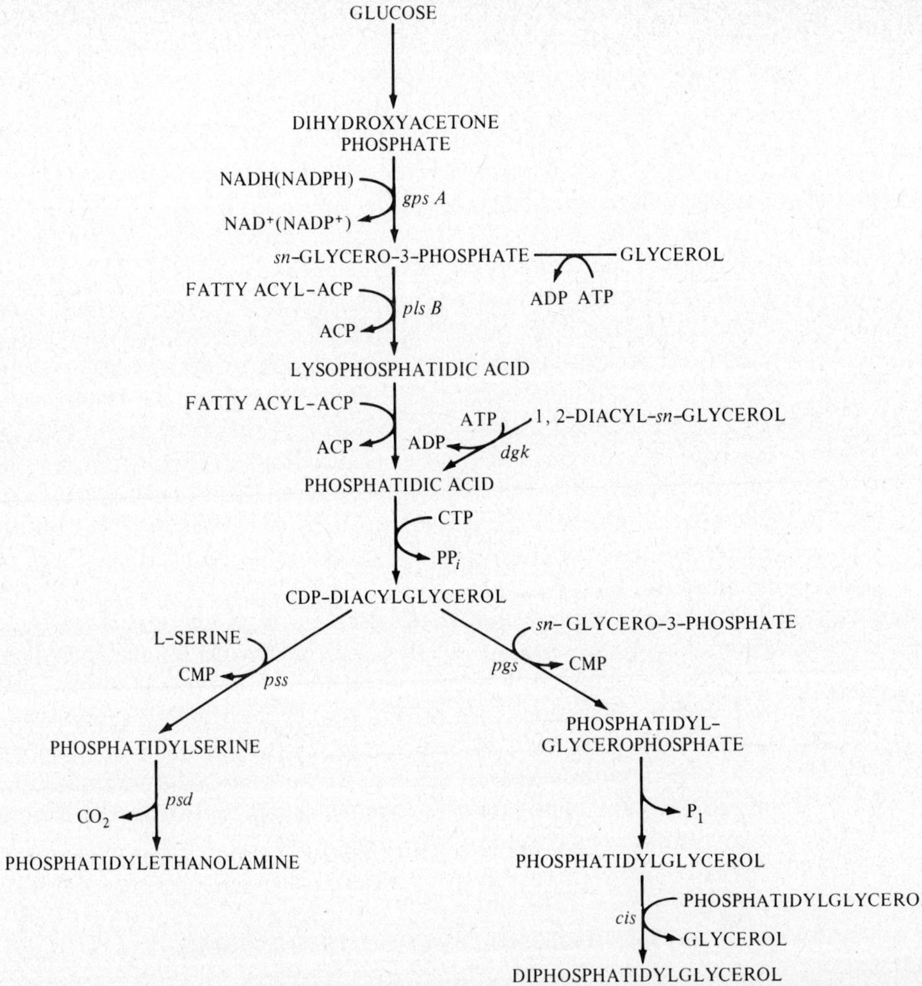

Figure 8.6 Biosynthetic pathways for *E. coli* membrane phospholipids. Various types of mutants are available; these are indicated by the genetic symbol alongside the enzymatic reactions. For a detailed discussion of the reactions in this branching pathway, see Leonard et al, 1981). (Reproduced with permission from J. E. Leonard, C. A. Lee, A. J. Apperson, S. S. Dills and M. H. Saier, Jr., "The Role of Membranes in the Transport of Small Molecules," in *Organization of Prokaryotic Cell Membranes,* B. K. Ghosh, ed., CRC Press, Boca Raton, FL, 1981.)

each). It is active with C_2-C_{14} ACP derivatives, but is not active with fatty acyl-ACP derivatives with chain lengths of sixteen carbons or greater. As a consequence, a fatty acid of sixteen carbon atoms is the largest fatty acid that can be made. The enzyme can not act on fatty acyl derivatives of coenzyme A. A second enzyme, β-ketoacyl-ACP synthase II, a homodimer of 88,000 molecular weight, is active with C-16 fatty acids containing an unsaturation between the 9 and 10 carbons. These two enzymes have been separated from one another and purified to homogeneity.

Once the acetyl (or acyl) group has been transferred to a cysteyl residue in the

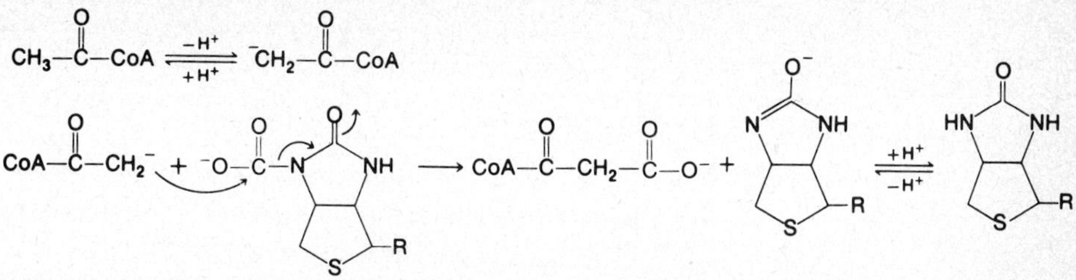

Figure 8.7 Mechanism of action of acetyl CoA carboxylase. Removal of a proton from the methyl group of acetyl CoA yields a carbanion which nucleophilically attacks the carboxyl group of carboxy biotin. (Reproduced with permission from D. E. Vance, "Metabolism of Fatty Acids and Triacyglycerols," in *Biochemistry,* G. Zubay, ed., Addison-Wesley, Reading, MA, 1983.)

synthase, condensation with malonyl-ACP can occur (Figure 8.2). The mechanism of this reaction involves decarboxylation of the malonyl-ACP derivative and nucleophilic attack by the resultant carbanion on the carbonyl of the acetyl-*S*-synthase derivative. Decarboxylation of malonyl CoA and nucleophilic attack on acetyl-ACP may occur by a concerted mechanism. A tetrahedral intermediate results. Regeneration of the carbonyl bond then occurs with transfer of electrons to the thiol group of the synthase. The synthase, therefore, serves as the leaving group, and the resultant β-keto acid becomes covalently bound to ACP. Because the reaction involves decarboxylation, it proceeds to completion.

The fourth enzyme in the reaction sequence catalyzed by the fatty acid synthase is β-ketoacyl-ACP reductase, an NADPH-dependent enzyme which is active with substrates with lengths of from 4 to 16 carbon atoms. Subsequently, one of the three β-hydroxyacyl-ACP dehydrases found in *E. coli* dehydrates the β-hydroxy acid to a 2,3-trans unsaturated acid. All three enzymes are specific for D-hydroxy acids. One acts exclusively on C_4, C_6, and C_8 acids, the second on C_6-C_{12} acids, and the third on C_{12}-C_{16} acids.

The final reaction giving rise to a saturated fatty acid is enoyl-ACP reductase. There may be two such enzymes in *E. coli,* one specific for NADPH, the other for NADH. Both enzymes act on substrates with C_4-C_{16} chain lengths. This reaction completes the biosynthetic sequence outlined in Figure 8.2, and the saturated acyl group can be transferred to the synthase to initiate another cyclic addition of a C_2 unit.

Repeated cycling of the fatty acid synthase reactions leads to the formation of the C_{16} saturated fatty acyl-ACP derivative, palmitoyl-ACP. Due to the specificity of the synthase, further chain elongation is not catalyzed. Either free palmitate or palmitoyl CoA is released from the fatty acyl synthase complex, preparing the enzyme for acetylation and the synthesis of another palmitate molecule.

Most bacteria have fatty acid synthases which resemble the *E. coli* enzyme. However, mycobacterial species synthesize high molecular weight synthases (MW = 2×10^6) consisting of multifunctional polypeptide chains. The complex contains 6 to 8 apparently identical subunits with a molecular weight of 300,000. This synthase complex can make long chain fatty acids of up to 24 carbons. The synthase is markedly stimulated by a methylated, acylated polysaccharide containing 6-*O*-

methylglucopyranosyl residues (MW = 4100) or a distinct polysaccharide containing 3-*O*-methylmannopyranosyl residues (MW = 2000). These polysaccharides cyclize, forming hydrophobic interiors that bind equimolar quantities of long-chain acyl CoA derivatives. Without these amphipathic polysaccharides, the long-chain acyl CoA products (particularly C_{22} and C_{24}) do not dissociate from the enzyme complex, and hence the activity is inhibited. The rate-limiting step may be dissociation of the product from the complex, mediated by the water-soluble, amphipathic, methylated polysaccharides. These polysaccharides, therefore, perform unique catalytic and regulatory functions in the mycobacterial cell, normally provided by proteins.

While plants contain ACP-dependent fatty acid synthases like that of *E. coli,* those of higher animals and fungi more closely resemble the mycobacterial complex. The yeast enzyme complex, for example, has a molecular weight of 2,300,000, and it consists of two different multifunctional polypeptides encoded by two distinct genes. The subunit structure of the yeast enzyme is A_6B_6. Subunit A (MW = 185,000) contains the phosphopantetheyl residue, the β-keto acyl synthase activity, and the β-keto acyl reductase activity. Subunit B (MW = 175,000) contains the remaining activities of the complex. One such activity transfers long chain fatty acyl groups from ACP to coenzyme A. Further, a single active site within polypeptide B may catalyze both malonyl and palmitoyl transacylations. A schematic representation of the structure of the yeast fatty acid synthase is shown in Figure 8.5.

The fatty acid synthase complex purified from mammalian liver is apparently a homodimer of about 500,000 molecular weight. Each giant polypeptide chain contains only one phosphopantetheyl residue. This single polypeptide chain apparently contains the ACP region and all of the activities required for fatty acid synthesis as well as a fatty acyl thioesterase that hydrolyzes the product from its covalent attachment site in the enzyme complex. In the presence of CoA, the product is transferred to this coenzyme, thus allowing retention of the energy maintained within the thioester bond.

Elucidation of the structures of fatty acid synthase complexes from different organisms has shown that while each activity may be associated with a separate polypeptide chain in some organisms (such as *E. coli*), they may coexist as *fused* polypeptide chains in other organisms. The evolution of multifunctional proteins from unifunctional proteins and of multicomponent enzyme complexes from unassociated protein species serves some obvious functions: First, it allows coordination of the complex and facilitates its regulation by external stimuli. Second, it insures stoichiometric synthesis of all catalytic functions in the complex and eliminates the need for more than one regulatory region in the nucleic acid determining the rates of transcription and translation. Finally, it may facilitate organization of the complex with other cellular constituents such as the membrane-associated enzymes of fat and phospholipid biosynthesis. In the last chapter we shall see that the enzymes involved in the biosynthesis of simple metabolites such as the amino acid, tryptophan, can also carry one or more catalytic activities, depending on the organism under study.

We used to think that if we knew one, we knew two, because one and one are two. We are finding that we must learn a great deal more about "and".
—SIR ARTHUR STANLEY EDDINGTON

BIBLIOGRAPHY

Bloch, K., and D. Vance, "Control Mechanisms in the Synthesis of Fatty Acids," *Annual Review of Biochemistry,* **46:** 263–298 (1977).

Florkin, M., "Biosynthesis of Fatty Acids and Glycerides," Chapter 59 in: *A History of Biochemistry. Part V. The Unraveling of Biosynthetic Pathways,* Comprehensive Biochemistry, Vol. 33A, Elsevier/North Holland, Amsterdam (1979).

Ginsburgh, C. L., P. N. Black, and W. D. Nunn, "Transport of Long-Chain Fatty Acids in *Escherichia coli, Journal of Biological Chemistry,* **259:** 8437–8443 (1984).

Gunstone, F. D., *An Introduction to the Chemistry and Biochemistry of Fatty Acids and Their Glycerides* (2nd Edition), Chapman and Hall, London (1967).

Leonard, J. E., C. A. Lee, A. Apperson, S. S. Dills, and M. H. Saier, Jr., "The Role of Membranes in the Transport of Small Molecules," in *Organization of Prokaryotic Cell Membranes, Volume I,* B. K. Ghosh, ed., CRC Press, Boca Raton, Fl., pp. 1–52 (1981).

Lynen, F., "On the Structure of Fatty Acid Synthetase of Yeast," *European Journal of Biochemistry,* **112:** 431–442 (1980).

Maloy, S. R., C. L. Ginsburgh, R. W. Simons, and W. D. Nunn, "Transport of Long and Medium Chain Fatty Acids by *Escherichia coli* K-12", *Journal of Biological Chemistry,* **256:** 3735–3742 (1981).

McGarry, J. D., and D. W. Foster, "Regulation of Hepatic Fatty Acid Oxidation and Ketone Body Production," in *Annual Review of Biochemistry,* **49:** 395–420 (1980).

Pawar, S., and H. Schulz, "The Structure of the Multienzyme Complex of Fatty Acid Oxidation from *Escherichia coli,*" *Journal of Biological Chemistry,* **256:** 3894–3899 (1981).

Pryde, E. H., ed., *Fatty Acids,* American Oil Chemists Society, Champaign, IL (1979).

Raetz, C. R. H., "Enzymology, Genetics, and Regulation of Membrane Phospholipid Synthesis in *Escherichia coli,*" *Microbiological Reviews,* **42:** 614–659 (1978).

Rock, C. O., and J. E. Cronan, Jr., "Regulation of Bacterial Membrane Lipid Synthesis," in *Current Topics in Membranes and Transport,* vol. *17, Membrane Lipids of Prokaryotes,* S. Razin and S. Rottem, eds., pp. 207–233 Academic, New York (1982).

Spratt, S. K., P. N. Black, M. M. Ragozzino, and W. D. Nunn, "Cloning, Mapping, and Expression of Genes Involved in the Fatty Acid–Degradative Multienzyme Complex of *Escherichia coli,*" *Journal of Bacteriology,* **158:** 535–542 (1984).

Vance, D. E., "Metabolism of Fatty Acids and Triacylglycerols," in *Biochemistry,* G. Zubay, ed., pp. 471–503, Addison-Wesley, Reading, MA (1983).

Volpe, J. J., and P. R. Vagelos, "Saturated Fatty Acid Biosynthesis and its Regulation," in *Annual Reviews of Biochemistry,* Vol. 42, pp. 21–60 (1973).

Wakil, S. J., J. K. Stoops, and V. C. Joshi, "Fatty Acid Synthesis and Its Regulation," in *Annual Reviews of Biochemistry,* Vol. 52, pp. 537–579 (1983).

Chapter 9

Amino Acid Biosynthesis

> *Man's mind stretched to a new idea never goes back to its original dimensions.*
> —OLIVER WENDELL HOLMES

In Chapter 4 the mechanisms by which enzyme cofactors function in catalysis were examined. These cofactors participate in a majority of reactions catalyzed by both biosynthetic and degradative enzymes. While it will not be possible to examine the numerous biosynthetic pathways responsible for the synthesis of the macromolecular precursors, it is instructive to consider a few representative examples. There are three principal reasons for doing so: first, to exemplify the utility of the coenzymes examined in Chapter 4 in facilitating reactions which can not be catalyzed with the limited biochemical machinery of native proteins; second, to reveal the precursor–product relationships that exist between the major carbohydrate catabolic pathways and the branching amino acid biosynthetic pathways; and, third, to compare the enzymic and regulatory aspects of a single pathway in evolutionarily divergent organisms. Such comparative studies provide insight into the evolutionary process which gave rise to variations in individual enzymes and their regulatory responses.

With these purposes in mind, we shall first discuss in general terms the biosynthetic families of amino acids, and then focus on three such pathways: (1) the pathway responsible for the synthesis of serine and the interconversion of this amino acid with cysteine, glycine, and the methyl group of methionine; (2) the pathway responsible for the incorporation of ammonia into α-ketoglutarate to give glutamate and glutamine; and (3) the pathway responsible for tryptophan synthesis.

The amino acid pathways are essentially the same in all living organisms capable of *de novo* synthesis of these compounds with only a few exceptions. It was the realization of this unifying principle that allowed application to microorganisms of the powerful tools of the biochemical geneticist to reveal the biosynthetic pathways present in all living organisms.

9.1 BIOSYNTHETIC FAMILIES OF AMINO ACIDS

Many heterotrophic bacteria can grow at the expense of a single carbohydrate, while certain photosynthetic bacteria can reproduce in the presence of inorganic compounds and carbon dioxide alone. Consequently, these organisms must be able to synthesize every essential cellular constituent from a simple sugar, or from carbon dioxide, respectively. The immediate precursors of the amino acids are just a few of the common metabolites of the carbohydrate degradative pathways. These include three glycolytic intermediates, 3-phosphoglycerate, phosphoenolpyruvate, and pyruvate; two Krebs cycle intermediates, α-ketoglutarate and oxaloacetate; and two intermediates of the pentose phosphate pathway, ribose-5-phosphate and erythrose-4-phosphate.

Figure 9.1 illustrates the precursor–product relationships of the main amino acid biosynthetic pathways without revealing the intermediate steps. There are six branching biosynthetic families for the syntheses of the 20 common amino acids found in proteins.

1. α-Ketoglutarate gives rise to glutamate which is the precursor of glutamine, proline, and arginine.
2. Oxaloacetate is the immediate precursor of aspartate, which then is utilized for the synthesis of asparagine, methionine, threonine, and lysine, and isolucine is derived from threonine.
3. 3-Phosphoglycerate gives rise to serine in a simple three-step process, and serine is then utilized as the precursor of cysteine and glycine. Moreover, the methyl group of methionine can arise from the β-hydroxymethyl group of serine.
4. Pyruvate gives rise to three of the aliphatic hydrophobic amino acids, alanine, valine and leucine; while
5. PEP plus erythrose-4-phosphate serve as precursors for the biosyntheses of the aromatic amino acids, phenylalanine, tyrosine, and tryptophan.
6. Finally, histidine is synthesized in a nonbranching pathway from ATP and ribose-5-phosphate.

9.2 THE SERINE FAMILY

The biosynthesis of L-serine from the glycolytic intermediate, 3-phospho-D-glycerate, occurs in three steps as shown in Figure 9.2. First, the 2-hydroxyl group is oxidized to a keto group with transfer of a hydride, the α-hydrogen of 3-phospho-D-glycerate, to NAD^+; second, the amino group of glutamate is transferred to the 2-keto group of the product, *O*-phosphohydroxypyruvate, in a pyridoxal phosphate-dependent transamination reaction; and, third, the phosphoryl moiety of the product of this second reaction, 3-phospho-L-serine, is cleaved to give L-serine and inorganic phosphate.

As is frequently observed for biosynthetic pathways, the first enzyme in this sequence, the dehydrogenase, is allosterically regulated in many microorganisms by the end-product of the reaction sequence, L-serine. The enzyme from *E. coli* is a tetramer of four identical subunits (subunit molecular weight = 41,000). A concen-

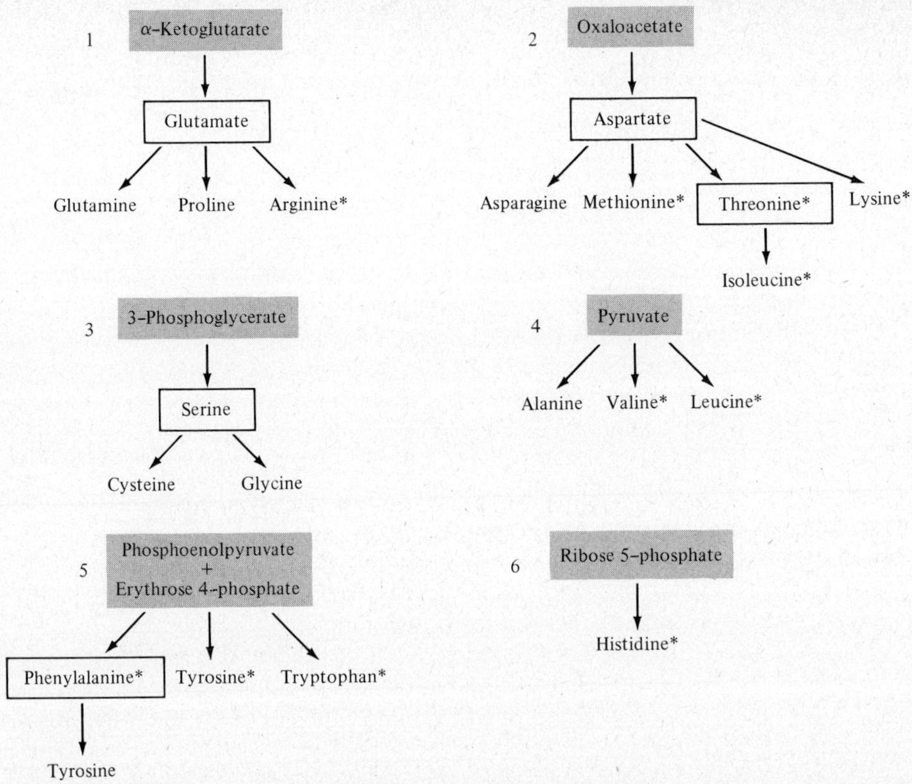

Figure 9.1 The six biosynthetic families of amino acids. In each case, common intermediates of glycolysis (families 3, 4, and 5), the Krebs cycle (families 1 and 2), and the pentose phosphate pathway (families 5 and 6) serve as precursors for the syntheses of the amino acids (lightly shaded compounds). As shown, common amino acids frequently serve as precursors of other amino acids (glutamate in family 1; aspartate and threonine in family 2; serine in family 3, and phenylalanine in family 5; darkly shaded compounds). Each arrow shown in the figure may represent a single step or several metabolic interconversions. These families of biosynthetic pathways are sometimes designated the glutamate family (family 1), the aspartate family (family 2), the serine family (family 3); the aliphatic-amino acid family (family 4); and the aromatic amino acid family (family 5). Only histidine is synthesized via a nonbranching pathway. The essential amino acids which cannot be synthesized by mammals include *arg, met, thr, ile, lys, val, leu, phe, tyr, trp,* and *his,* and these amino acids are indicated by an asterisk.

tration of 40 μM L-serine gives half maximal inhibition. The binding of serine to the allosteric regulatory site has been shown to produce its inhibitory effect by inducing a conformational change in the enzyme. In mammalian tissues L-serine has been shown to be a potent product inhibitor of the third enzyme of the sequence, the phosphatase. It has been postulated that the different location of the control point in mammalian cells results from additional biosynthetic functions of 3-phosphohydroxy-pyruvate and 3-phosphoserine.

Synthesis of glycine from L-serine then occurs in a single but complex step involving pyridoxal phosphate as the cofactor and tetrahydrofolic acid as the hydroxy-

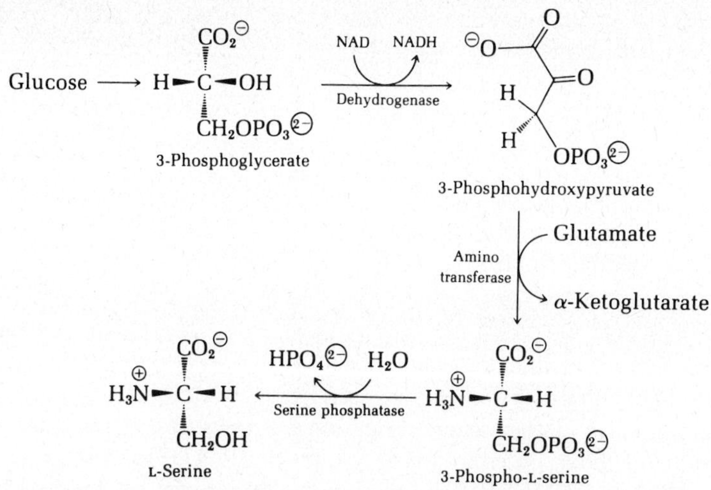

Figure 9.2 The biosynthetic pathway for the conversion of the glycolytic intermediate, 3-phospho-D-glycerate to the amino acid, L-serine. 3-Phosphoglycerate is first oxidized in an NAD^+-dependent reaction to the optically inactive compound, 3-phosphohydroxypyruvate. The enzyme that catalyzes this reaction is phospho-D-glycerate dehydrogenase (EC 1.1.1.95). Transfer of the α-amino group of glutamate to this keto acid gives 3-phospho-L-serine. Because this aminotransfer (transaminase-catalyzed) reaction occurs stereospecifically, only the L-isomer of 3-phosphoserine is produced. The pyridoxal phosphate-dependent enzyme which catalyzes this reaction is called phospho-L-serine aminotransferase (EC 2.6.1.52). Finally, 3-phospho-L-serine is hydrolyzed to L-serine, the biosynthetic product, in a reaction catalyzed by phosphoserine phosphatase (EC 3.1.3.3). Serine is also the precursor of cysteine and glycine biosyntheses as shown in Figure 9.1. Glycine is a biosynthetic precursor of purines and the heme tetrapyrole ring; and the one carbon unit obtained from serine (see below) is utilized in the syntheses of purines, thymine, methionine, histidine, and many methylated products. The serine pathway is therefore a highly branched pathway of central physiological significance.

methyl group acceptor. The enzyme, termed *serine hydroxymethylase* (E.C.2.1.2.1), catalyzes an aldol cleavage reaction which gives glycine and N^5,N^{10}-methylene FH_4 as products.

$$\text{L-serine} + FH_4 \xrightarrow{\text{PLP}} \text{glycine} + N^5,N^{10}\text{-methylene } FH_4 \quad (9.1)$$

In a subsequent step, N^5,N^{10}-methylene FH_4 can be reduced to N^5-methyl FH_4. The source of the hydride ion that nucleophilically attacks the methylene group, displacing an electron pair to N^{10}, is NADH:

$$N^5,N^{10}\text{-methylene } FH_4 + NADH + H^+ \rightarrow N^5\text{-methyl } FH_4 + NAD^+ \quad (9.2)$$

Finally, methionine synthase transfers the methyl group from N^5-methyl FH_4 to homocysteine. There are apparently two distinct methyl transferases in bacteria that catalyze this reaction. One is a coenzyme B_{12}-dependent enzyme, while the other functions by a completely different mechanism in the absence of coenzyme B_{12}. In either case, the reaction proceeds as follows:

$$N^5\text{-methyl } FH_4 + \text{L-homocysteine} \xrightarrow{(CoB_{12})} FH_4 + \text{L-methionine} \quad (9.3)$$

These three steps [equations (9.1)–(9.3)] serve to interconvert serine and glycine and to provide the methyl group for methionine.

9.3 BIOSYNTHESIS OF GLUTAMATE AND GLUTAMINE FROM α-KETOGLUTARATE

Perhaps the most central of the amino acids with respect to the amino acid biosynthetic pathways are glutamate and glutamine. These two amino acids result from reductive amination and ATP-dependent amidation reactions, respectively, using ammonia as the source of the amino and amido groups and NADPH as the source of reducing power. The use of NADPH rather than NADH might be expected for a reductive biosynthetic step involving one of the nicotinamide coenzymes. These two reactions can be thought of as *ammonium fixation* reactions. These reactions account for most of the ammonia assimilated by a living cell.

The enzymes catalyzing these two reactions are glutamate dehydrogenase and glutamine synthase, respectively (Figure 9.3). An additional reaction, catalyzed by glutamate synthase, takes the amido group from glutamine, and transfers it to α-ketoglutarate yielding two molecules of glutamate (Figure 9.3). The central role of these compounds in biosynthesis results from the fact that virtually all aminotransferases (transaminases) utilize glutamate as the amino donor while most amidotransferases utilize glutamine as the amido donor.

As shown in Figure 9.3, glutamate dehydrogenase catalyzes the reductive amination of α-ketoglutarate with ammonia. Although some organisms such as yeast have two glutamate dehydrogenases, one which functions in catabolism, the other in anabolism, only a single enzyme is present in enteric bacteria such as *E. coli,* and this enzyme functions primarily as a biosynthetic catalyst. The reaction proceeds via a Schiff's base intermediate in which the keto function of α-ketoglutarate is condensed with ammonia to yield an imine:

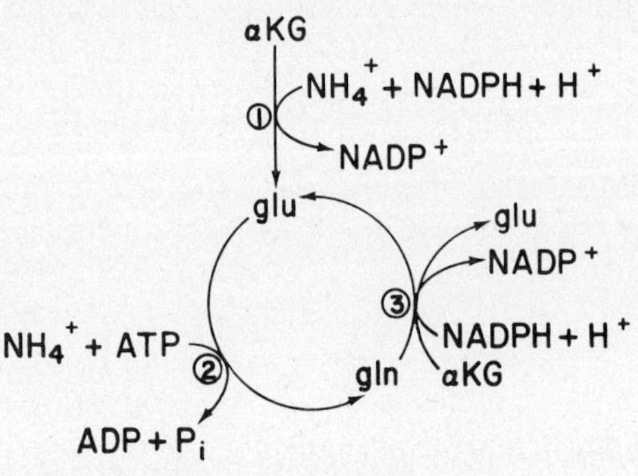

Figure 9.3 Pathways for the biosyntheses of L-glutamate (*glu*) and L-glutamine (*gln*) from α-ketoglutarate (αKG). The three enzymes catalyzing these reactions are: (1) glutamate dehydrogenase (EC 1.4.1.4), (2) glutamine synthase (EC 6.3.1.2), and (3) glutamate synthase (EC 2.6.1.53).

$$>C{=}NH$$

This intermediate is then reduced with a hydride ion from NADPH:

$$>C{=}NH + H^- + H^+ \rightarrow -\!\!\!>C{-}NH_2$$

The *E. coli* enzyme has a molecular weight of 300,000 and is a hexamer of six identical subunits. Because it has a high Km for both of its substrates (about 1 mM) this enzyme may not be catalytically active during growth in media containing low concentrations of ammonium ions. Thus, ammonia assimilation at low concentrations of ammonia is due exclusively to the reaction catalyzed by glutamine synthase although both enzymes are functional at high ammonia concentrations.

Glutamate synthase, which catalyzes the synthesis of two molecules of glutamate from one of α-ketoglutarate and one of glutamine, is a large, multimeric enzyme. In *E. coli* it has an aggregate molecular weight of 800,000 and probably consists of four catalytically active dimers. Each dimer is comprised of two nonidentical subunits having molecular weights of 53,000 and 135,000. Although it is an amidotransferase, it differs from all other such enzymes in being an iron–sulfur flavoprotein. The iron–sulfur centers associated with the large subunit are similar to those in the redox components of the electron transfer chain (see Chapters 4 and 7). While the roles of these prosthetic groups in the catalytic function (or functions) of this complex enzyme are not entirely understood, they presumably function in the coupled reduction of the imine of α-ketoglutarate and the oxidation of NADPH. It is possible that other proteins, such as components of the electron transfer chain, can serve as alternative electron donors.

The large subunit of glutamate synthase is known to bind glutamine, and it transfers the amido group of glutamine to α-ketoglutarate which is bound to the smaller subunit. In most amidotransferases, however, it is the smaller subunit that binds glutamine. The occurrence of a polypeptide chain that binds glutamine and extracts the amido group for reaction with the amido acceptor (in this case α-ketoglutarate) is typical of amidotransferases (see the next section on tryptophan biosynthesis). It is probable that the large subunit of glutamate synthase arose by the fusion of two structural genes, one encoding a protein which functioned exclusively in amidotransfer from glutamine, the other which participated exclusively in catalysis of the reduction of the imine of α-ketoglutarate to L-glutamate. In keeping with the catalytic activities of other amidotransferases, the α-ketoglutarate-binding subunit of glutamate synthase can catalyze ammonia-dependent amination of α-ketoglutarate.

As shown in Figure 9.3, glutamine synthase is responsible for the amidation of glutamate to glutamine. In most organisms at low ammonium concentrations it is this reaction that is primarily responsible for the incorporation of ammonia into organic matter. The initial product of the reaction is a tightly bound enzyme–substrate complex in which the γ-carboxyl group of glutamate is activated by formation of a mixed anhydride bond with the γ-phosphoryl moiety of an ATP molecule. In the second step, ammonia must nucleophilically attack the activated γ-carboxyl group, displacing the phosphoryl group which is released as inorganic phosphate. Creation of the mixed anhydride bond facilitates glutamine biosynthesis because the phosphate group attached to the carboxyl group is a good leaving group, while the anionic hydroxyl group of the carboxylic acid is not.

Because of the importance of glutamine synthase in ammonium fixation, it is not surprising that the enzyme is subject to control by multiple mechanisms involving covalent modification, cumulative allosteric inhibition by end-products of various biosynthetic reactions which are dependent on glutamine, and possibly, also, by reversible sulfhydryl oxidation which inactivates the enzyme. Moreover, the enzyme responsible for covalent modification of glutamine synthase is regulated by direct protein–protein interaction with a structural regulatory protein *P* which itself can be covalently modified. The remainder of this section will be devoted to a discussion of these regulatory interactions. The properties of the proteins which comprise the glutamine synthase regulatory cascade are summarized in Table 9.1.

Glutamine synthase from *E. coli* has a molecular weight of 600,000 and consists of twelve identical subunits, each of 50,000 molecular weight. These subunits are arranged in two symmetrical hexameric rings. Each subunit apparently possesses binding sites for each of the allosteric effectors. In *E. coli* these effectors include carbamyl-

TABLE 9.1 PROPERTIES OF THE PROTEIN CONSTITUENTS OF THE GLUTAMINE SYNTHASE REGULATORY CASCADE

Enzyme	Abbreviation	Molecular weight	Molecular forms	Reactions catalyzed	Allosteric activators	Allosteric inhibitors
Uridylyltransferase	UTase	160,000		P + 4 UTP → P(UMP)$_4$ + 4 P$_2$	αKG, ATP	Gln, P$_i$
				P(UMP)$_4$ + 4 H$_2$O → P + 4 UMP	Glu	α-KG, ATP
ATase regulatory protein	P	50,000 12,500 (subunit)	P	Activates adenylylation of GS	None	None
			P(UMP)$_4$	Activates de-adenylylation of GS	None	None
Adenylyltransferase	ATase	130,000		GS + 12 ATP → GS(AMP)$_{12}$ + 12 P$_2$	Gln, P$_i$	α-KG
				GS(AMP)$_{12}$ + 12 P$_i$ → GS + 12 ADP	α-KG, ATP	Gln
Glutamine synthase	GS	600,000 50,000 (subunit)	GS	Active form	None	Histidine, tryptophan, AMP, CTP, glucosamine-6-P, carbamyl-P, glycine, alanine
			GS(AMP)$_{12}$	Inactive form		

phosphate, glucosamine-6-phosphate, CTP, AMP, tryptophan, and histidine. All of these six compounds receive an amido group from glutamine during their biosyntheses and can consequently be thought of as end-product, feed-back inhibitors. Two additional inhibitors, glycine and alanine, only secondarily derive their amino groups from glutamine.

The covalent modification of glutamine synthase (GS) involves the ATP-dependent adenylylation of a tyrosyl residue near the C-terminus of each of the twelve subunits of this enzyme as summarized in Table 9.1:

$$\mathrm{GS(AMP)}_n + \mathrm{ATP} \xrightarrow{\mathrm{ATase}} \mathrm{GS(AMP)}_{n+1} + \mathrm{P}_2 \tag{9.4}$$

Because the adenylyl transfer reaction is only slightly exergonic, the reaction is readily reversible. However, adenylylation is accompanied by release of pyrophosphate which can be hydrolyzed by a cellular pyrophosphatase to two molecules of inorganic phosphate. This coupled reaction renders the adenylyl transfer reaction essentially irreversible.

Each additional AMP group covalently attached to the enzyme progressively inhibits its activity further because the affinities of the enzyme for its substrates decrease with increasing degrees of derivatization. The covalently modified enzyme is also more susceptible than the unmodified enzyme to negative feedback inhibition by the various biosynthetic end-products of pathways that utilize glutamine as an amidating agent. With all twelve subunits derivatized, the enzyme is essentially inactive under physiological conditions. Although the fully adenylylated enzyme exhibits activity with Mn^{++} instead of Mg^{++}, this activity is of doubtful physiological significance.

The deadenylylation of glutamine synthase is a phosphorolytic reaction using inorganic phosphate. It results in ADP production:

$$\mathrm{GS(AMP)}_{n+1} + \mathrm{P}_i \xrightarrow{\mathrm{ATase}} \mathrm{GS(AMP)}_n + \mathrm{ADP} \tag{9.5}$$

This reaction is catalyzed at a second active site associated with the adenylyl transferase. Like the adenylylation reaction, it is fully reversible since the reaction is only slightly exergonic. Hydrolysis of the byproduct, ADP, to AMP and inorganic phosphate, or rephosphorylation of ADP to ATP, removing ADP from the cytoplasmic pool of adenine nucleotides, pulls the equilibrium to the right.

The net result of the adenylylation and deadenylylation of glutamine synthase is pyrophosphorolysis of ATP:

$$\mathrm{ATP} + \mathrm{P}_i \xrightarrow[\mathrm{GS}]{\mathrm{ATase}} \mathrm{ADP} + \mathrm{P}_2 \tag{9.6}$$

While this reaction is also reversible, hydrolysis of the pyrophosphate produced renders the reaction irreversible. Continuous cycling of these two reactions [equations (9.4) and (9.5)] could therefore result in considerable energy loss to the cell. Regulatory constraints minimize such a cycling process because the adenylyltransferase is usually activated primarily either for adenylylation or for phosphorolytic deadenylylation of glutamine synthase at any one time. The activity expressed by the adenylyltransferase is based largely on the relative concentrations of glutamine and α-ketoglutarate in the cytoplasm and on the uridylylation state of a regulatory protein, designated P, which controls the activity of the adenylyltransferase by direct protein–protein interaction.

The cascade-type mechanism of regulation by which glutamine synthase activity is regulated is shown in Figure 9.4. This figure illustrates both the involvement of the P protein and of the glutamine (*gln*) to α-ketoglutarate (αKG) ratio in regulation. When the cell is faced with a deficiency of NH_4^+, the concentration of αKG increases while that of *gln* decreases. αKG stimulates the UTase to uridylylate a tyrosyl residue in each of the four subunits of the P protein:

$$P(UMP)_n + UTP \xrightarrow{\text{UTase}} P(UMP)_{n+1} + P_2 \tag{9.7}$$

The uridylylated P protein together with αKG phosphorolytically deadenylylates the adenylylated form of GS, converting the enzyme to its active state so that any ammonium ions present in the cytoplasm can be incorporated into organic matter. By contrast, when the concentration of NH_4^+ is excessive, the concentration of αKG decreases to low values while that of *gln* increases. The change in the ratio of these two sensors of nitrogen availability causes the uridylylation activity of the UTase to decrease while the $P(UMP)_n$ hydrolytic activity increases:

$$P(UMP)_{n+1} + H_2O \xrightarrow{\text{UTase}} P(UMP)_n + UMP \tag{9.8}$$

The generation of the free, nonuridylylated P protein and a high *gln* to αKG ratio promote adenylylation of GS, converting GS to the inactive conformation. The ratio of αKG to *gln* therefore serves as a sensor of organic nitrogen availability, a *second*

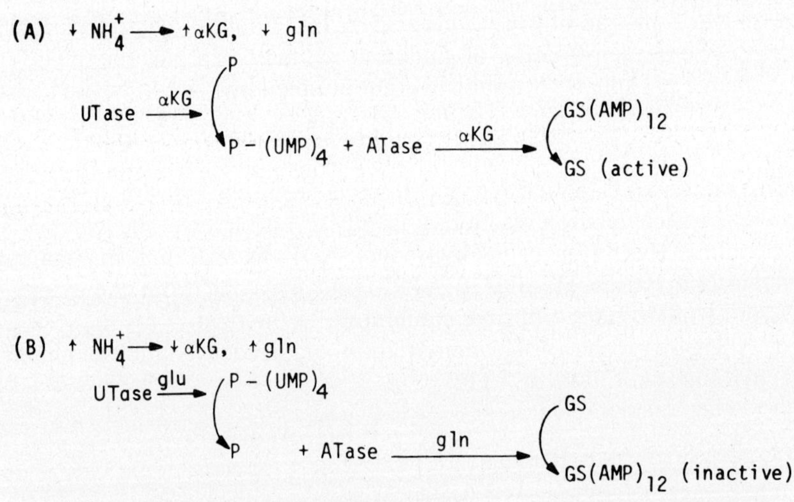

Figure 9.4 Proposed mechanism for the control of nitrogen metabolism by glutamine synthase in bacteria. (A) Ammonium deprivation increases the cellular concentration of α-ketoglutarate (αKG) and decreases the concentration of glutamine (*gln*). This leads to a cascade of events which causes glutamine synthase to exist in the nonadenylylated, active form. (B) Ammonium availability causes a decrease in the cellular concentration of α-ketoglutarate and a concomitant increase in the concentration of glutamine. The end result is adenylylation of glutamine synthase to the inactive state. The abbreviations used are as indicated in Table 9.1.

messenger or *alarmone,* by regulating the two opposing activities of the UTase and the ATase which function as constituents of a cascade system to regulate glutamine synthase (Table 9.1).

This cascade-type of regulation has several consequences relative to a simpler mode of control:

1. It allows for amplification, i.e., a single uridylyltransferase can control the activities of numerous glutamine synthase molecules.
2. It increases the number of compounds that can regulate glutamine synthase.
3. It allows greater sensitivity to a single regulatory agent, such as α-ketoglutarate or glutamine. The cytoplasmic messengers are α-ketoglutarate, glutamate, and glutamine. The proteins that sense the concentrations of these compounds are the uridylyl- and adenylyltransferases.

We have seen that in the glutamine synthase regulatory cascade, each of the two catalytic enzymes, the UTase and the ATase, catalyzes both the forward and reverse reactions for derivatization of its target protein. Evidence has been presented to suggest that two separate active sites in the ATase protein catalyze the two reactions. Possibly these two active sites resulted by an internal gene duplication generating a larger, two-domain protomer from a smaller one-domain protomer. Such an occurrence would allow the two similar domains to evolve with the acquisition of different but related catalytic functions. Moreover, it is quite possible that the ATase and UTase evolved from a common ancestor and share a similar subunit structure. If so, the UTase may also possess two distinct active sites, one for the uridylylation of the P protein and one for the hydrolysis of the uridylylated protein.

Finally, we have noted in Chapter 5 that the enzyme that catalyzes the synthesis of the important regulatory molecule of glycolysis, fructose-2,6-diphosphate, also catalyzes its hydrolysis. The protein kinase discussed in Chapter 6 which catalyzes the phosphorylation of a seryl residue in the *E. coli* isocitrate dehydrogenase is another example of a regulatory protein that catalyzes both the forward and reverse reactions. The incorporation in a single enzyme complex of both the forward and reverse catalytic activities regulating principal metabolic pathways seems to be a common theme. It may result in tighter regulatory control over processes preventing wasteful expenditure of metabolic energy by futile cycling.

9.4 BIOSYNTHESIS OF TRYPTOPHAN

Tryptophan is synthesized via a pathway that initially is common to the three aromatic amino acids, phenylalanine, tyrosine, and tryptophan. Seven enzyme-catalyzed steps are shared in a pathway that begins with condensation of phosphoenolpyruvate with erythrose-4-phosphate and gives rise to the common biosynthetic precursor, chorismate (Figure 9.1). Chorismate is then converted to L-tryptophan in a five-step reaction sequence involving four enzymes in *E. coli* but as few as two, and as many as seven, polypeptide chains in other organisms. In this section we shall discuss this latter well-characterized pathway which comprises the tryptophan-specific part of the biosynthetic sequence. It is of particular interest because of the unusual nature of the reactions catalyzed, the multifunctional nature of the enzymes involved, and the availability of comparative data which allow proposals with respect to the evolution of the genetic apparati that encode the enzymes of this pathway in different organisms.

The tryptophan biosynthetic pathway in *E. coli* has been more extensively studied than any other biosynthetic pathway. Mechanistic and regulatory characteristics of each enzymatic step are well understood. Nucleotide and aminoacyl sequences of the genes and gene products that encode and comprise the enzymes of tryptophan biosynthesis, respectively, have been determined, and the factors controlling transcription of the *trp* (tryptophan)-specific DNA into messenger RNA species, and the translation of the *trp* messenger RNA into the biosynthetic enzymes, have been thoroughly studied. Some of these subjects will be discussed in this section.

The pathway for the conversion of chorismate to L-tryptophan is illustrated in Figures 9.5 and 9.6, and some properties of the *E. coli* enzymes are summarized in Table 9.2. *Anthranilate synthase* (*AS*) is the first enzyme specific to tryptophan biosynthesis. This enzyme catalyzes nucleophilic attack (S_N2) by a free electron pair of the amide nitrogen of glutamine at the ring position between the carboxyl and enolpyruvyl groups. The protein consists of two nonidentical subunits. One, designated ASII, binds glutamine, possesses glutaminase activity, and probably functions to transfer the amide group of *gln* to the NH_3-binding site of ASI. Cleavage of the amide bond of glutamine is accompanied by the intermediate formation of a γ-glutamyl enzyme. This enzyme constituent is called *glutamine amidotransferase.* As with other glutamine amidotransferases, ammonia can replace *gln,* but the reaction with NH_3 is slow and requires high concentrations of NH_3. The reaction in which NH_3 replaces *gln* can be catalyzed by ASI alone. First, $:NH_3$, derived from the amido group of *gln,* attacks

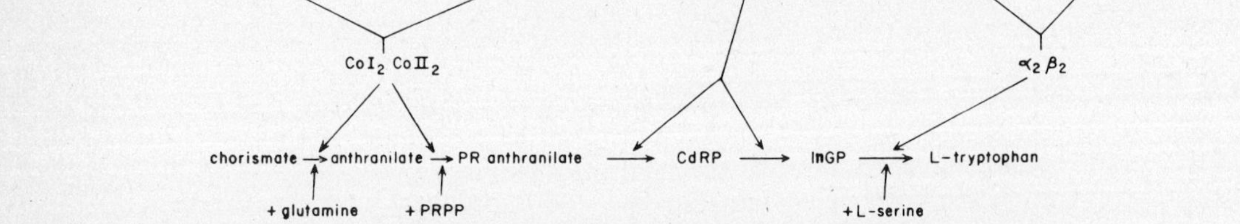

Figure 9.5 Gene structure of the tryptophan operon (top), enzyme constituents encoded by this operon (middle), and biosynthetic pathway for tryptophan (bottom). Numbers above the operon indicate the number of nucleotides downstream from the origin of transcription. (Reproduced with permission from C. Yanofsky, T. Platt, I. P. Crawford, B. P. Nichols, G. E. Christie, H. Horowitz, M. Van Cleemput, and A. M. Wu, *Nucleic Acid Research,* **29,** 6647–6668, 1981.)

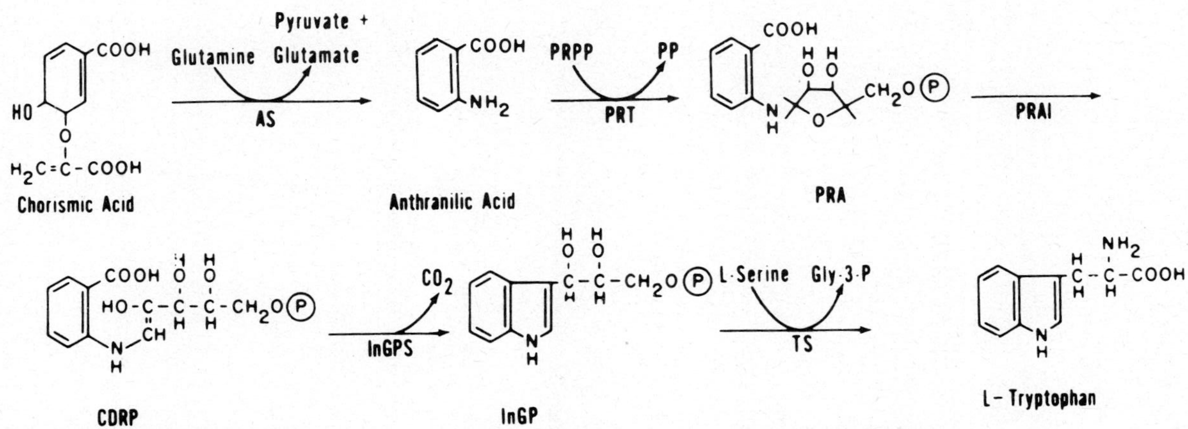

Figure 9.6 Biosynthetic pathway for tryptophan showing the structures of all biosynthetic intermediates. Abbreviations: AS, anthranilate synthase (the amidotransferase reaction is shown); PRPP, 5-phosphoribosyl pyrophosphate; PP, pyrophosphate; PRT, anthranilate phosphoribosyltransferase; PRA, *N*-phosphoribosylanthranilate; PRAI, phosphoribosylanthranilate isomerase; CDRP, 1-(*o*-carboxyphenylamino)-deoxyribulose phosphate; InGPS, indoleglycerol phosphate synthase; InGP, indoleglycerol phosphate; Gly-3-P, D-glycerldehyde-3-phosphate; TS, tryptophan synthase. (Reproduced with permission from I. P. Crawford, "Gene Rearrangements in the Evolution of the Tryptophan Synthetic Pathway," *Bacteriological Reviews,* **39:** 87–120, 1975.)

TABLE 9.2 ENZYMES AND CORRESPONDING GENE DESIGNATIONS FOR THE PROTEIN CONSTITUENTS OF THE TRYPTOPHAN BIOSYNTHETIC PATHWAY IN *E. COLI*

Enzymatic protein	Abbreviation	E.C. #	Number of amino acids	Universal gene designation	Gene in *E. coli*
Anthranilate synthase (large subunit, I)	ASI	E.C.4.1.3.27	520	E	E
Anthranilate synthase (small subunit, II)	ASII		531	G	D(G)
Anthranilate phosphoribosyl transferase	APRT	E.C.2.4.2.18		D	
Phosphoribosyl anthranilate isomerase	PRAI	E.C.4.1.1.48	452	F	C(F)
Indole glycerol phosphate synthase	InGPS			C	
Tryptophan synthase (β-subunit)	TSβ	E.C.4.2.1.20	396	B	B
Tryptophan synthase (α-subunit)	TSα		268	A	A

nucleophilically on the ring with elimination of the ring hydroxyl group. The second step catalyzed by ASI involves elimination of the ring enolpyruvyl group generating the aromatic ring of anthranilate. The byproduct is pyruvate.

As the enzyme which catalyzes the first unique step in *trp* biosynthesis, it is not surprising that AS is subject to allosteric feedback control by the end-product of this biosynthetic sequence, tryptophan. The allosteric binding site is associated with the large subunit, ASI. Binding of tryptophan to its allosteric site reduces the affinity of the catalytic site for chorismate. Since anthranilate synthases from all prokaryotic and eukaryotic organisms so far examined are sensitive to this feedback inhibition, and since in all cases both the amidotransfer and amination reactions are sensitive to regulation, it can be concluded that the evolutionary pressure to conserve this site has been considerable. It is worth noting that glutamine synthase and the first enzyme in chorismate biosynthesis are both sensitive to feedback regulation by tryptophan and therefore serve as secondary regulatory sites.

Anthranilate phosphoribosyl transferase (APRT) catalyzes the second reaction shown in Figure 9.5. In this reaction, the amino group of anthranilate displaces the pyrophosphate group (PP) of 5′-phosphoribosyl pyrophosphate (PRPP), giving rise to *N*-(5-phosphoribosyl)-anthranilate. In some bacteria such as *E. coli* and its close relatives, APRT and AS are associated in a single tetrameric enzyme complex with two dissimilar subunits. Anthranilate synthase II is fused to anthranilate phosphoribosyltransferase in a single polypeptide chain, and two of these polypeptide chains associate with two anthranilate synthase large subunits. It is probable that anthranilate is passed directly from the synthase active site to the phosphoribosyltransferase active site, thereby enhancing catalytic efficiency. Because of the tight coupling of the two subunits, all three catalytic subunits of the complex are subject to allosteric control by tryptophan. In other bacteria, these two functions are encoded by separate genes. It is possible that the enzymes catalyzing all five steps shown in Figure 9.5 are present in the cell as a single, loosely associated biosynthetic enzyme complex. The conditions of cell disruption may cause the enzyme constituents of the complex to dissociate.

Phosphoribosyl anthranilate isomerase (PRAI) first catalyzes an Amadori rearrangement of phosphoribosyl anthranilate in which the phosphoribosyl moiety becomes a phosphoribulosyl moiety (Figure 9.6). The furanose ring opens as a result of the loss of a proton from the C-2′ carbon of the ribosyl moiety and formation of a π double bond between C-1 and C-2. The formation of this carbon–carbon double bond displaces an electron pair from C-1 to the ring oxygen associated with C-4. This enol form, called enol-1-*O*-carboxyphenylamino-1-deoxyribulose phosphate can tautomerize to the 2-keto derivative. This step and the subsequent one are catalyzed by a two-domain polypeptide that possesses both catalytic activities (Table 9.2).

Indole glycerol phosphate synthase (InGPS) catalyzes the fourth step shown in Figures 9.5 and 9.6. This step involves the decarboxylative closure of the indole ring. The reaction mechanism may involve a single concerted process. In *E. coli* and other closely related bacteria, a single enzyme catalyzes steps 3 and 4. In other bacteria two smaller proteins encoded by two separate genes carry out these catalytic functions. When the two activities are fused as part of a single polypeptide chain, the enzyme is called indole glycerol phosphate synthase.

Tryptophan synthase (TS) catalyzes the final reaction giving tryptophan as the product. The enzyme consists of an $\alpha_2\beta_2$ tetramer containing two copies each of two nonidentical subunits. The two α-subunits catalyze indole glycerol phosphate (InGP) aldolysis, producing indole and glyceraldehyde-3-phosphate. Indole normally remains as an enzyme-bound intermediate, while the glyceraldehyde-3-P is displaced from the active site by serine. However, the half-reaction of aldolysis and dissociation of indole from the enzyme surface as well as tryptophan synthesis from indole and L-serine can be observed under certain conditions. Each of the two β-subunits of tryptophan synthase contains pyridoxal phosphate as a prosthetic group. Serine forms a Schiff's base linkage with the coenzyme, activating the serine for condensation with indole in a reaction that is essentially the reverse of the glycerol phosphate elimination reaction.

Comparative studies with a variety of bacteria have revealed considerable variation in the structures of the operons or regulons which encode the different proteins of the *trp* biosynthetic pathway. Some of this variation is shown in Figure 9.7.

In enteric bacteria such as *E. coli* and *Serratia,* all of the *trp* enzymes are encoded within a single operon, a single unit of transcription. Thus, for these bacteria, *trp* operon transcription gives rise to a single messenger RNA species from which all of the biosynthetic genes are translated. By contrast, in *Pseudomonas* and *Acinetobacter* the biosynthetic structural genes are constituents of three different operons. In *Bacillus,* the *trpG* gene encoding the amidotransferase is not encoded within the *trp* operon, and the protein that serves this function is a multifunctional protein that maps elsewhere on the bacterial chromosome. For example, it functions in the biosynthesis of *p*-amino benzoic acid as well as that of tryptophan.

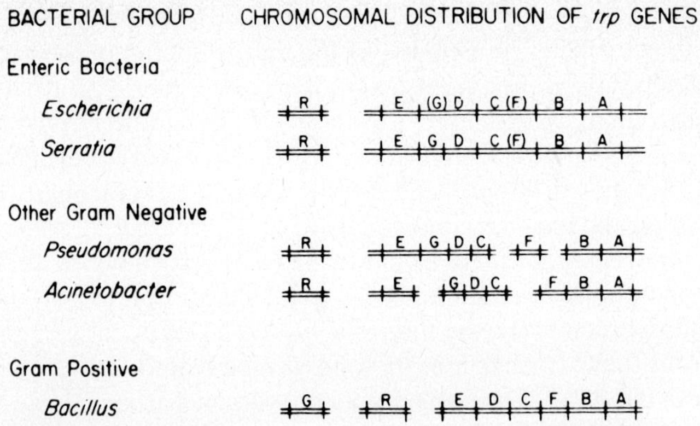

Figure 9.7 Tryptophan gene distribution in selected Gram-negative and Gram-positive bacterial genera. In two genera of the enteric bacteria, *Escherichia* and *Serratia,* all of the biosynthetic enzymes are encoded by genes within a single unit of transcription, the *trp* operon. In the other bacteria depicted, more than one operon encodes these genes. In all bacteria, the (*trpR*) gene, which encodes the tryptophan repressor that regulates the rate of transcription of the *trp* regulon, is encoded within a distinct unit of transcription. In *Escherichia* there are two fused biosynthetic genes, *trp(G)D* and *trpC(F),* while in *Serratia* only the *trpC(F)* gene is fused. The other bacteria portrayed do not possess fused genes. In two cases two distinct genes encode proteins which comprise the functional unit. *trpE* and *trpD* encode the two subunits of anthranilate synthase while the *trpA* and *trpB* genes encode the two polypeptide chains of trptophan synthase. Gene designations and the proteins encoded are as shown in Figure 9.5. (Reproduced with permission from I. P. Crawford, *Bacteriological Reviews,* **39:** 88–120, 1975.)

The *trpR* gene is a regulatory gene encoding the tryptophan repressor which controls expression of the other *trp* genes. The *trpE* gene is the first to be transcribed. It encodes the large subunit of anthranilate synthase. The *trp*(*G*)*D* gene in *E. coli* is a complex gene having its proximal third devoted to the glutamine amidotransfer function of anthranilate synthase and its distal two thirds to the anthranilate phosphoribosyltransferase function. The *trpD* and *trpG* genes are distinct, encoding separate proteins in *Serratia* species and many other bacteria. *trpC*(*F*) is also a complex gene in *E. coli* encoding the indole glycerol phosphate synthase (C) in its proximal half and the phosphoribosyl anthranilate isomerase (F) in its distal half. Mutations that abolish the activity of one of these domains frequently leave the other intact. In most bacterial species outside of the enteric bacterial group, the C and F genes are distinct, encoding separate proteins. Finally, *trpB* encodes the β-subunit of tryptophan synthase, while the *trpA* gene encodes the α-subunit of this tetrameric enzyme.

> *Flowers on the hillside*
> *bloomin' crazy,*
> *Crickets talkin' back and*
> *forth in rhyme,*
> *Blue river runnin' slow*
> *and lazy,*
> *I could stay with you*
> *forever and never*
> *realize the time.*
>
> —BOB DYLAN

BIBLIOGRAPHY

Arnstein, H. R. V., ed., *Amino Acid and Protein Biosynthesis,* University Park Press, Baltimore, MD (1978).

Chock, P. B., S. G. Rhee, and E. R. Stadtman, "Interconvertible Enzyme Cascades in Cellular Regulation," *Annual Reviews of Biochemistry,* **49:** 813–843 (1980).

Crawford, I. P., "Gene Rearrangements in the Evolution of the Tryptophan Synthetic Pathway," *Bacteriological Reviews,* **39:** 88–120 (1975).

Crawford, I. P., and G. V. Stauffer, "Regulation of Tryptophan Biosynthesis," *Annual Review of Biochemistry,* **49:** 163–195 (1980).

Ebner, K. E., ed., *Subunit Enzymes. Biochemistry and Function,* Marcel Dekker, New York (1975).

Florkin, M., *A History of Biochemistry. Part V. The Unraveling of Biosynthetic Pathways,* Comprehensive Biochemistry, Vol. 33B, Elsevier/North Holland, Amsterdam (1979).

Herrmann, K. M., and R. L. Somerville, eds., *Amino Acids: Biosynthesis and Genetic Regulation,* Addison-Wesley, Reading, MA (1983).

Lerner, J., *A Review of Amino Acid Transport Processes in Animal Cells and Tissues,* University of Maine, Orono Press, Orono, ME (1978).

Mora, J., and R. Palacios, eds., *Glutamine—Metabolism, Enzymology and Regulation, Proceedings of an International Symposium,* Academic, New York (1980).

Nyhan, W. L., *Abnormalities in Amino Acid Metabolism in Clinical Medicine,* Appleton-Century-Crofts, Norwalk, CT (1984).

Umbarger, H. E., "Amino Acid Biosynthesis and its Regulation," *Annual Review of Biochemistry,* **47:** 533–606 (1978).

Umbarger, H. E., "Biosynthesis of Amino Acids," in *Biochemistry,* G. Zubay, ed., pp. 825–871, Addison-Wesley, Reading, MA (1983).

Yanofsky, C., "Comparison of Regulatory and Structural Regions of Genes of Tryptophan Metabolism," *Molecular Biology and Evolution,* **1:** 143–161 (1984).

Yanofsky, C., T. Platt, I. P. Crawford, B. P. Nichols, G. E. Christie, H. Horowitz, M. Van-Cleemput, and A. M. Wu, "The Complete Nucleotide Sequence of the Tryptophan Operon of *Escherichia coli,*" *Nucleic Acids Research,* **9:** 6647–6668 (1981).

Index